MEDICAL
INTELLIGENCE
UNIT

Pancreatic Islet Transplantation Volume I:
PROCUREMENT OF PANCREATIC ISLETS

Editors:

Robert P. Lanza, M.D.
William L. Chick, M.D.

BioHybrid Technologies Inc.
Shrewsbury, Massachusetts
U.S.A.

R.G. LANDES COMPANY
AUSTIN

Medical Intelligence Unit

PANCREATIC ISLET TRANSPLANTATION
VOLUME I: PROCUREMENT OF PANCREATIC ISLETS

R.G. LANDES COMPANY
Austin

CRC Press is the exclusive worldwide distributor of publications of the Medical Intelligence Unit.
CRC Press, 2000 Corporate Blvd., NW, Boca Raton, FL 33431. Phone: 407/994-0555.

Submitted: April 1994
Published: July 1994

Production Manager: Deborah Molsberry
Copy Editor: Elinda McKenna

Please address all inquiries to the Publisher:
R.G. Landes Company, 909 Pine Street, Georgetown, TX 78626
or
P.O. Box 4858, Austin, TX 78765
Phone: 512/ 863 7762; FAX: 512/ 863 0081

ISBN 1-57059-133-4
CATALOG # LN9133

While the authors, editors and publisher believe that drug selection and dosage and the specifications
and usage of equipment and devices, as set forth in this book, are in accord with current recommend-
ations and practice at the time of publication, they make no warranty, expressed or implied, with
respect to material described in this book. In view of the ongoing research, equipment development,
changes in governmental regulations and the rapid accumulation of information relating to the biomedical sciences, the reader is urged to carefully review and evaluate the information provided herein.

Library of Congress Cataloging-in-Publication Data

Pancreatic islet transplantation series / editors, Robert P. Lanza, William L. Chick.
    p. cm.—(Medical intelligence unit)
    Includes bibliographical references and index.
    Contents: v. 1. Procurement of pancreatic islets—v. 2. Immunomodulation of pancreatic islets—v.
3. Immunoisolation of pancreatic islets.
    ISBN 1–57059–133–4 (v. 1).—ISBN 1–57059–134–2 (v. 2).—ISBN 1–57059–135–0 (v. 3)
    1. Islands of Langerhans—Transplantation. 2. Diabetes—Surgery.
  I. Lanza, R.P. (Robert Paul), 1956– . II. Chick, William L. (William Louis), 1938– . III. Series.
    [DNLM: 1. Islets of Langerhans Transplantaiton. 2. Pancreas—immunology. 3. Islets of Langer-
hans—immunology. 4. Organ Procurement. 5. Tissue Culture. WK 800 P188 1994]
RD599.5. I84P36 1994
617.5'570592—dc20
DNLM/DLC
for Library of Congress

         94-25951
         CIP

To Our Readers

R.G. Landes Company publishes four book series: *Medical Intelligence Unit, Molecular Biology Intelligence Unit, Neuroscience Intelligence Unit,* and *Biotechnology Intelligence Unit.* Our goal is to publish the most recent information in biomedical science for sophisticated researchers and physicians.

To achieve this goal we have accelerated our publishing program to conform to the fast pace in which information grows in biomedical science. The book you have in hand, like all titles in our series, was published *within 90 days of receipt of the manuscript.*

As you might expect, this causes a few problems for us; sometimes it makes our office more like a big city newspaper than a scholarly publisher. So as you look through this book you may see something that isn't just right. Please let us know. Or if you have an idea for improving our books, we'd like very much to hear from you. If the problem you describe hasn't already been discovered or if your idea is provocative enough to promote a discussion here, we'll give you a free book of your choice. Just list three titles in order of preference and we'll send you one, based on availability—with our thanks. Our address is printed on the copyright page of each of our books.

Elinda McKenna
Director of Operations
R.G. Landes Company

CONTENTS

CONTENTS

CONTENTS

CONTENTS

ABBREVIATIONS

2-DOG	2-deoxyglucose
ADP	adenosine diphosphate
AO	acridin orange
ATP	adenosine tryphosphate
BBs	Brockman bodies
BCS	bovine calf serum
BDS	Biological Detection System
BrdU	5-bromo-2'deoxyuridine
BSA	bovine serum albumin
BSS	balanced salt solution
CC	conventional culture
CCK	cholecystokinin
CPP	cryoprecipitated plasma
DMSO	dimethylsulfoxide
DTZ	diphenylthiocarbazone
EIN	equivalent islet numbers
FCS	fetal calf serum
GRF	growth hormone releasing factor
HBSS	Hanks balanced salt solution
hGH	human growth hormone
HIT	hamster insulinoma cell line
HS	human serum
ICC	islet cell-like clusters
IDDM	insulin-dependent diabetes mellitus
IFNγ	gamma interferon
MHC	major histocompatibility complex
MLIC	mixed lymphocyte islet coculture
NOD	nonobese diabetic (mice)
NGF	nerve growth factor
PCR	polymerase chain reaction
PI	propidium iodide
PL	placental lactogens
PP	pancreatic polypeptide
PPF	plasma protein fraction
PRL	prolactin
RIA	radioimmunassay
RIN	rat insulinoma
SGFP	silica gel filtered plasma
TCC	Technical Control Language
TDR	[³H] thymidine
TSH	thyroid stimulating hormone
TSQ	tolulene sulfonamide

EDITORS

Robert P. Lanza, M.D.
Director, Transplantation Biology
BioHybrid Technologies Inc., Shrewsbury, Massachusetts, USA
and
Clinical Associate Professor of Surgery, Tufts University
North Grafton, Massachusetts USA
Chapter 7

William L. Chick, M.D.
President and Scientific Director
BioHybrid Technologies Inc., Shrewsbury, Massachusetts USA
Chapter 7

CONTRIBUTORS

Rodolfo Alejandro, M.D.
Professor of Medicine
Diabetes Research Institute
University of Miami
Miami, Florida, USA
Chapter 9

Ziliang Ao, M.Sc., M.D.
Research Assistant
Department of Surgery
University of Alberta
Edmonton, Alberta, Canada
Chapter 8

Hector BeltrandelRio, M.D., Ph.D.
Post-Doctoral Fellow
Departments of Biochemistry and
  Internal Medicine
  and
  Gifford Laboratories for Diabetes
  Research
University of Texas Southwestern
  Medical Center
Dallas, Texas, USA
Chapter 15

Susan Bonner-Weir, Ph.D.
Investigator
Section on Islet Transplantation
and Cell Biology
Joslin Diabetes Center
Boston, Massachusetts, USA
Chapter 5, Part I

Reinhard G. Bretel, M.D.
Professor of Medicine
Third Medical Department & Policlinic
University of Giessen
Giessen, Germany
Chapter 13

David R. Chadwick, M.B., Ch.B.,
  F.R.C.S.
Lecturer in Surgery
Department of Surgery
Leicester University
Leicester Royal Infirmary
Leicester, United Kingdom
Chapter 3

CONTRIBUTORS

Thomas Cavanagh, B.S., M.T.
Research Investigator
Boehringer Mannheim Corporation
Indianapolis, Indiania, USA
Chapter 4

Alberto M. Davalli, M.D.
Visiting Scientist
Section on Islet Transplantation
  and Cell Biology
Joslin Diabetes Center
Boston, Massachusetts, USA
Chapter 5, Part I

Benigno J. Digon, III
Research Associate
Diabetes Research Institute
University of Miami
Miami, Florida, USA
Chapter 9

Francis E. Dwulet, Ph.D.
Senior Research Investigator
Boehringer Mannheim Corporation
Indianapolis, Indiania, USA
Chapter 4

Konrad F. Federlin, M.D.
Professor and Head
Third Medical Department and Policlinic
University of Giessen
Giessen, Germany
Chapter 13

Sarah Ferber, Ph.D.
Assistant Professor
The Claim Sheba Medical Center
Tel-Aviv University
Sackler School of Medicine
Tel-Hashomer, Israel
Chapter 15

Terry Fetterhoff, M.S.
Research Investigator
Boehringer Mannheim Corporation
Indianapolis, Indiania, USA
Chapter 4

John Gill, Ph.D.
Research Investigator
Boehringer Mannhein Corporation
Indianapolis, Indiania, USA
Chapter 4

Derek W.R. Gray, D.Phil, M.R.C.P,
  F.R.C.S.
Clinical Reader and Consultant Surgeon
Transplantation Surgery
Nuffield Department of Surgery
University of Oxford
and
John Radcliff Hospital
Headington, Oxford, United Kingdom
Chapter 2

Bernhard J. Hering, M.D.
Third Medical Department and
  Policlinic
University of Giessen
Giessan, Germany
Chapter 13

Jennifer Hollister, B.A.
Research Assistant
Section on Islet Transplantation and
  Cell Biology
Joslin Diabetes Center
Boston, Massachusetts, USA
Chapter 5 Part I

Paul R.V. Johnson, M.B., Ch.B.,
  F.R.C.S.
Lecturer in Surgery
Department of Surgery
Leicester University
Leicester Royal Infirmary
Leicester, United Kingdom
Chapter 3

Maria Koulmanda, M.Sc.
Chief Technical Officer
The Walter and Eliza Hall Institute of
  Medical Research
University of Melbourne
and
The Royal Melbourne Hospital
Victoria, Australia
Chapter 10

Willem M. Kühtreiber, Ph.D.
Senior Scientist
BioHybrid Technologies, Inc.
Shrewsbury, Massachusetts, USA
Chapter 7

Jonathan R.T. Lakey, B.Sc., M.Sc.
Graduate Student
Department of Surgery
University of Alberta
Edmonton, Alberta, Canada
Chapter 8, Chapter 12

Nick J.M. London, M.B., Ch.B., M.D.,
  M.R.C.P., F.R.C.S.
Lecturer in Surgery
Department of Surgery
Leicester University
Leicester Royal Infirmary
Leicester, United Kingdom
Chapter 3

Shawn C. Lonergan, M.S.
Director
Molecular Diagnotics Business
  Development
Boehringer Mannheim Corporation
Indianapolis, Indiania, USA
Chapter 4

Robert C. MacCarthy, Ph.D.
Manager
New Product Development
Boehringer Mannheim Corporation
Indianapolis, Indiania USA
Chapter 4

Willy J. Malaisse, M.D.
Professor and Director
Laboratory of Experimental Medicine
Brussels Free University
Brussels, Belgium
Chapter 5, Part II

Francine Malaisse-Lagae, M.D.
Senior Research Associate
Laboratory of Experimental Medicine
Brussels Free University
Brussels, Belgium
Chapter 5, Part II

Thomas E. Mandel, M.D.
Head
Transplantaton Unit
The Walter and Eliza Institute of
  Medical Research
University of Melbourne
and
The Royal Melbourne Hospital
Victoria, Australia
Chapter 10

CONTRIBUTORS

Daniel H. Mintz, M.D.
Scientific Director
Diabetes Research Institute
University of Miami
Miami, Florida, USA
Chapter 9

Christopher B. Newgard, Ph.D.
Associate Professor
Departments of Biochemistry and
    Internal Medicine
and
Gifford Laboratories for Diabetes
    Research
University of Texas Southwestern
    Medical Center
Dallas, Texas, USA
Chapter 15

Jens Hoiriis Nielsen, D.Sc.
Head
Department of Cell Biology-
    Immunobiology
The Hagedorn Research Institute
Gentofte, Denmark
Chapter 14

Ray V. Rajotte, Ph.D.
Director
Surgical-Medical Research Institute and
    Professor of Surgery and Medicine
Departments of Surgery and Medicine
University of Alberta
Edmonton, Alberta, Canada
Chapter 8, Chapter 12

Camillo Ricordi, M.D.
Professor of Surgery
Director, Division of Cellular
    Transplantation
Co-Director, Diabetes Research Institute
University of Miami School of Medicine
Miami, Florida, USA
Chapter 6, Chapter 9

Gavin S.M. Robertson, M.B., Ch.B., M.D.,
    F.R.C.S.
Lecturer in Surgery
Department of Surgery
Leicester University
Leicester Royal Infirmary
Leicester, United Kingdom
Chapter 3

Wolfgang J. Schnedl, M.D.
Post-Doctoral Fellow
Departments of Biochemistry and Internal
    Medicine
and
Gifford Laboratories for Diabetes Research
University of Texas Southwestern Medical
    Center
Dallas, Texas, USA
Chapter 15

Hans W. Sollinger, M.D., Ph.D.
Professor of Surgery and Pathology
Departments of Surgery and Pathology
University of Wisconsin Hospital
Madison, Wisconsin, USA
Chapter 1

CONTRIBUTORS

E. Donnall Thomas, M.D.
Emeritus Professor of Medicine
University of Washington
Director, Clinical Research Division
Fred Hutchinson Cancer Research Center
Seattle, Washington, USA
Foreword

Garth L. Warnock, M.Sc., M.D.,
    F.R.C.S.(C)
Director
Clinical Islet Transplant Program
Surgical-Medical Research Institute
and
Associate Professor of Surgery
Department of Surgery
University of Alberta
Edmonton, Alberta, Canada
Chapter 8, Chapter 12

Gordon C. Weir, M.D.
Head
Section on Islet Transplantation and
    Cell Biology
Joslin Diabetes Center
Boston, Massachusetts, USA
Chapter 5, Part I

Stephen White, M.B., Ch.B.
Lecturer in Surgery
Department of Surgery
Leicester University
Leicester Royal Infirmary
Leicester, United Kingdom
Chapter 3

James R. Wright, Jr., M.D.
Assistant Professor
Departments of Pathology and Surgery
Izaak Walton Killam Children's Hospital
Dalhousie University
Halifax, Nova Scotia, Canada
Chapter 11

Carlton J. Young, M.D.
Surgical Transplant Fellow
Department of Surgery
University of Wisconsin Hospital
Madison, Wisconsin, USA
Chapter 1

In 1949, Jacobsen and colleagues reported that mice could survive otherwise lethal irradiation if the spleen were protected by a lead shield. Shortly thereafter, Lorenz and coworkers showed that the same irradiation–protection could be achieved by an infusion of marrow cells. In 1955, Ford et al used cytogenetics to demonstrate that the marrow of an irradiated mouse protected by an infusion of marrow cells contained cells of donor, not host, origin. These experiments marked the beginning of the field of cell transplantation.

The field of solid organ transplantation had its beginning at almost the same time. In 1959, Schwartz and Damasek reported that 6-mercaptopurine was an immunosuppressive agent that could confer a form of tolerance. Following this demonstration, Hitchings and Ilion developed Imuran and Murray and Starzl and colleagues used these immunosuppressive agents along with superb surgical skills to open up the field of transplantation of kidney, heart and liver.

During the following two decades marrow grafting was applied with increasing success to diseases such as aplastic anemia, leukemia and a series of genetic diseases. The increasing knowledge of human histocompatibility typing, additional immunosuppressive agents and improved supportive care made the progress possible.

Yet, until quite recently transplantation of hematopoietic progenitor cells was the only form of cell transplantation being actively pursued. It had been known for more than 15 years that marrow grafting also involved grafting of donor pulmonary macrophages and Kupffer cells. Recently, Starzl and colleagues demonstrated that solid organ transplants also involved systemic "microchimerism" of donor cells, presumably dendritic cells. Clearly, transplantation of cells other than marrow stem cells can be achieved. Why not transplant other cells needed because of disease — liver cells, pancreatic islet cells, glial cells?

This series of presentations focuses on the transplantation of pancreatic islet cells. Despite the wealth of knowledge about diabetes and the availability of recombinant insulin, diabetes remains a major scourge of mankind. The present series demonstrates the wealth of scientific technology being brought to bear on the possibility of therapy by islet cell transplantation. Although the problem is formidable, progress in science often occurs with great rapidity. The investigators reporting here are to be congratulated on their vision and resourcefulness to insure continued progress in developing improved treatment for diabetics.

E. Donnall Thomas, M.D.

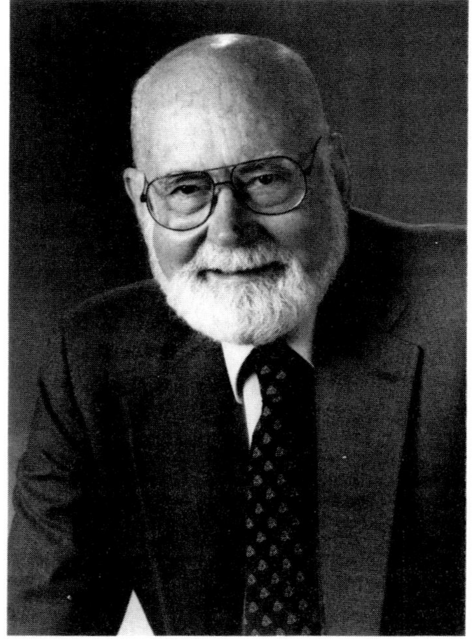

E. Donnall Thomas, M.D.
Nobel Laureate 1990

Dr. Thomas is one of the pioneers who ushered in the modern era of cell transplantation. In 1956, he performed the first human marrow transplant and was the first to treat acute leukemia by bone marrow transplantation while working at the Mary Imogene Bassett Hospital in Cooperstown, New York.

PREFACE

The modern era of clinical cell transplantation was ushered in approximately 40 years ago when E. Donnall Thomas performed his pioneering work using bone marrow transplantation as a therapy for leukemia. At approximately the same time, Joseph Murray and colleagues performed the first successful long-term renal transplant between identical twins at the Peter Bent Brigham Hospital in Boston. This technology was subsequently extended to transplantation between more distantly related and unrelated kidney donors through the use of immunosuppressive drugs such as Imuran and glucocorticoids and more recently cyclosporine A. To date, almost 400,000 patients worldwide have received life sustaining renal transplants.

Medical applications of transplantation technology have grown significantly during the past decade to include pancreas, heart and liver. In addition to transplanting whole organs, isolation and transplantation of cells and tissues with specific differentiated functions (e.g., beta cells which secrete insulin) represents an important conceptual and technological advance. It is readily apparent that transplantation of organs, tissues and cells into patients with a wide variety of serious disorders will constitute a major segment of the health care industry over the next several decades. The potential economic impact of transplantation, as a treatment for human disease, are enormous given the fact that the cost of a renal transplant is presently $35,000, while heart and liver transplants fall in the $100,000 to $200,000 range.

Further advancement and wider application of tissue and cell transplantation will require solving several problems including development of new strategies to overcome present formidable obstacles and to simplify implantation procedures. These problems include: (1) requirements for immunosuppressive drugs which expose patients to a wide variety of serious complications including cancer, infection, renal failure and osteoporosis; (2) lack of sufficient human donor tissue, which is so severe that patients may die while awaiting procurement of a matched donor organ; (3) requirements for extensive surgery such as transplantation of the whole pancreas with vascular anastomoses in diabetics when only 1-2% of the tissue produces insulin.

Resolution of these problems would open the door to widespread practical applications of cell and tissue transplantation. Diabetes mellitus is likely to be the initial major disease to which these advances will be applied for several reasons: (1) pancreatic islet transplantation is an area of current intense investigation, and would demonstrate improved treatment of a disorder currently affecting 80 million diabetics worldwide, at an estimated $92 billion annual cost for health care and lost wages in the U.S. alone; (2) pancreatic islets can be isolated from a wide variety of animal sources— animal insulins are fully active in man and have been used to treat diabetics for 70 years; and, (3) the quantity of differentiated islet tissue to be transplanted is within a reasonable range (<1 g).

The last several years of research and technology development have produced a dramatic advancement in islet isolation techniques, and in our knowledge of the human immune system, autoimmune disease, and immune rejection processes. This has resulted in a reliable source of human and animal islets, and in the development of procedures for immune modulation and immune isolation of donor islets that have the potential for preventing rejection of islet allografts and islet xenografts in patients without need for a life long regimen of generalized immunosuppression. This remarkable progress has furnished the stimulus for this series.

It appears increasingly likely that as we approach the 21st century islet transplantation will assume increasing importance as a treatment for diabetes. The resultant improvements in glycemic control will serve to prevent or to greatly retard the development of the dreaded complications of this disease which have claimed the health and life of millions.

We wish to express our indebtedness and gratitude to all our coauthors, who generously contributed their time and knowledge in the preparation of this series.We also thank Ms. Kathy Vairo for her valuable secretarial assistance.

Robert P. Lanza, M.D.
William L. Chick, M.D
March, 1994

CHAPTER 1

PANCREAS PROCUREMENT AND PRESERVATION

Carlton J. Young

Hans W. Sollinger

The steady evolution of pancreas transplantation has been exciting. In 1966, Drs. William Kelly and Richard Lillehei from the University of Minnesota performed the first successful human pancreas transplant. Their segmental duct-ligated transplant functioned for approximately two months. Following this, 13 more transplants were performed using the whole pancreas with a segment of duodenum and enteric drainage. Their results were modest. Since then, refinements in surgical technique followed. Gliedman in 1973 suggested exocrine pancreatic drainage by anastomosing the pancreatic duct to the recipient's ureter. In 1978, Dubernard used duct-injection for obliteration of exocrine tissue. However, by 1980 the International Pancreas Transplant Registry reported a one-year graft survival of only 21% and a patient survival of 67%. Because of these poor results, and complications secondary to the exocrine pancreas, further modifications were developed.

In 1982, Sollinger began using the bladder for drainage, which was later modified by Corry, who included a closed loop segment of duodenum for the anastomosis to the bladder. These refinements in surgical technique combined with the introduction of cyclosporine, and modified immunosuppressive therapy, as well as the ability to diagnose rejection, has increased both graft and patient survival rates to 80% and 90%, respectively, at one year. However, without advances in organ procurement and preservation, none of these advances could have been made.

PANCREAS PROCUREMENT

Of all the organs procured for transplantation, the pancreas is considered the most difficult. The ultimate success of a functioning graft is often predicated upon expertise by which the organ is recovered. Prior to 1990, transplant surgeons removed the entire pancreas or the liver, since combined removal was believed to compromise the quality of both organs. Presently in the United States, the majority of transplant centers perform combined liver-pancreas procurement.[1,2] In our experience, more than 95% of

Pancreatic Islet Transplantation Volume I: Procurement of Pancreatic Islets, edited by Robert P. Lanza, MD, William L. Chick, MD; ©1994 R.G. Landes Company.

multi-organ donors serve both as liver and pancreas donors. Isolated pancreas procurement is done only in instances where the liver is unsuitable for transplantation. In our center, the liver and pancreas are procured en bloc with a blood supply between the pancreas and the liver undisturbed during the procurement. This minimizes the risk of injury to the hepatic blood supply. This is especially important when aberrant hepatic artery anatomy exists.

The operative technique begins with a long midline incision extending from the sternal notch to the symphysis pubis. Bilateral cruciate extensions can be used when necessary. Prior to removing the organs a nasogastric tube is inserted and 250 mL of povidine iodine solution and 250 mL of amphotericin solution (50 mg amphotericin per liter of normal saline) are instilled into the nasogastric tube and milked into the duodenum. This helps facilitate a decrease in bacterial and fungal contamination.

The distal aorta and vena cava are encircled before the dissection begins, in case the patient becomes unstable. The falciform ligament is divided prior to splitting the sternum. This avoids injury to the liver. Additional room can be obtained by dividing the diaphragm bilaterally. Evaluation of the hepatic blood supply is accomplished by passing a hand through the foramen of Winslow with palpation of the porta hepatis. In approximately 16% of donors a replaced right hepatic artery will be palpated posterior and to the right of the portal vein. In 10-12% of patients the left hepatic artery will arise from the left gastric artery. If no vascular anomalies are appreciated, the gastrohepatic ligament is divided with a Bovie as well as the left triangular ligament of the liver. Dissection is then carried out along the greater curvature of the stomach, dividing the short gastric arteries. This allows for mobilization of the stomach which exposes the anterior surface of the pancreas. The left gastric artery is also divided. In those instances where exposure is difficult, the stomach can be removed by stapling across the distal esophagus and pylorus.

The proximal aorta is identified near the diaphragm and is encircled with an umbilical tape. At this time, complete vascular control has been obtained. Splenic attachments are freed, with the spleen remaining in continuity with the tail of the pancreas.

Mobilization of the pancreas is performed by excising the peritoneum posterior and lateral to the spleen and by using blunt and sharp dissection to free the pancreas from its posterior attachments. The inferior mesenteric vein is ligated and divided. The diaphragmatic crura and celiac lymphatics are divided with the electrocautery. The aorta, celiac axis, and superior mesenteric artery are then exposed. Care must be exercised to avoid injury to the left renal vein.

The hepatoduodenal ligament is then dissected after complete kocherization of the duodenum. The common hepatic duct is dissected, ligated, and divided as close to the pancreas as possible. The portal vein is then identified and isolated with an umbilical tape. In order to expose the mesenteric axis, the gastrocolic ligament is ligated and divided. The lateral peritoneal attachments of the colon are divided and the colon is moved caudally. The proximal jejunum is divided between staple lines, isolating the duodenum around the head of the pancreas. The superior mesenteric artery is ligated below the inferior border of the pancreas and divided, allowing the entire colon and small bowel to be placed inferiorly outside of the body. The liver, pancreas and both kidneys are now in full view.

Once the dissection is completed, a cannula is placed into the aorta and connected to a 2 L bag of Belzer-UW solution. The patient is then heparinized. Following this, the infra-diaphragmatic aorta is clamped. The portal vein is divided approximately 1.5 cm cephalad to the superior pancreatic margin and the aortic flush is started. Another cannula is placed into the distal portal vein and held in place with a forceps while the liver is flushed (Fig. 1.1). The IVC in the chest is divided to allow the efflux of blood and Belzer-UW solution. This procedure allows for rapid cooling of the liver. In

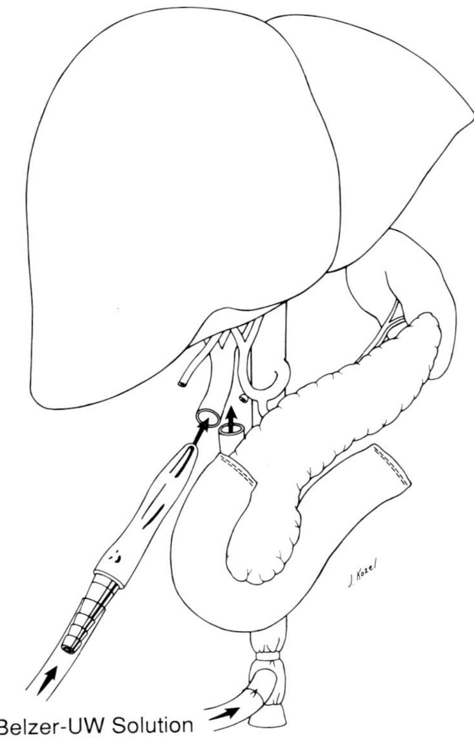

Fig. 1.1. Simultaneous in situ flush of aorta and portal vein with Belzer–UW solution during combined liver–pancreas procurement.

all, 2000 mL of Belzer-UW solution enters the aorta and 500-1000 mL enters the portal vein. Once flushing is completed the liver, duodenum, pancreas and spleen are removed en bloc and placed in a steel basin. Another 500 cc of Belzer-UW solution is then infused into the celiac axis and superior mesenteric artery.

As mentioned previously, separation of the liver and pancreas is performed after extrication. Not only does this method decrease the risk of vascular injury during dissection, but hepatic artery vasospasm, which can lead to posttransplant dysfunction of the liver, is avoided. The splenic artery is divided 1 cm beyond takeoff of the celiac trunk. The splenic artery stump is oversewn with a 6-0 prolene.

In those instances where the liver is not procured, a large Carrel patch comprising the celiac axis and superior mesenteric artery can be used for the pancreatic graft

(Fig. 1.2). Otherwise, the arterial supply to the pancreas must be reconstructed. In all procurements, the iliac arteries are harvested. Once the superior mesenteric artery and splenic arteries are cleared of surrounding tissue, a Y graft consisting of the donor common iliac artery, internal iliac artery and external iliac artery is used to reconstruct the arterial supply of the graft. In most instances, the internal iliac artery is anastomosed to the splenic artery and the external iliac artery is anastomosed to the superior mesenteric artery. This facilitates a better size matching of these vessels. In all cases, the liver will have a Carrel patch of aorta if it is harvested along with the pancreas. The kidneys are procured in the usual manner and stored in Belzer-UW solution.

Prior to performing the vascular reconstruction, the pancreatic graft must be prepared. The excess duodenum is separated from the pancreatic head by carefully ligating

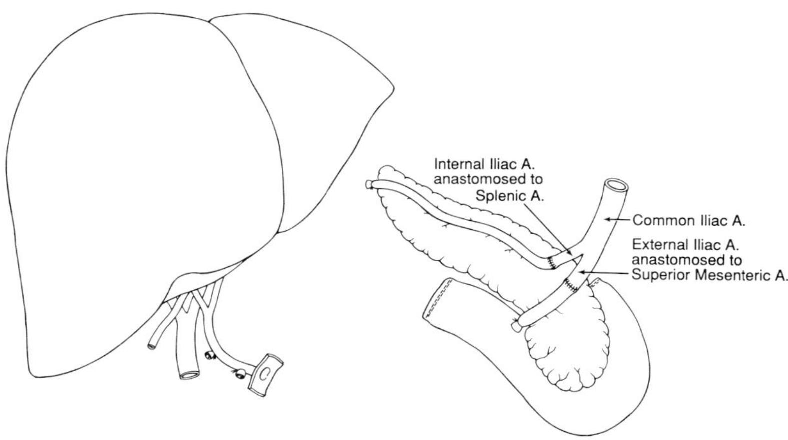

Fig. 1.2. Reconstruction of the pancreatic arterial blood supply with an iliac artery Y graft..

all blood vessels with 2-0 silk sutures. Once trimmed, the duodenal segment should measure approximately 10-12 cm in length. The ends are stapled and the excess duodenum is removed. The stapled ends are then oversewn with interrupted Lembert sutures using 3-0 silk sutures. The duodenal contents are aspirated and sent for culture. We have found gram stains to be less helpful, and therefore have been omitted. Lymphatics in the area of the celiac axis are carefully ligated. Potential bleeding points are also ligated. The spleen is then removed by carefully ligating and dividing tissue and vessels connecting it to the tail of the pancreas. The bifurcated iliac graft is then anastomosed using 5-0 or 6-0 prolene. Careful handling of the pancreas must be foremost, as rough handling may lead to posttransplant pancreatitis.

PRESERVATION

Excellent pancreatic graft preservation is important for several reasons. First, increased preservation times are needed for logistic reasons. Second, longer preservation times allow the performance of lymphocytotoxic crossmatches and elective scheduling of the operation. And third, the quality of the preservation will affect short- and long-term graft

outcome after transplantation. Preservation of endocrine and exocrine function for at least 30 hours is possible with Belzer-UW solution.

Early preservation solutions such as Collins' solution and its modifications were most widely used prior to the development of silica gel filtered plasma (SGFP), by the University of Minnesota. Following this, Belzer-UW solution became available in 1986. Despite transplanting the pancreas in less than 10 hours following preservation with Collins' solution, many cases of severe pancreatic edema and posttransplant pancreatitis were observed.

Presently, most transplant centers in the United States and Europe are using either Minnesota SGFP or Belzer-UW solution. Both solutions provide up to 30 hours of safe preservation; however, the Belzer-UW solution can be used as a universal flush solution for safe preservation of liver, kidney and pancreas.[3] The key ingredients of the Belzer-UW solution are shown in Table 1.1. Each ingredient serves a specific purpose at maintaining cellular integrity during hypothermia. Hypothermia suppresses the rate of cell death but does not prevent the process.[4] It also aids the organ to withstand anoxia and ischemia; however, no matter how successful the induction and maintenance of hypothermia may be, the final measure of success is the function of the graft. The kidney can be supported artificially until it resumes normal function, but organs such as the liver, heart and lungs must resume life support immediately.

Most methods of liver and pancreas preservation are adaptations of kidney preservation techniques. Unlike the kidney, the liver and pancreas are extremely sensitive to warm ischemia. Systems such as the sodium-potassium Na,K-ATPase pump are very sensitive to hypothermia. The loss of this ion exchange pump results in cell swelling and death. Liver and pancreatic islet cells are vulnerable to various oncotic support agents such as mannitol, which can permeate the cell membrane and cause cell death and swelling. Because of the delicate nature and vulnerability of these preparations, hypothermic preservation remains a formidable and complex problem.

In 1967, Belzer[5] attempted continuous hypothermic perfusion of kidneys with a variety of solutions. Early attempts to perfuse kidneys with fresh plasma were unsuccessful, as the kidneys developed an increasing perfusion pressure after 24 hours. Freezing, thawing and filtration of plasma produced a perfusate, cryoprecipitated plasma (CPP), which consistently yielded successful preservation for 72 hours. This process removed unstable lipoproteins of formed aggregates that cause blockage of the capillaries and a subsequent rise in perfusion pressure. CPP, however, is not stable and cannot be prepared in advance, and is also difficult to prepare. For this reason, other perfusates were developed.

Silica gel filtered plasma (SGFP) is prepared by treating plasma with silica to remove unstable lipoproteins and other lipid materials. This perfusate is shelf stable and yields preservation of kidneys for up to 72 hours. The addition of human serum albumin or a plasma protein fraction (PPF) to a type of saline solution yields preservation up to 72 hours. Southard[4] sought to improve on these results by developing a perfusate that would suppress hypothermia, reduce cell swelling, maintain normal tissue potassium concentrations and stimulate ATP synthesis both during and after transplantation. Results have been good in kidney preservation, but the same success has not been seen in liver and pancreas perfusion techniques.

Rapid core cooling of transplant allografts is accomplished by vascular flushout. This is necessary, as warm ischemia has been shown to cause the depletion of ATP and the accumulation of protons and lactic acid from anaerobic glycolysis. Hypothermia does not prevent this process, but it does slow the process whereby organ viability is maintained.

Table 1.1. Composition of Belzer–UW solution*

Substance	Amount
K^+–lactobionate (mM)	100
KH_2PO_4 (mM)	25
$MgSO_4$ (mM)	5
Raffinose (mM)	30
Adenosine (mM)	5
Glutathione (mM)	3
Insulin (U/L)	100
Bactrim (ml/L)	0.5
Dexamethasone (mg/L)	8
Allopurinol (mM)	1
Hydroxyethyl starch (gm/L)	50

*This solution is brought to ph 7.4 at room temperature with NaOH. The final concentrations are: Na = 30 ± 5 mM; K^+ = 120 ± 5 mM; mOsm/L = 320 ± 5. Bactrim = trimethoprim (16mg/mL) and sulfamethoxazole (80 mg/mL).

Hypothermia directly affects intracellular enzymes. Most normothermic animals have enzymes that show a 1.5-2.0-fold decrease for every 10°C decrease in temperature. This effect is analogous to van't/Hoff's rule: $Q10=(K2-K1)$ to $10/(t2-t1)$ where $Q10$ is the van't/Hoff coefficient for a 10° change in temperature and $K1$ and $K2$ are the reaction rates at temperatures $t1$ and $t2$, respectively. Therefore, for an enzyme pathway with a $Q10$ of 2, the metabolic rate is suppressed by about 12-13-fold when the temperature is decreased from 37°C to 0°C.[6]

Belzer cited five specific functions a preservation solution must accomplish.[6]

1. Minimize Hypothermic-Induced Cell Swelling

The extracellular milieu that bathes cells has a sodium concentration 10-20 times that of the intracellular environment. The reverse is true for potassium. These concentrations are maintained by the Na,K-ATPase pump, which is found in virtually all animal cells. The pump operates as an anti-port, actively pumping three sodium ions out against this electrochemical gradient for every two potassium ions going into the cell.[7] This pump effectively makes sodium an impermeant outside the cell that counteracts the colloid osmotic pressure derived from the intracellular protein and other impermeable ions.

The colloid osmotic force derived from the intracellular proteins and impermeable ions is about 110-140 mOsm/kg.[8] Macromolecules themselves contribute very little to the osmolarity of the cell interior, since despite their large size, each one counts only as a single molecule and there are relatively few of them compared to the large number of small molecules in the cell. However, these macromolecules are highly charged and they attract many inorganic ions of opposite charge. As a result, these counter-ions do make a major contribution to intracellular osmolarity. Also, the cell contains a high concentration of small organic molecules such as sugars, amino acids and nucleotides to which the plasma membrane is impermeable. These substances also attract counter-ions. Nevertheless, the osmolarity of the extracellular fluid is due mainly to small inorganic ions. If it were not for the sodium-potassium. ATPase pump, an equilibration of these ions would occur within and outside the cell. The Donnan Effect is also at work within these cells. The presence of these charged macromolecules and metabolites attract these ions causing the total concentration of inorganic ions to be greater inside than outside the cell at equilibrium.

If the cell had no mechanism to control its osmolarity, the higher total concentration of solutes inside the cell would eventually lead to water crossing the plasma membrane by osmosis, leading to cell rupture. The Na,K-ATPase pump controls the intracellular osmolarity by pumping out inorganic ions so the cytoplasm contains a lower total concentration of inorganic ions than the extracellular fluid, thereby compensating for the presence of excess intracellular organic solutes.

Admittedly, the basis for cell integrity rests in the activity of this pump to maintain cellular osmolarity and to prevent cell swelling. Anaerobic-hypothermic preservation suppresses the activity of this pump and decreases the membrane potential of the plasma membrane.[9] In turn, sodium enters the cell down the electrochemical gradient, while potassium exits. This results in the aforementioned cell swelling and death. Therefore, any cell preservation solution should seek to minimize this effect by increasing the extracellular potassium concentration.

2. Prevention of Intracellular Acidosis

Ischemia stimulates glycolysis and glyconeolysis (Pasteur Effect), which increases the production of lactic acid and hydrogen ions.[6] The resultant tissue acidosis damages cells, induces lysosomal instability, activates lysosomal enzymes, and alters mitochondrial properties. Flushout solutions must therefore prevent intracellular acidosis as well as prevent expansion of the interstitial space. Alkalinizing the flushout with buffering agents improves storage of liver and pancreatic grafts.

The suppression of cell swelling necessitates the use of an effective impermeant.

Glucose, the main impermeant of Collins' solution, is not effective with the liver or pancreas, since it readily enters cells. Mannitol also readily enters cells. This is one reason why cold storage solutions which depend on glucose or mannitol are not useful in long-term liver or pancreatic preservation. The Belzer-UW solution uses K^+–lactobionate, which achieves these goals.

3. Prevention of Expansion of the Intracellular Space

Addition of substances which increase the colloid osmotic pressure of the flushout prevents rapid expansion of the interstitial space during the flushout period. This allows for the complete washout of blood elements, with retention of normal interstitial spaces.[6] In the Belzer-UW solution, raffinose, a saccharide with a large relative molecular mass (594 daltons), is added for osmotic support. Hydroxy-ethyl starch, a stable, non-toxic colloid, is also added to prevent expansion of the extracellular space.

4. Oxygen-Derived Free Radicals

The development of oxygen-derived free radicals during cold storage may play an important role in cell damage during reperfusion. A free radical is any molecule that has an odd number of electrons. Free radicals, which can occur in both organic, (quinones), and inorganic molecules (O_2-) are highly reactive, and therefore, transient. They are generated in vivo as the by-products of normal metabolism or the result of ionizing radiation or by xenobiotics, i.e., environmental agents including photo chemicals, pollutants, hyperoxia, and pesticides.[10]

Oxygen-derived free radicals produced by activated phagocytes are microbicidal and can inadvertently cause tissue damage. Irradiation of organisms with electromagnetic radiation (x-rays, gamma rays, protons, neutrons) generate primary radicals by transferring their energy to cellular components like water. These primary radicals include OH and H, which then undergo secondary reactions with dissolved oxygen or cellular solutes.

Intracellular sources of free radicals encompass a wide variety of soluble cell components which are capable of undergoing oxidation reduction reactions in a neutral aqueous milieu. Also, numerous enzymes generate free radicals during the catalytic activity. Xanthine oxidase generates oxygen-free radicals during the reduction of oxygen to peroxide. The relative proportion of O_2- and H_2O to release from the active site depends on the pH, O_2 concentration, and substrate concentration. Human xanthine oxidase in vivo serves as a NAD+ dependent dehydrogenase and produces no free radical intermediates. Proteolytic modification of the enzyme during purification or during in vivo ischemia converts the enzyme from the dehydrogenase form to O_2-, producing the oxidized form.[10]

Other sources of oxygen-derived free radicals can occur throughout the cell. The mitochondrial electron transport chain, endoplasmic reticulum, and nuclear membrane electron transport system are but a few of those sites. Their detailed descriptions are beyond the scope of this text, but each contributes to the overall cellular concentration of oxygen-derived free radicals at varying degrees.

There are several varying sites of action by free radicals. The plasma membrane is the critical site, since extracellular free radicals must cross the membrane before they can react with other cell components. The unsaturated fatty acids present in the membrane (phospholipids, glycolipids, glycerides and sterols) and the transmembrane proteins contain oxidizable amino acids which are susceptible to free radical damage. Protein-containing amino acids tryptophan, tyrosine, phenylalanine, histadine, methionine, and cysteine can undergo free radicalmediated amino acid modification. Nucleic acids and DNA are also at risk from these substances.[11] The cell, however, has intrinsic defenses. These defenses include both low molecular weight free radical scavengers and complex enzyme systems. These defenses serve to lower the steady state concentrations of free radical species to acceptable levels. Two of the more common enzyme scavengers are catalase and superoxide dismutase. Catalase lowers the steady state concentration of H_2O_2, which is a precursor of more potent radical species. Thus, the cytotoxic potential of H_2O_2 is in large part a function of intracellular catalase and peroxidase activity to scavenge H_2O_2. Superoxide dismutases are metalloproteins that are primarily located within the mitochondria, where a large portion of O_2- radicals are produced. They function to convert oxygen-derived free radicals into water and oxygen. They are so effective that only micromolar (μM)concentrations of these species are measured within mitochondria and in the cytosol.

In addition to the above, ischemia results in the depletion of ATP and a rise in AMP, whose catabolism results in a build-up of hypoxanthine. Hypoxanthine can then be oxidized by either xanthine dehydrogenase or oxidized leading to more oxygen-derived free radicals. Also, as mentioned above, cells produce oxygen-free radicals all throughout the cell and are also bombarded by them constantly.

Allopurinol, a xanthine oxidase inhibitor, is a main ingredient in the Belzer-UW solution. Its effect is to decrease the activity of xanthine oxidase and therefore subsequently decrease the production of oxygen-derived free radicals.

5. Preservation and Regeneration of ATP

Adenosine triphosphate (ATP) rapidly degrades during hypothermic storage, and this degradation results in the formation of end products which in the plasma membrane are freely permeable. Organ reperfusion necessitates the rapid regeneration of the sodium pump activity as well as other energy-requiring steps. ATP production is coupled to the electron transport chain, which is slowed during hypothermic storage. The primary effect of hypothermia is the suppression of the rate of translocation of adenosine nucleotides across the inter-mitochondrial membrane.[6] Here the exchange of an external adenosine diphosphate (ADP) for an internal ATP is accomplished. However, at 10°C or less, this process is limited, with a resultant decrease in the rate of oxidative phosphorization and ATP production.

In an effort to maintain a normal ratio of adenine nucleotides, adenylate kinase converts 2 ADP to 1 ATP and 1 AMP. The accumulation of AMP and the eventual decrease in ATP stimulates catabolic reactions, leading to the breakdown of AMP to the oxypurines (adenosine, inosine and hypoxanthine). These end products are freely permeable to the plasma membrane and equilibrate with the extracellular milieu.[12] These series of reactions appear to explain the loss of adenosine nucleotides during hypothermic storage. By adding adenosine to the preservation solution, the loss of intracellular adenosine, which is needed for the regeneration of ATP during reperfusion, can be decreased.

CONCLUSION

The Belzer-UW solution has been successful in preserving livers, kidneys and pancreata for up to 30 hours. This solution is a vast improvement over prior cold storage solutions. It has enabled liver transplantation to be performed on a semi-elective basis, while kidney and pancreas transplantation can be performed on an elective basis.

As discussed previously, there are several key areas in hypothermic cell preservation. The Belzer-UW solution is presently based on lactobionate (molecular weight 358) and raffinose (molecular weight 504) which act as impermeants to suppress hypothermia-induced cell swelling. The lactobionate anion is used in place of the freely permeable chloride anion and raffinose in place of glucose and mannitol, which act as impermeants in Collins' solution and hypertonic citrate, respectively. These sugars are effective impermeants in the kidney, but the liver shows free permeability to these small carbohydrates. Thus, the lack of effectiveness of these solutions for prolonged preservation of the liver and pancreas is not unexpected.

Phosphate acts as a buffer to minimize changes in pH during storage. While magnesium sulfate acts as a membrane stabilizer and reduced glutathione as an anti-oxidant. Adenosine is included as a precursor for the resynthesis of adenine nucleotides, allopurinol as a free radical scavenger and xanthine oxidase inhibitor, and hydroxy-ethyl starch as a colloid for oncotic support. This solution is also effective, as stated, in pancreas and kidney preservation, and can be used as the sole flushing solution for all intra-abdominal organs prior to harvesting.

The careful procurement and preservation of pancreatic grafts is imperative in obtaining excellent graft function. En bloc extrication of liver, pancreas and duodenum with later separation avoids vascular injuries and decreases procurement time. Careful dissection and handling of the pancreatic graft is necessary to avoid post-transplant complications. Also, using a preservation solution such as Belzer-UW solution will provide long-term cold storage of these grafts with subsequent excellent graft function.

REFERENCES

1. Sollinger HW, Vernon WB, D'Alessandro AM, Kalayoglu M, Stratta RJ, Belzer FO. Combined liver and pancreas procurement with Belzer-UW solution. Surgery 106: 685-691, 1989.
2. Marsh CL, Perkins JD, Hayes DH, et al. Combined hepatic and pancreatico-duodenal procurement for transplantation. Diabetes 38:231, 1989.
3. Kalayoglu M, Sollinger HW, D'Alessandro AM, Stratta RJ, Hoffmann RM, Pirsch JD, Belzer FO. Successful extended preservation of the liver for clinical transplantation. Lancet 1:617-619, 1988.
4. Southard JH, Belzer FO. Organ preservation. Flye MW (ed): Principles of Organ Transplantation. W. B. Saunders Company, Philadelphia, 1989, 194-213.
5. Belzer FO, Ashby BS, Dunphy JE. Twenty-four hour and 72-hour preservation of canine kidneys. Lancet 2:536, 1967.
6. Belzer FO, Southard JH. Principles of short-term preservation by cold storage. Transplantation 45:673, 1988.
7. Alberts B, Bray B, Lewis J, Raff M, Roberts K, Watson JD (eds.): Molecular Biology of the Cell, Second Edition. Garland Publishing, Inc., New York, 1989, pages 304-309.
8. MacKnight ABC, Leaf A. Regulation of cellular volume. Physiological Review 57:570, 1977.
9. Martin DR, Scott DF, et al. Primary cause of unsuccessful liver and heart preservation: cold sensitivity of the ATP ace system. Annals of Surgery 175:111, 1972.
10. Freeman BA, Crapo JD. Biology of disease: free radicals in tissue injury. Laboratory Investigation 47:412, 1982. 16
11. Myers LS, et al. Free radical damage of nucleic acids and their components. Pryor WA (ed.): Free Radicals in Biology, Volume 14, New York Academy Press, 1981, 95.
12. Southard JH, Lutz MF, et al. Stimulation of ATP synthesis in hypothermically perfused dog kidneys by adenosine and PO_4. Cryobiology 21:13, 1984.

CHAPTER 2

APPROACHES TO PANCREATIC TISSUE DISPERSION

Derek W.R. Gray

The goal of pancreatic islet isolation is to separate islet tissue from the surrounding exocrine pancreas while preserving tissue viability. In most techniques the aim is to keep the islet structure intact during the isolation procedure, rather than reduce the tissue to single cells, although the latter approach is also possible.[1] This deceptively simple aim represents a new departure in tissue separation techniques, since the need to separate one intact organ (the islet) from within another organ (the pancreas) while maintaining structural integrity is a unique requirement. Bearing this in mind it is perhaps understandable that progress in pancreatic islet isolation techniques has been a slow and fitful progression over many years. The islet isolation process falls naturally into two stages: dispersion of the pancreatic tissue followed by purification. It is the purpose of this chapter to discuss aspects of the dispersion stage.

SPECIES DIFFERENCES

The techniques that have been used for islet isolation have been derived from experiments performed on numerous species of animal, and it is pertinent to first remember that considerable differences exist between the anatomical structure of the pancreata of these species. Although the different endocrine cells of pancreas are always clustered together, the relationship to the exocrine tissue varies considerably. The clearest example of separation of the exocrine and endocrine tissue is seen in teleost fish, where the islet tissue is located separately from the exocrine tissue in one or more Brockman bodies. Most experiments have been performed using rodent pancreas from rat, mouse, hamster and guinea pig. These species all have the islets scattered throughout the pancreas, which is a relatively diffuse organ within the mesogastrium and periduodenal tissues. The exocrine tissue has a relatively loose structure with a small quantity of collagen fibrils binding the acinus to acinus and acinus to islet. The peri-pancreatic tissue is poorly developed and thin, and the islets tend to be large, varying from 25 μm to 350 μm diameter, with maximum tissue volume held in islets of around 150-200 μm.

Pancreatic Islet Transplantation Volume I: Procurement of Pancreatic Islets, edited by Robert P. Lanza, MD, William L. Chick, MD; ©1994 R.G. Landes Company.

The islets are rounded, compact, and separated from the surrounding exocrine tissue by a distinct peri-islet capsule which becomes most obvious after the fixation shrinkage artefact seen on paraffin embedded histological sections.

In species such as the dog and pig, the pancreas is naturally much larger, weighing 20-30 grams in the middle sized dog and 100-400 grams depending on the age of the pig. In these species, the exocrine tissue is more densely packed, with considerably more collagen binding acini together, surrounding vessels and forming a peri-pancreatic capsule, particularly in the pig. Islets tend to be smaller, in the dog islets vary from 25-200 μm diameter, with maximum tissue volume held in islets of 90-125 μm diameter. Pig islets tend to be slightly larger, varying from 25 μm to 300 μm in diameter, with the maximum tissue volume held in islets with a diameter of 100 to 200 μm. In the dog the islets tend to be more irregular, interdigitating into the surrounding tissues, with a less complete peri-islet capsule. In the pig the islets are more or less rounded but the peri-islet capsule is often poorly developed and incomplete.

Human and monkey islets tend to be rounded, and can be very large (range 25 μm to 500 μm diameter) with the maximum tissue volume held in islets of 100-250 μm diameter.[2] The exocrine tissue is compact but the fibrous tissue content varies enormously, sometimes being very thick type 3 collagen in the interlobular tissue and peri-vascular tissue with a variable quantity of type 1 and type 3 collagen binding the acini and islets together.[3]

In addition to framework differences there are considerable variations in the arrangement of the pancreatic duct or ducts and the relationship to the bile duct. In man and monkeys, the pancreatic drainage is largely by a duct into the terminal bile duct with a smaller accessory duct draining directly into the duodenum. The dog and pig have a basically similar arrangement to the human, although the layout of the pancreatic lobes differs considerably. Rodents have multiple pancreatic ducts entering the length of the bile duct, while the rabbit has a single pancreatic duct entering the jejunum some 25 cm distal to the entry point of the bile duct in the duodenum.

The Development of Pancreatic Islet Dispersion Techniques

The first description of a technique for separation of islets from exocrine was a process of microdissection, using the pancreas of several species, but most successfully the obese mouse, where the islets are easily visible by stereo microscopy of the unstained pancreas.[4] Although useful for providing islets for biochemical experiments the number of islets obtainable was limited to 50 or so. The advance that started the push towards islet transplantation was the discovery that guinea pig pancreatic tissue could be dispersed by a combination of ductal distension using a balanced salt solution and then scissor chopping the tissue and exposing it at 37°C to a crude enzymic extract from the bacterium clostridium histolyticum, which had collagenase activity.[5] The enzyme acted on the tissue to encourage disintegration of the interacinar adhesion, andwhen combined with fairly vigorous agitation and trituration through syringe and wide-bore needle, produced dispersion of the pancreas into mainly single acini, with larger, denser intact islets that could be retrieved by hand-picking. The same digestion technique was subsequently applied to the pancreas of the rat,[6] and when combined with a density gradient separation[7] allowed for the first time the isolation of islets in large enough numbers for the purpose of transplantation.[8] Approximately 200 islets were obtainable from the adult rat pancreas, and up to 6 donors were often used to obtain enough islets for a single transplant.

For the next few years the method of digestion was standardized for production of islets from the rat and guinea pig pancreas.[8] For the mouse pancreas it was found to be difficult and unnecessary to distend the pancreas, and the tissue was simply chopped into large pieces and then exposed to collagenase. Yields of 50 islets or so per pancreas were usual.[9] Early attempts to isolate islets from human pancreas applied the same method, and success was claimed,[10] although no details of the tissue preparation were given and it is now clear that the purity, intact islet content and viability of the tissue produced was probably very poor. Looking back, it is likely that the density of the tightly packed human exocrine tissue prevented adequate distension of the tissue, and subsequent chopping or mincing of the tissue was still insufficient to allow penetration so that proper cleavage of the islets from exocrine tissue was not obtained. The same result occurred when the rodent isolation technique was applied experimentally to dog or pig pancreas. The result from pig pancreas was particularly poor using the rodent technique.[11]

Considerable research was undertaken into alternative techniques for distending the pancreas using the dog model, with some improvement in results in the dog[12] but not the human pancreas. The inability to isolate purified islets led some groups to abandon attempts to purify the islet tissue altogether, and to simply distend the tissue by direct collagenase injection, chop the tissue mechanically and lightly digest the tissue to reduce the average particle size. The dispersed tissue was then injected without further purification.[13] This approach proved to be surprisingly successful in the dog model, where it was possible to inject the large volume of tissue obtained into the spleen, which was large enough to accept the tissue without major complications.[13] The first repeatably successful islet transplants in a large animal model were obtained using this crude preparation technique,[13-18] and long-term normoglycemia resulted following autotransplantation in totally pancreatectomized dogs, allowing metabolic studies.[19,20] The good results using unpurified dispersed pancreas autotransplantation in the dog model encouraged clinicians to try the same approach in patients, with disastrous results,[21] and the attempt to perform human transplantation was abandoned. Some groups took the approach of mechanical dispersion of pancreatic tissue to extremes, using high speed mechanical chopping devices[22] or pressing the tissue through sieves[23,24] to obtain

dispersion. The tissue obtained was then transplanted without subsequent purification, and success was claimed in both dog[25] and pig[22] models, although it turns out that these reports have not been repeatable by others.

Few advances came until the technique of injecting collagenase into the pancreatic duct was developed, first in the dog[26,27] and subsequently applied to the human pancreas.[28] With hindsight, it is hard to understand why this apparently logical development took so long; possibly it was due to a fixation on the use of intraductal distension as a physical method for dispersing the pancreas (as in the rodent technique), while failing to realize it could be a route of delivery of the collagenase enzyme to allow more efficient enzymic dispersion. The intraductal collagenase technique has now become the preferred approach for dispersing the pancreas of all species, although interestingly there are reports of earlier techniques still in use[29] and the claim for superiority of the intraductal collagenase technique is not entirely undisputed.[30] The intraductal collagenase technique has also been applied back to rodent islet isolation, with improvements in the yield of islets to over 1000 islets per rat pancreas and over 300 islets per mouse pancreas,[31] allowing single donor islet autotransplantation.

INTRADUCTAL COLLAGENASE DIGESTION—CURRENT CONCEPTS

It has become abundantly clear to all those working in the field of islet isolation that the key to the second or purification stage of islet isolation is to get the first stage of digestion right; that is to cleave the islets cleanly away from the islet tissue, but to maintain the viability and structure of the islet tissue. There are two basic tenets that underlie most of the successful techniques for islet isolation:

Trauma = Tissue Death

Complexity = Tissue Loss

What is meant by this aphorism is that techniques for islet retrieval should be as gentle with the tissue as possible, to avoid reducing tissue viability and have as few stages as possible for handling the tissue, since each transfer of tissue results in tissue loss. However, this latter concept does not exclude the use of complex and sophisticated machinery, for example to automate or control the digestion process, but the actual number of separate processes and transfers that the tissue is subjected to should be reduced to a minimum. Despite the latter aim there are still numerous stages that the tissue must go through. We shall examine what is known about each stage and its effect on the digestion process, in logical order, with particular reference to the technique of human islet isolation, making reference to experimental studies in animals where appropriate.

Donor Factors

A number of variables may be imagined to affect successful islet isolation from the cadaveric human pancreas, including donor age, sex and weight, all of which might alter the fibrous tissue content of the pancreas gland. Human cadaveric donors are subject to a number of stresses arising out of the conditions that led to brain death and subsequent management of the brain dead cadaveric donor. These include major swings in blood pressure, temperature, oxygenation, hydration and treatment with various pressor agents, intravenous fluids and drugs. The duration of stay on the intensive care unit, allowing the above variables to act, might also be an adverse factor. The role of homeostatic mechanisms, including hormonal and cytokine release, are largely unknown, however it is certain that many brain-dead donors have major derangements of glucose metabolism in the absence of a history of previous diabetes. Insulin treatment for hyperglycemia is often required. The data regarding the influence of the above variables is fairly sparse and to some extent conflicting. Some studies have commented on the relatively poor results obtained using pancreata from younger donors (<20 years),[32,33] although this has not been the experience of all centers.[34] There is general agreement that results are not as good from donors where there has been significant hyperglycemia, where perhaps the important factor is the lowest blood sugar achieved during the admission rather than the highest blood sugar recorded.[34]

Warm and Cold Ischemia

During the donation procedure, minor or even major warm ischemia of the pancreas is common, followed by a period of cold ischemia after removal and transport of the organ, prior to the digestion process. The effect of both warm and cold ischemia on the islet isolation process has been studied both in experimental animal systems and by analysis of the results of islet isolation from human pancreas. In rodent models early studies suggested relatively little effect of warm ischemia[35-37] and cold ischemia was suggested to have little effect up to 24 hours if pulsatile hypothermic perfusion was used.[38] More recent studies in the rodent have shown both warm and cold ischemia impair the yield of islet obtainable using the intraductal collagenase technique,[39] and warm ischemia was shown to affect islet yield in the dog.[40] Cold ischemia was shown to impair the islet isolation process, resulting in reduced yields in a dog intraductal islet isolation model.[41,42] However, the use of UW solution to flush the pancreas was reported to improve the yield in one study,[43] but not in another, where the use of cold collagenase solution injected intraductally to cool the gland was found to produce a great improvement in islet yield.[44] For the human pancreas, cold ischemia times greater than 6-8 hours have been reported to result in reduced islet yields,[45,34] but cold ischemia up to 20 hours has been reported to make no significant difference by others.[33]

Cooling by Vascular Perfusion or Ductal Distension

At organ donation the pancreas may be cooled either by flushing via the vascular system or by direct surface cooling. In rodents and dogs both techniques appear to produce good results in the immediately processed pancreas,[44] but in both the rat and the dog the use of an intravascular flush of the pancreas was associated with inferior results if the pancreas was stored before islet isolation.[44] One logical reason why islet isolation using the intraductal collagenase technique might not work as well after intravascular flush is if tissue edema develops, which might physically prevent the desired distribution of the injected collagenase within the tissue. The type of solution used for the intravascular flush would be expected to have a significant effect on the development of edema; for example UW solution has been shown to produce less pancreatic swelling[46] and has been suggested to improve the yield of islets obtainable when used as an intravascular flush in one canine study[43] although this was not confirmed in another study.[44] Recent studies of the use of UW solution as an intravascular flush before human islet isolation have shown no advantage over "nonosmotic" solutions such as hypertonic citrate solution; indeed the UW treatment has been suggested to inhibit the digestion process, requiring a higher collagenase concentration.[47] This inhibitory effect is most marked if UW solution is used to make up the collagenase for intraductal digestion, (although this is an illogical approach, since the digestion stage is performed at warm temperatures and UW solution is a cold storage solution that is probably quite toxic at warm temperatures). The exact nature of the effect of UW solution on collagenase digestion and the component responsible remains speculative, although it is interesting to note that UW solution has considerable chelating power for calcium[48] (see the role of calcium below).

An alternative approach which combines rapid cooling with placement of the collagenase into the tissue is to inject cold collagenase solution into the duct.[44] The gland can later be rewarmed, either by surface warming if the gland is small enough (for example in the rodent) or by re-injecting warmed collagenase into the duct. This approach was effective in the dog pancreas, where it produced better results than intravascular cold flush[44,49] and has been advocated particularly for isolation of islets from the human pancreas from young donors.[50] It is the standard technique for rodent islet isolation using intraductal collagenase.[51,52]

REQUIREMENTS FOR PANCREAS DIGESTION

COLLAGENASE

There can be few components of a supposedly scientific technique more imbued with a sense of mystique than the collagenase used for pancreatic islet isolation. Different batches of commercially produced collagenase enzyme are tested and pronounced excellent by some groups, while the same batch is labeled as rubbish by others. One batch of collagenase may give excellent results for a time then mysteriously become useless, with no identifiable cause other than being "past the sell-by date." The problem of deciding which concentration of collagenase to use is also part of the same conundrum. The currently used commercial preparations are obtained from semi-purified extracts of clostridium histolyticum cultures, but the exact details of the culture and extraction processes are kept secret. The preparations certainly contain bacterial collagenase activity, usually expressed as collagen digestion units/mg, but they also contain several other enzymes, mostly varieties of proteases. The impurities are not retained because of an inability to purify the collagenase. Purified extracts including completely pure collagenase enzyme are available, but unfortunately completely purified collagenase does not produce good islets,[53] and we have evidence that the efficacy of islet releasing action, at least for the rat pancreas, correlates best with both collagenase and protease content.[54]

There can be little doubt that the development of a standardized collagenase preparation, with all the components from a pure source, would be a great boon to the development of islet transplantation. Arguably one of the biggest barriers to such development is the lack of a standardized laboratory-based islet production assay that will accurately predict utility when applied to a human pancreas or the pancreas of other species. It is possible that a rodent-based assay could be the basis for such a standard, but the work to prove applicability to human and the pancreas of other species has not been done. Currently several groups, both commercial and University based are working on the problem. One approach has been to try and produce an efficient islet producing preparation by combining various enzymes that are already available in purified form.[55] The combination of pure collagenase with a blend of neutral collagenase and elastase has seemed to produce the best results so far. Another approach has been to produce huge batches of commercial collagenase, identify the batch with the best islet producing characteristics, then analyse the components of the batch by physically separating the components, identifying them then mixing back the components stepwise to show which are essential for islet producing activity. Clearly, this latter approach is beyond the resources of the average research laboratory and has been undertaken by the Boehringer Company. Some progress has been reported (see chapter 4) and all working in the field will wish them success.

OTHER ADDITIVES

The question of "What is the ideal solution?" as a vehicle for delivery of collagenase has hardly been addressed. Obviously, the solution used must be able to provide a suitable environment for collagenase activity, while maintaining tissue viability during the digestion phase. Traditionally Hank's balanced salt solution has been used for this purpose, but there is virtually no data on whether this is ideal. Pure collagenase is certainly a calcium dependant enzyme, as can be proven by the addition of chelating substances such as EDTA, which stop the digestion process reliably in all species (Gray, D. 1983, unpublished data). However, the actual concentration of free calcium ions needed to allow digestion to proceed may be quite small, and for digesting the pancreas of some species, for example the rat, the absence of added calcium in the collagenase makes little difference and presumably there are sufficient calcium ions within the tissue to allow normal digestion. However, for pancreata from other species, this source of calcium may not be sufficient. Hanks solution normally contains 2 mM/L calcium, which is certainly sufficient for digestion of rat and possibly dog pancreata. The addition of higher concentrations of calcium to Hank's solution for digestion of human pancreas was originally introduced from our own laboratory on admittedly limited unpublished data. The requirement for extra calcium has never been proven to be necessary although some experimental studies have supported the addition,[56] and the extra calcium does not appear to have deleterious effects on tissue viability. The argument may therefore be put as "Why not put it in?," scientifically unsatisfactory as this may be.

TEMPERATURE CONTROL

A crucial factor for the efficiency of collagenase activity is the rapid attainment of working temperature. Collagenase activity rises in linear fashion with rising temperature and peaks at 43°C then falls off rapidly, presumably due to denaturation.[54] However, another consideration must be the viability of the tissue, which would be expected to be in jeopardy at temperatures above 43°C. Usually the pancreas gland is at low temperature before the initial injection of collagenase and the final temperature after injection is dependent on the starting temperature, the temperature of the injected solution and the volume injected. We have used temperatures up to 41°C for the injected solution, with success,[57] but the mechanism is probably to speed up the attainment of working temperature. It may well be that the reported advantage of perfusion techniques is based on the more rapid and reliable attainment of working temperature, rather than improved distribution of the collagenase enzyme.

DELIVERY OF ENZYME

If the requirement for intraductal enzyme delivery is taken as correct and most centers now agree this is so, then the question arises whether this is best achieved by a single injection (so called loading technique) or by constant perfusion. If the loading technique is used,[28] the pressure of injection and therefore rate of delivery may also be varied. There is little data on which is best, although there is limited data to support low pressure injection.[58] The only true comparison between constant perfusion and loading technique that has been performed on the human pancreas came down in favor of perfusion.[59] However, the need for more complex apparatus and increased volumes of expensive collagenase is a considerable inhibitor to the constant intraductal perfusion technique, and most centers still use a single loading injection of the collagenase at fairly high concentration, e.g., 3-6 mg/mL.[60-62]

Mechanism of Action

Studies of the distribution of intraductally injected collagenase have used two techniques to examine the distribution within the gland. We have injected contrast mixture into the duct in increasing volumes, varying pressure or by constant infusion into porcine pancreas, determining the distribution by radiography.[58] This method allowed only the gross distribution of the contrast material to be determined and showed that intraductal injection allowed remarkably uniform distribution of the contrast mixture throughout most of the gland, although some lobules would fail to fill, and remained unfilled despite further injection. Injection up to 1 mL/gm of tissue produced a complete "white-out" of all the distended lobules (Fig. 2.1), and little advantage was discernable by using constant perfusion rather than single injection.

The second technique, used by ourselves[58] and others,[30] has been to combine or replace the collagenase with india ink and examine the distribution by light microscopy. We found that there was relatively selective distribution of the injected ink throughout the exocrine tissue, permeating throughout the acini, and most of the islet tissue was relatively unstained (Fig. 2.2). Occasional islets showed penetration of the ink into the periphery. Another group using the same technique found more penetration into the islets than we found and concluded that there was relatively little selectivity of collagenase distribution after intraductal injection.[30]

The effect of intraductal collagenase has also been followed for human pancreata by multiple biopsies during the digestion stage and staining for collagen.[63,64] These studies have emphasised the large variation in quantity and distribution of collagen between different human pancreata. The main effect of the intraductal collagenase was first to remove the fine fibrils of collagen that bind acinus to acinus and acinus to islet. At this stage the effect on the thicker collagen surrounding large vessels and in the interlobular septae was relatively minor, and could only be removed by considerably prolonging the digestion. The effect on the collagen fibrils within the islet was variable: sometimes the fibrils were left intact, sometimes they appeared to be removed. The collagen fibrils often formed a "capsule" around the islet, and often this would be removed along with the interacinar collagen. The conclusion from these studies was that the intraductal collagenase digestion technique does indeed work by removing the collagen framework of the pancreas, but has the most effect on the inter-acinar structure but it also removes the islet structure if left too long. Removal of the collagen from the interlobular septae and larger vessels takes much longer digestion time.

A reasonable interpretation of the above studies would be that intraductal collagenase digestion is relatively non-selective in terms of sparing islets from the digestion process, and that prolonging the digestion to the point at which all the structural framework comprising the lobular septae and vascular supporting tissue are broken down will result in overdigestion of the islet tissue. The implication is that the digestion process should be used only to digest the fine inter-acinar collagen, while the coarser interlobular septae should be broken down by mechanical means.

Mechanical Aspects

From the last discussion it follows that there is a necessary mechanical stage in the digestion process to break down the remaining inter-lobular fibrous septae, including the fibrous capsule that surrounds the gland. Early techniques used a coarse tissue chopper at this stage,[26] which does release the

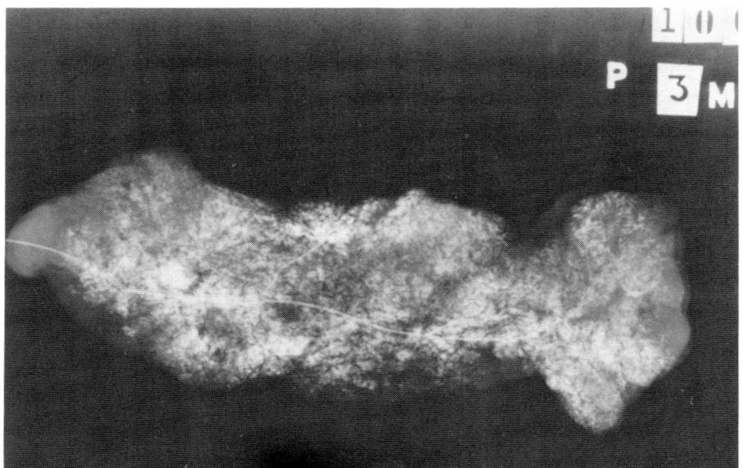

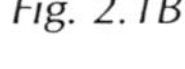

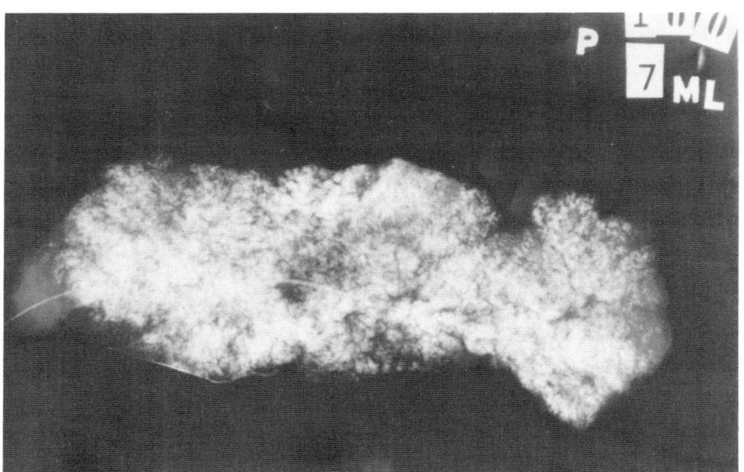

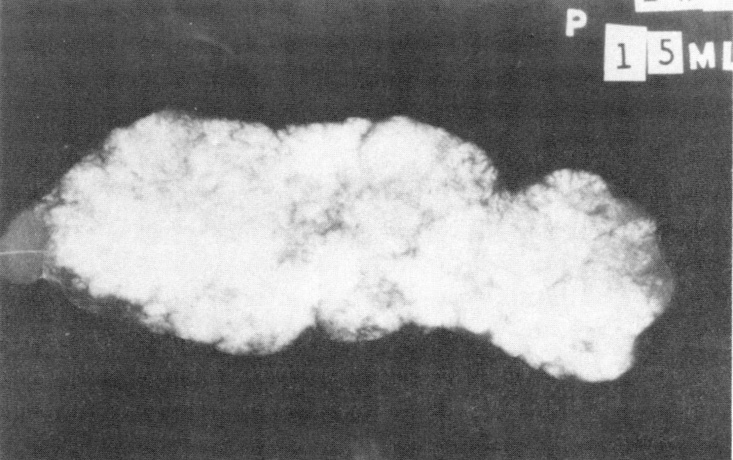

Figs. 2.1A–2.1C. X-rays of cynomolgus monkey pancreas following injection of progressive quantities (3,7 and 15 mLs) of dilute contrast medium into the pancreatic duct. Despite good general dispersion of the contrast throughout the gland some lobules, even some quite centrally placed, remain poorly injected.

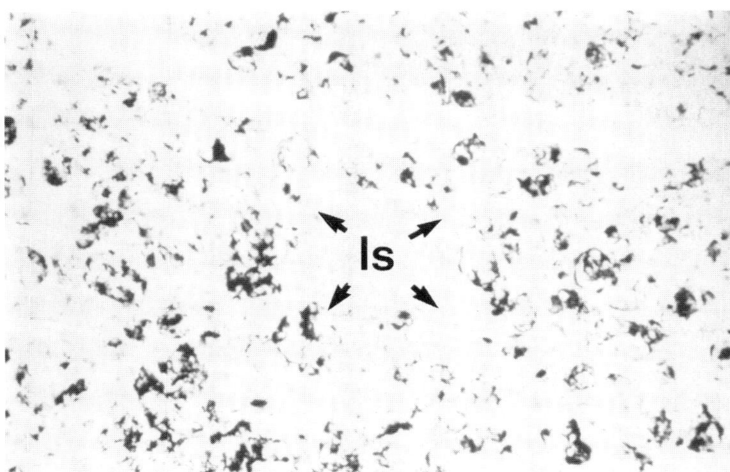

Fig. 2.2. Light micrograph of rat pancreas following intraductal injection of india ink suspension. There is relative sparing of the islet tissue (Is) whilst the exocrine pancreas is diffusely infiltrated with ink particles. Magnification approx. x 200.

digested tissue, but produces free strands of chopped fibrous tissue that tend to stay with the digest and produce problems for further processing. The technique that seemed most successful for the human pancreas was a combination of teasing the glandular tissue, to rupture the fibrous septae, and shaking the tissue gently with the forceps to release the digested acini and islets, leaving the fibrous tissue skeleton behind.[28] The problem with this approach was knowing when to stop the digest, cool the gland and begin the mechanical dispersion process. One advance, made possible by the introduction of dithizone stain for rapid identification of islets,[65] was to repeatedly biopsy the gland[60] (or to regularly examine biopsies taken from the gland after collagenase digestion which were incubated alongside the main tissue). The digestion was halted when free islets were first seen. We have adapted this technique, by regularly teasing a portion of the gland during the incubation, shaking the tissue gently and then immediately examining the fragments released into the fluid using dithizone stain. The teasing and shaking process is commenced once free islets are seen but the digestion is carried on, examining further samples regularly to confirm the islets are still being released intact, stopping the digestion if any fragmentation of the islets is seen.

The automation of the intraductal collagenase technique was a logical step,[66] the problem was the method to be used for breaking down the interlobular and capsular fibrous tissue, while the pancreas was located within a digestion chamber. The method chosen was a combination of vigorous shaking combined with placing 4 or 5 glass marbles within the chamber, which presumably tear the inter-acinar tissue by striking blows at the gland. This technique is described in detail elsewhere (chapters 6 and 9).

CONCLUDING REMARKS

Although advances have been made in the process of pancreatic islet isolation the digestion phase remains a difficulty, giving variable results particularly from the human pancreas. In part the variability is undoubtedly due to pre-donation factors and physical/structural variables within the pancreas, discussed in detail above. This is emphasised by the regular success which can be obtained from non-human primate pancreata if all the variables can be controlled. However, the digestion process is ultimately dependent on a "good" collagenase lot. The search for a standardized collagenase preparation must be seen as a priority for further progress in human islet isolation (see chapter 4). The correct digestion of the pancreatic tissue is vital for the success of the next stage, which is purification of the islets from the exocrine tissue. I'd like to hijack a maxim from the performing theater to express this: "If it ain't on the page—it ain't on the stage!!"

ACKNOWLEDGMENTS

I am grateful to Mr. Robert Sutton for provision of Figures 2.1 and 2.2. The work from the Nuffield Department of Surgery described in this chapter was supported by grants from the British Diabetes Association and the Juvenile Diabetes Foundatian, International.

REFERENCES

1. Pipeleers DG, Pipeleers-Marichal MA. A method for the purification of single A, B and D cells and for the isolation of coupled cells from isolated rat islets. Diabetologia 1981; 20:654-663.
2. Hellman B. Actual distribution of the number and volume of the islets of Langerhans in different size classes in non-diabetic humans of varying ages. Nature 1959; 184:1498-1499.
3. McShane P, Gray DWR, Hughes D, Morris PJ. Collagen type in human and rat pancreas. Localisation and relation to digestion. Diab Med 1990;7 (suppl 2):17A.
4. Hellerstrom C. A method for the microdissection of intact pancreatic islets of mammals. Acta Endocrinol 1964; 45:122-132.
5. Moskalewski S. Isolation and culture of the islets of Langerhans of the guinea pig. Gen Comp Endocrinol 1965; 5:342-353.
6. Ballinger WF, Lacy PE. Transplantation of intact pancreatic islets in rats. Surgery 1972; 72:175-186.
7. Scharp DW, Kemp CB, Knight MJ, Ballinger WF, Lacy PE. The use of ficoll in the preparation of viable islets of Langerhans from the rat pancreas. Transplantation 1973; 16:686-689.
8. Lacy PE, Kostianovsky M. Method for the isolation of intact islets of Langerhans from the rat pancreas. Diabetes 1967; 16:35-39.
9. Morrow CE, Sutherland DE, Steffes MW, Najarian JS, Bach FH. H-2 Antigen Class: Effect on mouse islet allograft rejection. Science 1983; 219:1337-1339.
10. Najarian JS, Sutherland DE, Matas AJ, Steffes MW, Simmons RL, Goetz FC. Human islet transplantation: a preliminary report. Transplant Proc 1977; 9:233-236.
11. Sutherland DE, Steffes MW, Bauer GE, McManus D, Noe BD, Najarian JS. Isolation of human and porcine islets of Langerhans and islet transplantation in pigs. J Surg Res 1974; 16:102-111.
12. Downing R, Scharp DW, Ballinger WF. An improved technique for the isolation and identification of mammalian islets of Langerhans. Transplantation 1980; 29:79-83.
13. Mirkovitch V, Campiche M. Absence of diabetes in dogs after total pancreatectomy and intrasplenic autotransplantation of pancreatic tissue. Transplant Proc 1977; 9:321-323.
14. Kolb E, Rucker R, Largiader F. Intraportal and intrasplenic autotransplantation of pancreatic islets in the dog. Eur Surg Res 1977; 9:419-426.
15. Kretschmer GJ, Sutherland DE, Matas AJ, Najarian JS. Preliminary experience with allotransplantation of pancreatic fragments to the spleen of totally pancreatectomized dogs. Transplant Proc 1979; 11:537-542.
16. Hanson SL, Sutherland DE, Field MJ, Rabe F, Najarian JS. Comparison of techniques for pancreatic islet transplantation in dogs. Surg Forum 1981; 32:383-385.
17. Mehigan DG, Zuidema GD, Cameron JL. Pancreatic islet transplantation in dogs: critical factors in technique. Am J Surg 1981; 141:208-212.
18. DuToit DF, Reece-Smith H, McShane P, Denton T, Morris PJ. A successful technique of segmental pancreatic autotransplantation in the dog. Transplantation 1981; 31:395-396.
19. Alderson D, Walsh TN, Farndon JR. Islet cell transplantation in diabetic dogs: studies of graft function and storage. Br J Surg 1984; 71:756-760.
20. Walsh TN, Fitzpatrick JM, Alderson D, Alberti KG, Farndon JR. Diurnal insulin and glucose profiles following transplantation of fresh and cryopreserved canine pancreatic islets. Br J Surg 1989; 76: 1287-1290.

21. Mehigan DG, Bell WR, Zuidema GD, Eggleston JC, Cameron JL. Disseminated intravascular coagulation and portal hypertension following pancreatic islet autotransplantation. Ann Surg 1980; 191:287-293.

22. Wise MH, Gordon C, Johnson RW. Renal subcapsular and intrasplenic transplantation of porcine islets of Langerhans. (Abstract). Br J Surg 1982; 69:285-286.

23. Hinshaw DB, Jolley WB, Hinshaw DB, Kaiser JE, Hinshaw K. Islet autotrans-plantation after pancreatectomy for chronic pancreatitis with a new method of islet preparation. Am J Surg 1981; 142:118-122.

24. Toledo-Pereyra LH, Rowlett AL, Lodish M. Autotransplantation of pancreatic islet cell fragments into the renal capsule prepared without collagenase. Am Surg 1984; 50:679-681.

25. Toledo-Pereyra LH, Bandlien KO, Gordon DA, Mackenzie GH, Reyman TA. Renal subcapsular islet cell transplantation. Diabetes 1984; 33:910-914.

26. Horaguchi A, Merrell RC. Preparation of viable islet cells from dogs by a new method. Diabetes 1981; 30:455-458.

27. Noel J, Rabinovitch A, Olson L, Kyriakides G, Miller J, Mintz DH. A method for large-scale high-yield isolation of canine pancreatic islets of Langerhans. Metabolism 1982; 31:184-187.

28. Gray DWR, McShane P, Grant A, Morris PJ. A method for isolation of islets of Langerhans from the human pancreas. Diabetes 1984; 33:1055-1061.

29. Burghen GA, Murrell LR. Factors influencing isolation of islets of Langerhans. Diabetes [Suppl 1] 1989; 38:129-132.

30. Van Suylichem PT, Wolters GH, Van Schilgaarde R. Peri-insular presence of collagenase during islet isolation procedures. J Surg Res 1992; 53:502-509.

31. Gotoh M, Maki T, Kiyoizumi T, Satomi S, Monaco AP. An improved method for isolation of mouse pancreatic islets. Transplantation 1985; 40:437-438.

32. Ricordi C, Alejandro R, Zeng Y, et al. Human islet isolation and purification from pediatric-age donors. Transplant Proc 1991; 23:783-784.

33. Yao QX, Yao Z, Heintz R, et al. Effect of donor age and cold ischemia time on yield, purity and function of human islets isolated from fifty four consecutive pancreas donors. Transplant Proc in press.

34. Benhamou PY, Watt PC, Mullen Y, et al. Human islet isolation in 104 consecutive cases: factors affecting isolation success.. Transplantation in press.

35. Henriksson C, Claes G, Petvrsson NG. Viability of the islets of Langerhans after warm ischemia as judged by isologous transplantation. Acta Chir Scand 1977; 143: 323-327.

36. Slater DN, Bardsley D, Mangnall Y, Smythe A, Fox M. Pancreatic ischaemia: sensitivity and reversibility of the changes. Br J Exp Pathol 1975; 56:530-536.

37. Matas AJ, Sutherland DE, Payne WD, Kretschmer GJ, Steffes MW, Najarian JS. Islet transplantation: the critical period of donor ischemia in neonatal rats. Transplantation 1977; 23:295-298.

38. Toledo-Pereyra LH, Valgee KD, Castellanos J, Chee M. Hypothermic pulsatile perfusion: its use in the preservation of pancreases for 24 to 48 hours before islet cell transplantation. Arch Surg 1980; 115:95-98.

39. Ohzato H, Gotoh M, Monden M, Yamamoto H, Kawai M, Mori T. Influence of warm and cold ischemia before islet isolation. Diabetes [Suppl 1] 1989; 38:270-271.

40. Nakamura M, Miyata M, Yumiba T, et al. Influence of ischemia on isolated islet function of dogs. Jpn J Surg 1989; 38:271-271.

41. Hesse UJ, Sutherland DE, Gores PF, Najarian JS. Experience with 3, 6, and 24 hours' hypothermic storage of the canine pancreas before islet cell preparation and transplantation. Surgery 1987; 102:460-464.

42. Heise JW, Casanova D, Field MJ, Munn SR, Najarian JS, Sutherland DE. Cold storage preservation of pancreatic tissue prior to and after islet preparation in a dog autotransplantation model. J Surg Res 1989; 47:30-38.

43. Zucker PF, Bloom AD, Strasser S, Alejandro R. Successful cold storage preservation of canine pancreas with UW-1 solution prior to islet isolation. Transplantation 1989; 48:168-170.

44. Munn SR, Kaufman DB, Field MJ, Viste AB, Sutherland DE. Cold-storage preservation of the canine and rat pancreas prior to islet isolation. Transplantation 1989; 47:28-31.

45. Warnock GL, Ellis DK, Cattral M, Untch D, Kneteman NM, Rajotte RV. Viable purified islets of Langerhans from collagenase-perfused human pancreas. Diabetes [Suppl 1] 1989; 38:136-139.

46. Wahlberg JA, Love R, Landegaard L, Southard JH, Belzer FO. 72-hour preservation of the canine pancreas. Transplantation 1987; 43:5-8.

47. Contractor H, Robertson GM, Chadwick D, James RFL, Bell PRF. The effect of UW solution and its components on the collagenase digestion of the porcine and human pancreas. Transplant Proc in press.

48. Burgmann H, Reckendorfer H, Sperlich M, Doleschel W, Spieckermann PG. The calcium chelating capacity of different protecting solutions. Transplantation 1992; 54:1106-1108.

49. Ohzato H, Gotoh M, Monden M, Dono K, Kanai T, Mori T. Improvement in islet yield from a cold-preserved pancreas by pancreatic ductal collagenase distention at the time of harvesting. Transplantation 1991; 51:566-570.

50. Socci C, Davalli AM, Vignali A, et al. A significant increase of islet yield by early injection of collagenase into the pancreatic duct of young donors. Transplantation 1993; 55:661-663.

51. Sutton R, Peters M, McShane P, Gray DWR, Morris PJ. Isolation of rat pancreatic islets by ductal injection of collagenase. Transplantation 1986; 42:689-691.

52. Gotoh M, Maki T, Satomi S, Porter J, Bonner-Weir S, O'Hara CJ, Monaco AP. Reproducible high yield of rat islets by stationary in vitro digestion following pancreatic ductal or portal venous collagenase injection. Transplantation 1987; 43:725-730.

53. Traverso LW, Abou-Zamzam AM. Activation of pancreatic proteolytic enzymes by commercial collagenase. Transplantation 1978; 25:226-227.

54. McShane P, Sutton R, Gray DWR, Morris PJ. Protease activity in pancreatic islet isolation by enzymatic digestion. Diabetes [Suppl 1] 1989; 38:126-128.

55. Wolters GHJ, Vos-Scheperkeuter GH, Van Suylichem PTR, Lin H-C, Van Schilfgaarde R. Influence of the collagenase/protease ratio and concentrations on pancreatic tissue dissociation. Transplant Proc in press.

56. Dono K, Gotoh M, Ohzato H, Monden M, Mori T. Addition of calcium to the preservation solution enhances the benefit of ductal collagenase solution at the time of harvesting. Transplant Proc 1992; 24:1000-1001.

57. Sutton R, Hammonds P, Hughes D, Clark A, Gray DW, Morris PJ. Isolation of islets from human pancreas using increased incubation temperatures and variable density gradients. Horm Metab Res [Suppl] 1989; 25:35-36.

58. Sutton R Experimental studies in pancreatic islet transplantation. D.Phil. Thesis, Oxford University, 1989.

59. Warnock GL, Ellis D, Rajotte RV, Dawidson I, Baekkeskov S, Egebjerg J. Studies of the isolation and viability of human islets of Langerhans. Transplantation 1988; 45:957-963.

60. London NJ, Lake SP, Wilson J, Bassett D, Toomey P, Bell PR, James RF. A simple method for the release of islets by controlled collagenase digestion of the human pancreas. Transplantation 1990; 49:1109-1113.

61. Ricordi C, Tzakis AG, Carroll PB, et al. Human islet isolation and allotrans-plantation in 22 consecutive cases. Transplantation 1992; 53:407-414.

62. Scharp DW, Lacy PE, Santiago JV, et al. Results of our first nine intraportal islet allografts in type 1, insulin-dependent diabetic patients. Transplantation 1991; 51:76-85.

63. McShane P, Gray DWR, Hughes D, Morris PJ. Collagen types in human and rat pancreas: localisation and relation to digestion. Diabetic Medicine (Suppl 2) 1990;7:17A.

64. Van Deijnen JHM, Hulstaert CE, Wolters GHJ, Van Schilfgaarde R. Significance of the peri-insular extracellular matrix for islet isolation from the pancreas of rat, dog, pig, and man. Cell Tissue Res 1992; 267:139-146.

65. Latif ZA, Noel J, Alejandro R. A simple method of staining fresh and cultured islets. Transplantation 1988; 45:827-830.

66. Ricordi C, Lacy PE, Finke EH, Olack BJ, Scharp DW. Automated method for isolation of human pancreatic islets. Diabetes 1988; 37:413-420.

CHAPTER 3

Approaches to Islet Purification

Nick J.M. London

Paul R.V. Johnson

Gavin S.M. Robertson

David R. Chadwick

Stephen White

At the present time, density gradient centrifugation is the most effective method of islet purification. The purification of islets by density gradient centrifugation of the collagenase-digested rodent pancreas is now possible on a routine basis, and with recent advances, islet purification from the pancreata of large animals and humans, although not routine, is frequently possible. This chapter discusses the rationale behind islet purification, describes the theoretical basis of the density gradient purification of islets, outlines the techniques currently used for islet purification and finally, examines future advances.

RATIONALE BEHIND ISLET PURIFICATION

It is pertinent to begin by questioning whether it is necessary to produce highly purified islet preparations. The potential advantages include increased safety, improved islet engraftment and reduced immunogenicity of the graft.[1] The risks of the intraportal embolization of dispersed, unpurified pancreatic tissue have been a cause for concern since two deaths were reported from hepatic necrosis[2,3] and one from disseminated intravascular coagulation[4] after islet autotransplantation in the early 1980s. In addition, one patient developed portal hypertension that required decompression via a mesocaval shunt.[5] Although there have not been any serious complications from unpurified islet autotransplantation in recent years,[6,7] it is not a corollary that dispersed pancreas allotransplantation is without risk, and indeed, a splenic rupture has recently been reported after dispersed pancreas allotransplantation.[8] The risks of dispersed intraportal allotransplantation may be greater than for autotransplantation because many of the pancreata processed for islet autotransplantation have marked acinar tissue destruction[9] and the total volume of collagenase-digested tissue produced for dispersed pancreas autotransplantation (e.g. 5 mL)[10] tends to be less than for dispersed allograft transplantation (e.g. 40 mL).[11] Also, the intrahepatic inflammatory response produced by the transplantation of allogeneic dispersed tissue is

Pancreatic Islet Transplantation Volume I: Procurement of Pancreatic Islets, edited by Robert P. Lanza, MD, William L. Chick, MD; ©1994 R.G. Landes Company.

likely to be greater than with autografts. For these reasons, we would agree with Gores and Sutherland[12] that although islet purification is not essential for clinical allograft success, purified islets are desirable.

There are very few experimental studies pertaining to the effect of contaminating exocrine tissue on islet engraftment and function. It has been shown that purified, but not unpurified rat islets reversed diabetes after intraperitoneal transplantation,[13] and exocrine contamination has also been shown to impair islet implantation in the renal subcapsular space.[14] Only one published study has addressed the effect of exocrine contamination on the function of intraportal islet grafts[15] and concluded that for rat isografts, the only adverse effect of increasing exocrine contamination was a reduced insulin response during IVGTT at 3 months.

Surprisingly, the immunogenicity of highly purified versus impure preparations has received little attention. Gotoh et al [16] reported that the survival of mouse renal subcapsular islet allografts was reduced by the presence of contaminating lymph nodes, vascular tissue and ductal elements, while in a similar model, Gores et al[17] found that a partially purified islet graft containing a moderate amount of acinar tissue was rejected at the same rate as a purified preparation. However, in the latter experiment both the pure and acinar-contaminated preparations contained lymph nodes and ductal elements. A reasonable conclusion from these two studies is that the acinar component of exocrine tissue does not increase graft immunogenicity to the same extent as lymph nodes, vascular tissue and ductal elements. A canine study that compared the outcome of intrasplenic islet allotransplantation using either highly purified or unpurified islets strongly suggested an immunological advantage for the highly purified preparation.[18] Two in vitro studies using human islets[19,20] have shown that crude islet preparations provoke a greater response in a mixed lymphocyte islet coculture (MLIC) system than purified islets. This latter finding may be due to the fact that collagenase-digested human exocrine tissue expresses MHC class II.[19] It should be noted that although purer preparations may be less susceptible to rejection, this effect is relative and not absolute, and even highly purified beta-cells can incite an immune response via indirect presentation of antigen.[21]

Further reasons to purify islet preparations are that effective immunomodulation in animal models requires the use of highly purified islet preparations[22,23] and contaminating exocrine tissue markedly reduces the survival of islets in tissue cultures.[24] In summary therefore, unpurified islet transplantation can be dangerous, may not markedly impair islet implantation, but probably does increase the immunogenicity of the graft.

THEORY OF DENSITY GRADIENT PURIFICATION

Cell separation by centrifugation is based on differences in density or differences in velocity of sedimentation. The two major determinants of the rate of sedimentation of a cell in a particular medium are its diameter and the difference in density between it and the medium.[25] Velocity sedimentation is achieved by centrifuging cells for a predetermined time in a gradient with a density as remote as possible from that of the cells.[26] It separates cells primarily on the basis of differences in cell diameter and to a lesser extent on differences in density. Density-dependent, or isopycnic separation is achieved by centrifugation for sufficient time or force to cause cells to arrive at the location in the gradient where their densities are equal to that of the gradient. The densities of cells from most tissues overlap much more than their diameters and because isopycnic centrifugation requires greater forces than velocity sedimentation, velocity sedimentation is superior to isopycnic separation for most cell types.[26] It is interesting to note however that Pretlow and Pretlow[26] found that pancreatic acinar cells are one of the few cell types that can be efficiently purified by isopycnic centrifugation. Although it is possible to use isopycnic and velocity centrifugation sequentially,[27] no form of sedimentation or combination of sedimentation techniques, regardless of the gradient medium used, can separate cells of the same diameter *and* density.

SPECIFIC PROBLEMS POSED BY ISLET PURIFICATION

The reason that islet purification has proved so difficult is that both the density and the diameter of acinar tissue and to a lesser extent islets, changes from one preparation to another.[28] Islets normally vary in diameter from 15-500 μm and in addition the diameter of islets and acinar tissue is critically dependent upon the collagenase digestion stage of the isolation process. This intrinsic variation in islet diameter combined with the effect of collagenase digestion means that we have no control over endocrine and acinar tissue size distribution. Because of these highly variable and overlapping tissue diameters it is not possible to purify islets from acinar tissue using velocity sedimentation and we are forced to accept the disadvantages of isopycnic centrifugation. Velocity sedimentation has however been used after isopycnic centrifugation[27] to separate ductal, vascular and lymphoid fragments (mostly less than 100 μm diameter) from the islet preparation.

There are a number of possible causes for variable acinar tissue density. Firstly, it is possible that acinar tissue density depends on the secretory status of the acinar cells. Pancreatic acinar cells belong to a small group of cells (parotid cells, cardiac myocytes, mature mast cells) with densities far greater than the normal range for mammalian cells.[26] These cells share in common very active cytoplasmic protein synthesis and storage. In the case of mast cells it has been shown that immature mast cells with fewer cytoplasmic granules are considerably less dense than mature mast cells.[29] It is likely therefore that acinar cells that have recently degranulated will be less dense than their granulated counterparts. Secondly, the density of acinar cells may be affected by the size of the aggregates formed[30] by the collagenase digestion of the pancreas, and finally, acinar tissue density may be reduced by cellular swelling and edema.

Recent studies from our laboratory[31] have shown that the single most important factor affecting the density of acinar tissue during islet isolation is acinar tissue swelling and edema, acinar tissue degranulation is relatively unimportant. Acinar cell swelling can be provoked by a number of insults. Thus, it is well described that acinar tissue is more sensitive to the effects of ischemia[32] and mechanical trauma[33] than endocrine tissue. Indeed, Schwartz and Traverso[33] observed at electron microscopy that mechanically damaged acinar cells rapidly developed electron-luscent vacuoles. Hypothermia leads to tissue edema[34] and collagenase digestion has been shown to influence cell membrane permeability and to cause cell swelling.[35]

There are additional problems faced by those attempting to purify islets. Damaged acinar tissue releases proteolytic enzymes that exacerbate cell aggregation—a process that is known to alter tissue density and greatly impair the results of density gradient centrifugation.[26] The attachment of even the smallest fragment of acinar tissue to an islet (uncleaved islet) increases its density so that it approaches that of acinar tissue proper. Finally, in order to produce islets of 90% purity it is necessary to purify the pancreatic digest 90-fold, whereas to produce monocytes or lymphocytes of 90% purity from the buffy layer of blood requires only a 10-fold and 3-fold purification respectively. Considering the obstacles outlined above, it is not surprising that islet purification remains a difficult problem!

TECHNIQUES FOR IMPROVING DENSITY GRADIENT ISLET PURIFICATION

Broadly speaking, techniques for optimizing islet purification can be divided into physical and chemical. We will firstly consider physical parameters. Although in theory, velocity sedimentation is preferable to isopycnic separation,[26,30] because of the overlapping diameters of islets and acinar tissue isopycnic separation is the preferred method for islet purification (*vide supra*). For cell separation to be optimized by density gradient centrifugation it is essential that certain experimental conditions are controlled. Thus, it is important that acceleration and deceleration are not too rapid or else swirling will occur. 'Wall effects' result from the fact that the walls of conventional centrifuge tubes are not parallel to the force vectors[26] and cells become relatively more concentrated at the periphery of the centrifuge tube. This leads to cell aggregation which is detrimental because aggregated cells will not separate from each other and the density of an aggregate is the mean density of its component cell types.[36] Wall effects can be reduced by bottom loading and cell aggregation can be reduced by rapid processing, using 3-10% bovine serum albumin (BSA), by lowering the pH and working at 4°C.[36]

Temperature may affect the results of density gradient purification[37] and we have shown that the results of human islet purification using BSA are the same at 4°C and 22°C while porcine islet purification is more efficient at 4°C.[38] In addition, it should be remembered that the viscosity of density media greatly increases at lower temperatures and that it will therefore take longer for cells to reach buoyant equilibrium. A final consideration of great practical importance is the concept of gradient capacity[26] or 'overloading'. It has been appreciated for many years that the introduction of excessive cells into a density gradient system can cause the gradient to become unstable.[39] In the case of islet purification this leads to excessive quantities of acinar tissue appearing in the less dense layers of the gradient. Unfortunately it is not possible to calculate the gradient capacity[26] and it has therefore to be determined empirically by experimentation.

Continuous gradients offer many theoretical advantages over discontinuous gradients.[40] The disadvantages of discontinuous gradients include a lower effective cell load,[36] the accumulation of cells at interfaces impeding the movement of cells to other regions[41] and the concentration of cells at interfaces can lead to aggregation.[26] It has recently been demonstrated that large-scale continuous density gradients can be established on the COBE 2991 processor[42,43] and this therefore is the preferred technique for large-scale islet purification. It has been shown that compared to discontinuous gradients on the COBE 2991, continuous gradients improve human islet yield by 26%

and also improve islet viability.[44] The use of the COBE 2991 cell processor[45] offers many other advantages. These include the ability to process a large volume of pancreatic digest in an enclosed sterile system, the complete absence of wall effects and the ability to unload the gradient without decelerating, thereby minimizing swirling.

A further area of relevance to the purification of islets is the question of top versus bottom loading of the pancreatic digest onto the gradient. Top loading has the potential advantages of keeping the digest in a physiological medium for the maximum possible time and minimizing centrifugal forces. There are however a number of disadvantages with top loading, these include increased cell aggregation,[46] inversion causing 'streaming'[26] and wall effects. In the case of islet separation, due to their relatively small number and large size, islets in the upper interfaces may be dragged down by the large volume of acinar tissue traveling into the denser regions of the gradient. Many of these disadvantages of top loading are not relevant to continuous gradients on the COBE 2991 cell processor and for these reasons we prefer to top load onto the COBE 2991 cell processor[42] and bottom load in tubes.[47]

Chemical methods for improving the purification of human islets by isopycnic centrifugation aim to increase or maintain acinar tissue density while leaving islet density relatively unaltered. As mentioned above, acinar tissue discharge is a relatively unimportant cause of reduced acinar tissue density and it is not therefore surprising that attempts to minimize acinar tissue discharge by the administration of agents such as somatostatin to organ donors have not improved islet purification in the human.[48] The major cause of variable islet purification efficiency is variable acinar tissue density consequent upon acinar tissue swelling and edema.[31] One approach to this problem has been described by van der Burg et al[49,50] who greatly improved the results of canine islet purification by collecting and washing the pancreatic digest in (UW) solution prior to density gradient centrifugation. These findings have been confirmed in the human[51] and for some isolations the results of density gradient purification are further improved by storing the digest in UW solution (at 4°C) for one hour prior to centrifugation. The beneficial action of UW storage results largely from the presence of the extracellular impermeant anion lactobionate[31] and the colloid hydroxyethyl starch.[52] Although it is possible to use UW solution at the collagenase delivery and pancreas digestion stages of porcine[27,53] and canine islet isolation,[53] this is not the case in the human[54] where UW solution is profoundly toxic at 37°C.

The most commonly used gradient media for islet isolation are Ficoll,[55] Euroficoll,[56] Ficoll-Diatrizoic acid[57] and hyperosmolar bovine serum albumin (BSA).[45,58] We have found that for some human islet isolations Euro-Ficoll gives better results than BSA, while on other occasions BSA is preferable.[59] Hyperosmolar (500 mOsm/kg/H_2O) bovine serum albumin density gradients improve human[28] and porcine[38] (400 mOsm/kg/H_2O) islet purification (Fig. 3.1). This phenomenon has been reported for other cell types[60] and in the case of islet purification[1*] (*these experiments were performed by Professor Douglas Walcerz and Dr. Mike Taylor at the Medical Cryobiology Unit, Cambridge, UK.) resulted from the hypertonic environment *differentially* increasing the density of acinar tissue more than endocrine tissue (Fig.

3.2). Olack et al have described improved islet purification using Euro-Ficoll.[56] Euroficoll is hypertonic (562 mOsm/kg/H_2O) and contains high concentrations of glucose (160 mM) and potassium (91 mM), and a low concentration of sodium (8 mM). Although the contribution of all of these biochemical parameters to the improved results using this modified Ficoll gradient are at present unknown, we have investigated the effect of increasing glucose and pH on porcine islet isolation. Using BSA continuous gradients (Fig. 3.3), we found that purification is improved by increasing glucose concentration. However, at glucose concentrations as high as 160 mM tissue fragmentation is problematic and 50 mM would therefore seem preferable. We have investigated the effect of pH by storing pancreatic digest in solutions of increasing pH (Table 3.1) for 20 minutes prior to continuous BSA density gradient purification (Fig. 3.4). It can be seen (Fig. 3.4) that increasing the pH from 7.45 to 8.45 does not significantly affect islet purification. Further improvements in the purification of islets by density gradient centrifugation will not result from the production of new density gradient media, but rather from the continued modification of the biochemical composition of the solvents in which established gradient media are dissolved. Thus it is well described for other

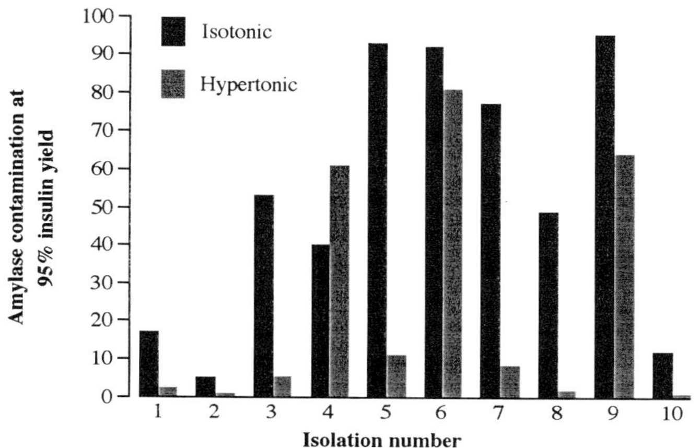

Fig. 3.1. Continuous bovine serum albumin (BSA) density gradients from 10 consecutive human islet isolations were run at 290 mOsm/Kg/H_2O (isotonic) and 500 mOsm/Kg/H_2O (hypertonic). The amylase contamination at 95% insulin yield was calculated and compared. The median (range) amylase contamination at 290 mOsm/Kg/H_2O was 51% (5-95) versus 6.4% (1-81) at 500 mOsm/Kg/H_2O (p = 0.025, Wilcoxon paired rank test).

Fig. 3.2

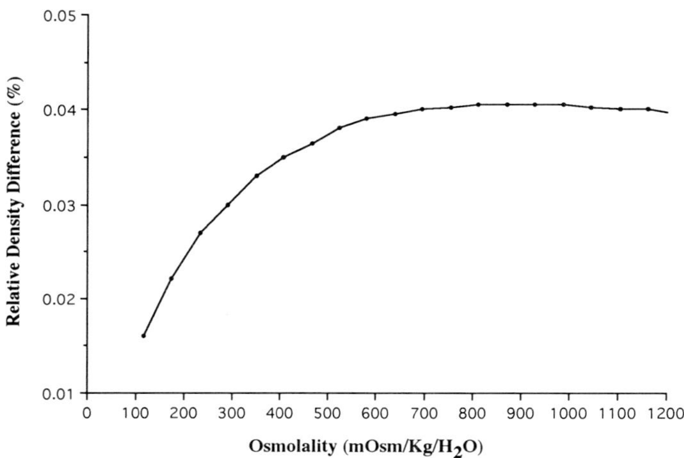

Fig. 3.2. Results of experiments to investigate the differential effect of hypertonicity on human islets and exocrine tissue. Islets and spherical clumps of exocrine tissue from five human islet preparations were placed into a microscopic cryostage and exposed to increasingly hypertonic saline solutions. The volume changes were recorded and analyzed by computerized videotape. The relative density difference between islets and exocrine tissue was then calculated at increasing osmolalities. It can be seen that by 500 mOsm the maximum density difference is very nearly attained.

Fig. 3.3. The effect of increasing the glucose concentration of BSA gradients on the purification of seven consecutive porcine islet isolations. Standard BSA contains 2 mM glucose and this was compared with 5 mM, 50 mM and 160 mM glucose. The results are expressed as the change in percent of amylase contamination at a 60% insulin yield. Purification using glucose concentrations of 50 mM was significantly better than 2 mM (p = 0.036) and the same trend was apparent at 160 mM glucose (p = 0.063). At 160 mM glucose both islet and exocrine tissue appeared fragmented.

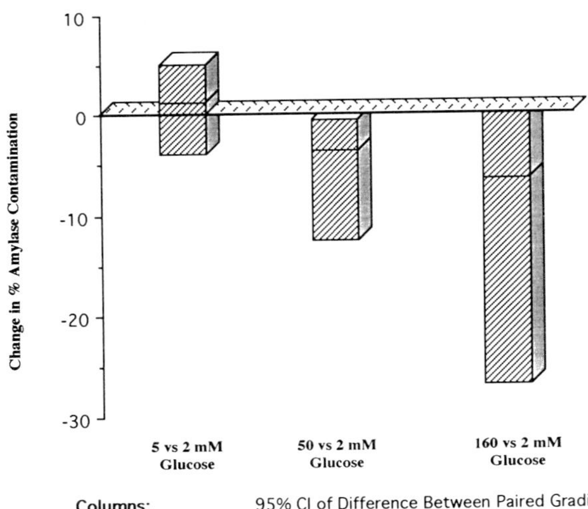

Fig. 3.3

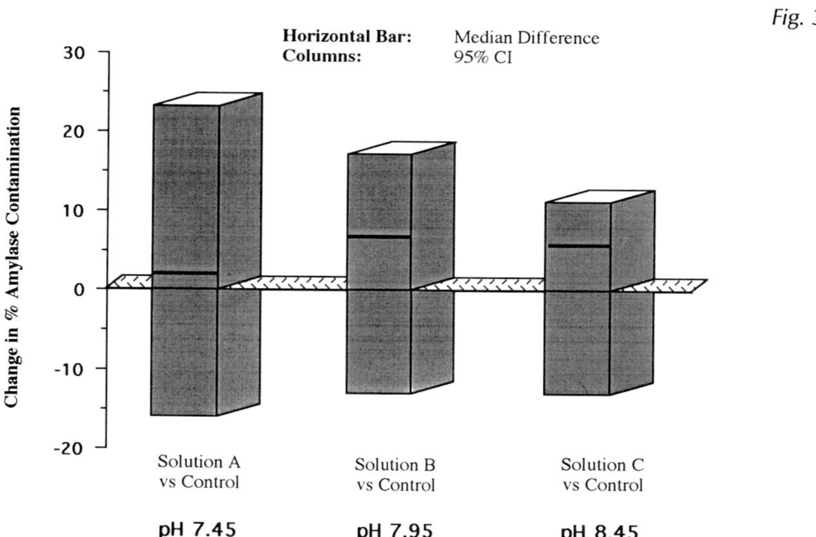

Fig. 3.4. The effect of increasing pH on the purification of porcine islets. Pancreatic digest from seven consecutive pancreata was stored for 20 minutes in four solutions (Table 3.1) prior to purification on continuous BSA gradients. The control solution is our standard storage solution and the other three solutions have had their pH adjusted and controlled by the addition of HEPES. The results are expressed as percent of amylase contamination at a 60% insulin yield and compared to the control solution. Increasing the pH did not significantly affect islet purification.

Table 3.1. The composition of storage solutions used to study the effect of pH on porcine islet purification

	Control Solution	Solution A	Solution B	Solution C
Lactobionate	115	115	115	115
Raffinose	30	30	30	30
$MgSO_4$	5	5	5	5
H_2PO_4	25	25	25	25
Na^+	20	30	44	54
K^+	140	140	140	140
HEPES*	—	35	35	35
pH	**7.45**	**7.45**	**7.95**	**8.45**
Osmolality (mOsm/kg/H_2O)	323	355	358	364

Values are in mM/L, unless otherwise stated
*Total Concentration of HEPES (Acid + Base).

cell types[61] that changes in ionic content, glucose concentration and pH can markedly affect cell density. These modifications may however produce an unphysiological environment,[41] and consequently their effect on islet viability must be determined. A recent promising approach has been the construction of density gradients by the addition of extra hydroxyethyl starch or Percoll to University of Wisconsin solution.[50] In the human, the challenge is to produce solutions that will minimize acinar tissue swelling without compromising islet yield and viability.

OUTLINE OF METHODS

GENERAL

Islet purification is critically affected by all of the isolation stages that preceded it. Thus, warm[57,62] and cold[63] ischemia should be kept to an absolute minimum. Animal pancreata should not receive in situ vascular flush[63] and if the human pancreas is subject to a vascular flush, then UW solution is the preferred perfusate if a cold ischaemic time of more than 6 hours is anticipated.[63] However, UW solution offers no advantages for human islet purification with cold ischaemic times of less than 6 hours.[64] Collagenase is best administered via the pancreatic duct,[65,66] and in animals, if a period of prolonged cold ischemia is anticipated, then the collagenase can be dissolved in UW solution and injected immediately after excision of the pancreas.[67] Delivery of collagenase in UW solution in the human pancreas greatly reduces islet yield and viability[54] and the collagenase should be administered in Hank's solution immediately after excision of the pancreas.[68] The collagenase digestion phase is most simply performed using a stationary digestion-filtration method for the rodent pancreas,[69] whereas for large animal and human pancreata an automated method is preferable.[70] It is essential for efficient density gradient purification that the islets liberated by the collagenase digestion phase are entirely free of acinar tissue (cleaved).

WHICH DENSITY GRADIENT MEDIUM?

At the present time the most commonly used gradient media for rodent islet purification are Ficoll[71] and BSA (305 mOsm/kg/H_2O),[69] for canine islet purification Ficoll,[72] Euro-Ficoll,[73] BSA (400 mOsm/kg/H_2O)[74] and Dextran,[75] for porcine islet purification, Ficoll,[76] Euro-Ficoll[77] and Ficoll-Diatrizoic acid,[27] and for human islet isolation, Ficoll,[55] Euroficoll,[56] Ficoll-Diatrizoic acid[57] and BSA.[45]

PREPARATION OF GRADIENT MEDIA

In order to produce consistent results with any one gradient medium it should be produced in a precise and reproducible manner. Particular attention should be paid to electrolyte composition, pH, osmolality and density. Although electrolyte concentrations can be measured using ion specific electrodes, flame photometry is more accurate. Density should be measured using a digital densitometer. Osmolality measurements must be performed with a vapor pressure osmometer because freezing point depression osmometry is inaccurate for concentrated solutions of Ficoll and BSA.[78,79]

PRELIMINARY MEASUREMENT OF TISSUE DENSITIES

Small scale linear continuous gradients constructed from the chosen density gradient medium[80] allow the precise characterization of tissue density[40] in that particular medium. This information can then be used to determine the optimum isolation densities for small scale discontinuous gradients in tubes or the optimum density range for large scale continuous gradients on the COBE 2991 cell processor. Because BSA exerts a minimal osmotic effect it is possible to construct a linear continuous density gradient in the absence of an osmotic gradient and the findings are therefore relevant to the situation in a BSA discontinuous gradient (where there is also not an osmotic gradient). Higher concentrations of Ficoll however bind water thereby increasing osmotic activity. Thus, although it is possible to construct a linear density gradient there is also an osmotic gradient which affects tissue density distribution.[4] This means that the findings from a Ficoll continuous gradient are not precisely relevant to the situation in a discontinuous Ficoll gradient (where although there is an osmotic gradient, it is not continuous). The information obtained from the Ficoll continuous gradient does however allow a good estimate of the densities required for discontinuous gradients. It should be stressed that when testing a new gradient medium it is wise to construct a continuous gradient with a wide density range and having determined the approximate tissue densities to narrow the density range such that the islets equilibrate towards the upper third of the gradient. Details concerning the construction of small-scale continuous gradients have previously been provided.[31,38,51,64,81]

DENSITY GRADIENT CENTRIFUGATION

Rodent islets are most easily purified in small tubes using discontinuous gradients whose densities have been determined using the technique described above. Round-bottomed tubes cause less physical trapping of islets in the digest pellet than conical tubes. Although large animal and human islets can be purified using large centrifuge tubes,[70] the Cobe 2991 cell processor is preferable. Continuous gradients offer both theoretical and practical advantages[44] and we will therefore restrict the description to these gradients. A detailed description of the techniques has previously been provided.[25,42,81] The pancreatic digest should be kept at 4°C in UW solution prior to gradient isolation and for some human islet isolations it is worthwhile storing the digest in UW solution for 1 hr.[51]

For detailed instructions concerning the safe use of the COBE 2991 cell processor the reader should consult the manual provided by the manufacturers (COBE Laboratories, Colorado, USA). It is firstly necessary to construct a glass gradient maker that can be autoclaved. The chambers of the gradient maker should be identical and have a capacity of 300 mL each. The autoclaved gradient maker is placed on a magnetic stirrer with a magnetic flea in the high density chamber and the connection between the two chambers closed. The outlet tubing from the gra-

dient maker is connected via a silicone pump segment to the blood-processing set.

Having chosen the density of the high and low density media based on the results of mini-continuous gradients, 270 mL of high density medium is placed into the high density chamber and 150 mL of low density medium into the low density chamber of the gradient maker. With the COBE 2991 *not* running and all the limbs of the processing bag occluded with clips, 120 mL of high density medium, i.e., until the levels in the gradient maker chambers are the same is pumped on at 30 mL/min. While doing this, the air in the tubing goes to waste before diverting the density gradient medium into the processor bag. The centrifuge bowl is then spun at 1200 rpm, and air vented into the waste bag from the processing bag.

The COBE 2991 is then set running at 1500 rpm and the continuous gradient generated and pumped onto the COBE 2991 processor. As the last of the density gradient medium is just leaving the gradient maker the pump is turned off, the connection between the chambers closed and the pancreatic digest (maximum 40 mL) which is suspended in a total volume of 100 mL UW (e.g. 40 mL of digest plus 60 mL UW) poured into the high density chamber. The pump is then turned on and the pancreatic digest pumped onto the gradient at 30 mL/min. If a tissue interface appears above the continuous gradient, the pump is turned off until it disappears and then restarted again. As the last of the digest leaves the chamber, the chamber is flushed with 80 mL UW solution. It is *essential* that any air that has entered the bag is carefully vented off to waste by *slowly* releasing the pressure on the clip on the waste line. The centrifuge speed is slowly increased to 2000 rpm and again air carefully vented off.

The centrifuge is run until all the tissue has entered the continuous gradient (usually 5 min) and the gradient unloaded using the superout mode. The first 150 mL is discarded. Then, 11 fractions of 30 mL each are collected into 50 mL conical tubes by intermittently interrupting the collection using the *'hold'* button and the *'continue'* button. A small sample from each fraction is then stained with dithizone so that it can be decided which fractions should be combined to form the final islet preparation.

FUTURE PROSPECTS

Further improvements in the purification of islets by isopycnic density gradient centrifugation will not result from the production of new density gradient *media*, but rather from the continued modification of the biochemical composition of the *solvents* in which established gradient media are dissolved. There are a number of alternative approaches to islet purification, including differential sedimentation at unit gravity,[82] filtration,[83] the use of Velcro to remove acinar tissue,[84] centrifugal elutriation,[85] cryopreservation,[86] gamma irradiation,[87] anti-acinar cytotoxic antibodies,[88] tissue culture,[89] the selective destruction of acinar cells by laser energy,[90] magnetic microspheres coated with anti-acinar cell monoclonal antibodies,[91] and fluorescence-activated cell sorting.[92] The latter two techniques seem to hold the greatest promise. A particular advantage of fluorescence-activated cell sorting is that it will separate uncleaved islets, and although problematical, it appears to be a worthwhile line of investigation.

ACKNOWLEDGMENTS

We are grateful to the British Diabetic Association, the Juvenile Diabetes Foundation, the Medical Research Council and the Trent Regional Health Authority for funding our work.

REFERENCES

1. Gray DW. The role of exocrine tissue in pancreatic islet transplantation. Transpl Int 1989; 2:41-45.
2. Cameron JL, Mehigan DG, Broe PJ, Zuidema GD. Distal pancreatectomy and islet autotransplantation for chronic pancreatitis. Ann Surg 1981; 193:312-317.
3. Toledo-Pereyra LH, Rowlett AL, Cain W, Rosenberg JC, Gordon DA, MacKenzie GH. Hepatic infarction following intraportal islet cell autotransplantation after near total pancreatectomy. Transpl 1984; 38:88-89.
4. Mittal VK, Toledo-Pereyra LH, Sharma M, et al. Acute portal hypertension and disseminated intravascular coagulation following pancreatic islet autotransplantation after subtotal pancreatectomy. Transplantation 1981; 31:302-304.
5. Memsic L, Busuttil RW, Traverso LW. Bleeding esophageal varices and portal vein thrombosis after pancreatic mixed-cell autotransplantation. Surgery 1984; 95:238-242.
6. Farney AC, Najarian JS, Nakhleh RE, et al. Autotransplantation of dispersed pancreatic islet tissue combined with total or near-total pancreatectomy for treatment of chronic pancreatitis. Surgery 1991; 110:427-437.
7. Farney AC, Sutherland DER. Islet autotransplantation. In: Ricordi C, ed. Pancreatic islet cell transplantation; 1892-1992. One century of transplantation for diabetes. Austin: R.G.Landes, 1992:291-312.
8. Gores PF, Najarian JS, Stephanian E, Lloveras JJ, Kelley SL, Sutherland DER. Transplantation of unpurified islets from a single donor with 15-deoxyspergualin immunosuppression. Transplant Proc 1994; 26:574-575.
9. Najarian JS, Sutherland DER, Baumgartner D. Total or near total pancreatectomy and islet transplantation for treatment of chronic pancreatitis. Ann Surg 1980; 192:526-539.
10. Fontes PA, Rilo HL, Carroll PB, et al. Human islet isolation and transplantation in chronic pancreatitis using the automated method. Transplant Proc 1992; 24:2809.
11. Gores PF, Najarian JS, Stephanian E, Lloveras JJ, Kelley SL, Sutherland DE. Insulin independence in type I diabetes after transplantation of unpurified islets from single donor with 15-deoxyspergualin. Lancet 1993; 341:19-21.
12. Gores PF, Sutherland DER. Commentary. Cell Transplantation 1993; 2:291-293.
13. Payne WD, Sutherland DER, Matas AJ, Gorecki P, Najarian JS. DL-ethionine treatment od adult pancreatic donors. Amelioration of diabetes in multiple recipients with tissue from a single donor. Ann Surg 1979; 189:248-256.

14. Gray DW, Sutton R, McShane P, Peters M, Morris PJ. Exocrine contamination impairs implantation of pancreatic islets transplanted beneath the kidney capsule. J Surg Res 1988; 45:432-442.

15. Downing R, Morrissey S, Kiske D, Scharp DW. Does the purity of intraportal islet isografts affect their endocrine function? J Surg Res 1986; 41:41-46.

16. Gotoh M, Maki T, Satomi S, Porter J, Monaco AP. Immunological characteristics of purified pancreatic islet grafts. Transplantation 1986; 42:387-390.

17. Gores PF, Mayoral J, Field MJ, Sutherland DE. Comparison of the immunogenicity of purified and unpurified murine islet allografts. Transplantation 1986; 41:529-531.

18. Kneteman NM, Evans MG, Cattral MS, Warnock GL, Rajotte RV. A comparison of canine renal and islet transplantation with cyclosporine: assessment of islet immunogenicity. Transplant Proc 1989; 21:3366-3367.

19. Ulrichs K, Muller Ruchholtz W. Mixed lymphocyte islet culture (MLIC) and its use in manipulation of human islet alloimmunogenicity. Horm Metab Res Suppl 1990; 25:123-127.

20. Zeevi A, Rilo HLR, Fontes PA, Carroll PB, Behboo R, Ricordi C. Effect of purity and culture on human islet immunogenicity in vitro. Transplant Proc 1994; (in press)

21. Stock PG, Ascher NL, Chen S, Field J, Bach FH, Sutherland DE. Evidence for direct and indirect pathways in the generation of the alloimmune response against pancreatic islets. Transplantation 1991; 52:704-709.

22. Lacy PE, Davie JM. Effect of culture on islet rejection. Diabetes 1980; 29 (Suppl 1):93-97.

23. Falqui L, Finke EH, Carel JC, Scharp DW, Lacy PE. Marked prolongation of human islet xenograft survival (human-to-mouse) by low-temperature culture and temporary immunosuppression with human and mouse anti-lymphocyte sera. Transplantation 1991; 51:1322-1324.

24. Sever CE, Demetris AJ, Zeng J, et al. Composition of human islet cell preparations for transplantation. Acta Diabetologica 1992; 28:233-238.

25. London NJM, James RFL, Bell PRF. Islet Purification. In: Ricordi C, ed. Pancreatic islet cell transplantation. 1892-1992. One century of transplantation for diabetes. Austin: R.G.Landes, 1992:113-123.

26. Pretlow TG, Pretlow TP. Sedimentation of cells: an overview and discussion of artefacts. In: Pretlow TG, Pretlow TP, eds. Cell separation: methods and selected applications Volume 1. San Diego: Academic Press, 1982:41-60.

27. Hering BJ, Gramberg D, Emst E, Kirchhof N, Bretzel RG, Federlin K. Isokinetic gradients: A new approach to reduce islet graft immunogenicity. Transplant Proc 1993; 25:959-960.

28. London NJM, Toomey P, Contractor H, Thirdborough ST, James RFL, Bell PRF. The effect of osmolality and glucose concentration on the purity of human islet isolates. Transplant Proc 1992; 24:1002.

29. Pretlow TG, Cassady IM. Separation of mast cells in successive stages of differentiation using programmed gradient sedimentation. Am J Pathol 1970; 61:323-333.

30. Pretlow TG, Weir EE, Zettergren JG. Problems connected with the separation of different kinds of cells. Int Rev Exp Pathol 1975; 14:91-204.

31. Chadwick DR, Robertson GSM, Rose S, et al. Storage of porcine pancreatic digest prior to islet purification: the benefits of UW solution and the role of its individual components. Transplantation 1993; 56:288-293.

32. Medvetskii EB, Keisevich LV. Electron-microscopic and autoradiographic study of the pancreas at different stages of postmortem ischemia. Bull Exp Biol Med 1978; 85:670-679.

33. Schwartz BD, Traverso LW. Morphological changes in pancreatic fragments prepared for transplantation by collagenase treatment. Transplantation 1984; 38:273-280.

34. Southard JH, Van Gulik TM, Ametani MS, et al. Important components of the UW solution. Transplantation 1990; 49:251-257.

35. Burg MB, Grollman EF, Orloff J. Sodium and potassium flux of separated renal tubules. Am J Physiol 1964; 206:483-491.

36. Shortman K. Physical procedures for the separation of animal cells. Ann Rev Biophys Bioeng 1972; 1:93-130.

37. Legge DG, Shortman K. The effect of pH on the volume, density and shape of erythrocytes and thymic lymphocytes. Br J Haemotol 1968; 14:321-333.

38. Chadwick DR, Robertson GSM, Toomey P, et al. Pancreatic islet purification using bovine serum albumin: the importance of density gradient temperature and osmolality. Cell Transplantation 1993; 2: 355-361.

39. Brakke MK. Density gradient centrifugation and its application to plant viruses. Adv Virus Res 1960; 7:193-224.

40. de Duve C. Tissue fractionation, past and present. J Cell Biol 1971; 50:20d-55d.

41. Leif RC. Buoyant density separation of cells. In: Weid GL, Bahr GF, eds. Automated cell identification and cell sorting. New York: Academic Press, 1970:21-96.

42. Robertson GSM, Chadwick DR, Contractor H, James RFL, London NJM. The optimization of large scale density gradient human islet isolation. Acta Diabetologica 1993; 30:93-98.

43. London NJM, Robertson GSM, Chadwick DR, et al. Purification of human pancreatic islets by large scale continuous density gradient centrifugation. Horm Metab Res 1993; 25:61.

44. Hering BJ, Eckhard M, Klitscher D, Brandhorst H, Bretzel RG, Federlin K. Media specifically designed for isopycnic human islet purification. Transplant Proc 1994; (in press)

45. Lake SP, Bassett PD, Larkins A, et al. Large-scale purification of human islets utilizing discontinuous albumin gradient on IBM 2991 cell separator. Diabetes 1989; 38 (Suppl 1):143-145.

46. Harwood R. Cell separation by gradient centrifugation. Int Rev Cytol 1974; 38:369-403.

47. Fritschy WM, van Suylichem PTR, Wolters GHJ, van Schilfgaarde R. Comparison of top and bottom loading of a dextran gradient for rat pancreatic islet purification. Diabetes Res 1992; 19:91-95.

48. Chadwick DR, Robertson GSM, Rose S, et al. Does exocrine enzyme discharge influence islet purification? Horm Metab Res 1993; 25:53.

49. van der Burg MP, Gooszen HG, Ploeg RJ, et al. Pancreatic islet isolation with UW solution: a new concept. Transplant Proc 1990; 22:2050-2051.

50. van der Burg MP, Guicherit OR, Frolich M, Bruijn JA, Gooszen HG. Islet preservation during isolation: a new concept in cell transplantation. Transplant Proc 1992; 24:2840-2841.

51. Robertson GSM, Chadwick D, Contractor H, et al. Storage of human pancreatic digest in University of Wisconsin solution significantly improves subsequent islet purification. Br J Surg 1992; 79:899-902.

52. Robertson GSM, Chadwick DR, Davies J, et al. The effectiveness of components of University of Wisconsin solution in improving human pancreatic islet purification. Transplantation 1994; 57:346-349.

53. Arbet-Engels C, Darquy S, Capron F, Reach G. The use of a modified University of Wisconsin solution for rat and porcine islet cryopreservation. Transplant Proc 1992; 24:2790.

54. Toomey P, Contractor H, James RFL, London NJM. Cold storage of the human pancreas prior to islet isolation; . Presented at the third International Congress on Pancreas and Islet Transplantation; Lyon 1991;

55. Warnock GL, Ellis D, Rajotte RV, Davidson I, Baekkeskov S, Egebjerg J. Studies of the isolation and viability of human islets of Langerhans. Transplantation 1988; 45:957-963.

56. Olack B, Swanson C, McLear M. Islet purification using Euro-Ficoll gradients. Transplant Proc 1991; 23:774-776.

57. Brandhorst H, Klitscher D, Hering BJ, Federlin K, Bretzel RG. Influence of organ procurement on human islet isolation. Horm Metab Res 1993; 25:51-52.

58. Vives M, Sarri Y, Conget I, et al. Human islet function after automatic isolation and bovine serum albumin gradient purification. Transplantation 1992; 53:243-245.

59. Chadwick DR, Robertson GSM, Contractor H, et al. Human islet purification: a prospective comparison of Euro-Ficoll and bovine serum albumin density gradients. Acta Diabetologica 1993; 30:57-59.

60. Boyum A. Isolation of human blood monocytes with Nycodenz, a new non-ionic iodinated gradient medium. Scand J Immunol 1983; 17:429-436.

61. Kneece WC, Leif RC. The effect of pH, potassium, sodium, bicarbonate, and chloride ions and glucose on the buoyant density distribution of human erythrocytes in bovine serum albumin gradients. J Cell Physiol 1971; 78:185-200.

62. Corlett MP, Scharp DW. The effect of pancreatic warm ischemia on islet isolation in rats and dogs. J Surg Res 1988; 45:531-536.

63. Kneteman NM, Lakey JRT, Warnock GL, Rajotte RV. Pancreas procurement and preservation: impact on islet recovery and viability. In: Ricordi C, ed. Pancreatic islet cell transplantation. 1892-1992. One century of transplantation for diabetes. Austin, Georgetown: R.G.Landes company, 1992: 72-81.

64. Robertson GSM, Chadwick D, Thirdborough S, et al. Human islet isolation - A prospective randomised comparison of pancreatic vascular perfusion with hyperosmolar citrate or University of Wisconsin solution. Transplantation 1993; 56:550-553.

65. Horaguchi A, Merrell RC. Preparation of viable islets cells from dogs by a new method. Diabetes 1981; 30:455-458.

66. Gray DW, McShane P, Grant A, Morris PJ. A method for isolation of islets of Langerhans from the human pancreas. Diabetes 1984; 33:1055-1061.

67. Mellert J, Hering BJ, Hopt UT, et al. Exchange of pancreata and islets between centers for experimental islet transplantation in the pig. Transplant Proc 1991; 23:2435-2436.

68. Socci C, Davalli AM, Vignali A, et al. A significant increase of islet yield by early injection of collagenase into the pancreatic duct of young donors. Transplantation 1993; 55:661-663.

69. Lake SP, Anderson J, Chamberlain J, Gardner SJ, Bell PR, James RF. Bovine serum albumin density gradient isolation of rat pancreatic islets. Transplantation 1987; 43:805-808.

70. Ricordi C, Lacy PE, Finke EH, Olack BJ, Scharp DW. Automated method for isolation of human pancreatic islets. Diabetes 1988; 37:413-420.

71. Scharp DW, Kemp CB, Knight MJ. The use of Ficoll in the preparation of viable islets of Langerhans from the rat pancreas. Transplantation 1973; 16:686-689.

72. Alejandro R, Latif Z, Polonsky KS, Shienvold FL, Civantos F, Mint DH. Natural history of multiple intrahepatic canine islet allografts during and following administration of cyclosporine. Transplantation 1988; 45:1036-1044.

73. Scharp DW, Marchetti P, Swanson C, Newton M, McCullough CS, Olack B. The effect of transplantation site and islet mass on long-term survival and metabolic and hormonal function of canine purified islet autografts. Cell Transplantation 1992; 1:245-254.

74. Alejandro R, Strasser S, Zucker PF, Mintz DH. Isolation of pancreatic islets from dogs. Semiautomated purification on albumin gradients. Transplantation 1990; 50:207-210.

75. Kaufman DB, Morel P, Field MJ, Munn SR, Sutherland DE. Purified canine islet autografts. Functional outcome as influenced by islet number and implantation site. Transplantation 1990; 50:385-391.

76. Ricordi C, Socci C, Davalli AM, et al. Isolation of the elusive pig islet. Surgery 1990; 107:688-694.

77. Marchetti P, Finke EH, Gerasimidi Vazeou A, Falqui L, Scharp DW, Lacy PE. Automated large-scale isolation, in vitro function and xenotransplantation of porcine islets of Langerhans. Transplantation 1991; 52:209-213.

78. Bach MK, Brashler JR. Isolation of subpopulations of lymphocyte cells by the use of isotonically balanced solutions of Ficoll. Exp Cell Research 1970; 61:387-396.

79. Williams N, Kraft N, Shortman K. The separation of different cell classes from lymphoid organs. Immunology 1972; 22:885-899.

80. Brakke MK. Density gradient centrifugation:a new separation technique. J Am Chem Soc 1951; 73:1847-1848.

81. London NJM, Robertson GSM, Chadwick DR, James RFL, Bell PRF. Adult Islet Purification. In: Ricordi C, Warnock GL, eds. Methods in Cellular Transplantation. Austin: R.G.Landes, 1994: (in press)

82. Dobroschke J, Langhoff G, Seyed Ali S, Kunze HH, Schwemmle K. Isolation of human islets of Langerhans. In: Federlin K, Bretzel RG, eds. Islet isolation, culture and cryopreservation. New York: Thieme-Stratton Inc, 1981:32-39.

83. Lorenz D, Wolff H, Lippert H, Hahn HJ, Abri O, Zander E. Clinical experience in islet transplantation. In: Thiede A, Deltz E, Engemann R, Hamelmann H, eds. Microsurgical models in rats for transplantation research. Berlin-Heidelberg: Springer Verlag, 1985:359-367.

84. Kuhn F, Schulz HJ, Lorenz D, et al. Morphological investigations in human islets of Langerhans isolated by the Velcro-technic. Biomed Biochim Acta 1985; 44:149-153.

85. Scharp D, Lacy P, Ricordi C, et al. Human islet transplantation in patients with type I diabetes. Transplant Proc 1989; 21:2744-2745.

86. Evans MG, Rajotte RV, Warnock GL, Procyshyn AW. Cryopreservation purifies canine pancreatic microfragments. Transplant Proc 1987; 19:3471-3477.

87. Nason RW, Rajotte RV, Procyshyn AW, Pedersen JE. Purification of canine pancreatic islet cell grafts with radiation. Transplant Proc 1986; 18:174-181.

88. Soon-Shiong P, Heintz R, Terasaki P. An immunological method of islet cell purification using anti-acinar cell monoclonal antibodies. Transplant Proc 1988; 20:61-63.

89. Matas AJ, Sutherland DER, Kretschmer G. Pancreatic tissue culture: depletion of exocrine enzymes and purification of islets for transplantation. Transplant Proc 1977; 9:337-339.

90. Brunicardi FC, Suh E, Kleinman R, et al. Selective photodynamic laser treatment of dispersed pancreatic tissue for islet isolation. Transplant Proc 1992; 24:2796-2797.

91. Fujioka T, Terasaki PI, Heintz R, et al. Rapid purification of islets using magnetic microspheres coated with anti-acinar cell monoclonal antibodies. Transplantation 1990; 49:404-407.

92. Jiao L, Gray DW, Gohde W, Flynn GJ, Morris PJ. In vitro staining of islets of Langerhans for fluorescence-activated cell sorting. Transplantation 1991; 52:450-452.

CHAPTER 4

COLLAGENASE SELECTION

Thomas J. Cavanagh

Terry J. Fetterhoff

Shawn C. Lonergan

Francis E. Dwulet

John F. Gill

Robert C. McCarthy

Progress in pancreatic islet transplantation is in part delayed by irreproducible islet recoveries from collagenase-mediated pancreatic dissociation. Irreproducible islet recovery is a consequence of many factors, including collagenase variability. Collagenase is a preparation of many different proteolytic enzymes concentrated from bacterial culture supernatant. Individual enzyme activities and concentrations vary with bacterial strain, culture conditions and age of the culture. This results in significant variation between each lot of commercial collagenase. The efficacy of each collagenase lot is further dependent upon the species of pancreas donor and the method of dissociation. Consequently, investigators must prescreen individual lots of collagenase to ensure efficacy prior to purchasing large amounts of a single lot. Typically, investigators screen 2-5 lots before finding a suitable lot,[1] incurring in this process unnecessary expense and consuming valuable donor organs. In addition, loss of enzyme activity appears over time, necessitating qualification of new lots at six month intervals.

It is essential to minimize the influence of donor and procedural variables when evaluating a new lot of collagenase. In this chapter we will describe guidelines for screening collagenase which may improve accuracy, decrease the costs associated with prescreening, and offer some advantage towards the pursuit of higher islet yields.

COLLAGENASE

Collagenase, commonly used for isolation of pancreatic islets, is a partially purified material derived from the fermentation of *Clostridium histolyticum*. This partially purified material is known to contain numerous enzyme activities (see Table 4.1 for summary).[2,3] The most critical components present in crude preparations are thought to be the collagenases and other general proteases which are responsible for degradation of the interstitial matrix in which islets are embedded.[4] In this section, we present a current summary of the knowledge regarding crude collagenase. For more detailed information on collagenase enzyme components, please refer to earlier reviews.[5-7]

Pancreatic Islet Transplantation Volume I: Procurement of Pancreatic Islets, edited by Robert P. Lanza, MD, William L. Chick, MD; ©1994 R.G. Landes Company.

Table 4.1. Enzyme activities in crude *C. histolyticum* collagenase

Proteases	Other Enzymes
Collagenase	β-D-Galactosidase
Clostripain	β-N-Acetyl-D-Glucosaminidase
Trypsin	α-L-Fucosidase
Neutral Protease	Phospholipase
Elastase	Neuraminidase
Aminopeptidase	Hyaluronidase

Crude Clostridial collagenase is isolated from culture supernatant by salt precipitation methods and commercially supplied as lyophilized powders containing key proteolytic enzymes as well as media components, pigments and other precipitated cellular materials. Collagenase preparations are heterogeneous with respect to color, texture, bulk density and, more importantly, in levels of specific enzyme activities. Typical heterogeneity is seen in several commercial collagenase preparations using SDS-PAGE analysis (Fig. 4.1). In general, 20 to 30 separate components can be observed by this method. To date, only a handful of these protein bands are characterized as to their enzymatic identity. The major effort over the past 30 years was in the purification and characterization of collagenolytic components. Table 4.2 summarizes many of the reported purification protocols. These results consistently show a heterogeneity of collagenase

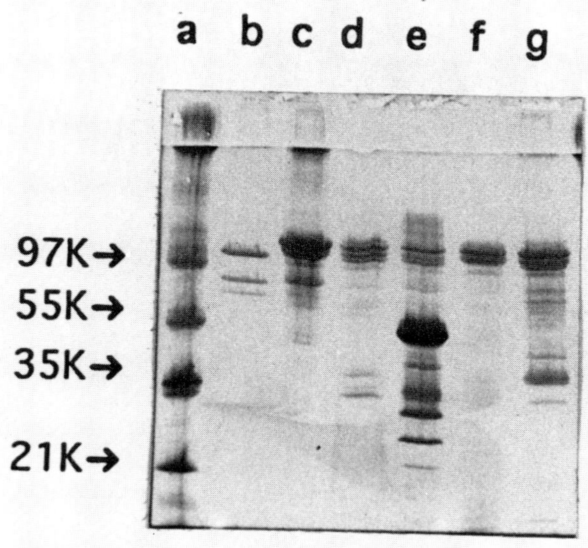

Fig. 4.1. SDS-polyacrylamide slab gel electrophoresis (8-25% gradient) of crude collagenases from various suppliers. (a) protein standards (phosphorylase b, 97,400; glutamate dehydrogenase, 55,400; lactate dehydrogenase, 36,500; trypsin inhibitor, 20,100), (b & c) Sigma, (d) Serva, (e) Seromed, (f & g) Boehringer Mannheim.

enzyme forms. There are as many as six distinct species present in crude Clostridial collagenase preparations. Taken in its entirety, these results reveal that all purified collagenase fractions can be characterized based upon their substrate specificity. The most definitive report on this subject by Bond and Van Wart[17] describes two classes of enzyme activity. Class I collagenases have a higher activity towards high molecular weight collagen while Class II collagenases prefer low molecular weight collagen fragments. These activities appear to be complementary[25] and are reported to act synergistically on native collagen.[11]

It is generally accepted that a major hurdle for the ultimate success of islet transplantation is resolution of the lot variability of collagenase preparations.[21] All commercial sources of collagenase commonly used in islet isolation exhibit lot to lot variability (see Fig. 4.2). Currently, commercial suppliers of collagenase characterize their preparations for specific activity of certain proteolytic enzymes. For example, Boehringer Mannheim provides a certificate of analysis

Table 4.2. Heterogeneity of Clostridial collagenase. Chromatographic fractionation of crude collagenase preparations have historically resulted in the identification of a number of enzymatic components with collagenolytic activity

Separation Methods	Collagenase Forms	Designation
DEAE-Cellulose[8]	3	A, B, C
DEAE-Sephadex[9]	3	I, II, III
DEAE-Cellulose[10]	2	I, II
SE-Cellulose[11] DEAE-Cellulose	3	A-α, B-α, B-β
DEAE-Cellulose[12] DEAE-Cellulose[13]	2 2	A, B A, B
DEAE-Cellulose[14] IEF	4	I, II, IIIa, IIIb
SP-Sephadex[15] DEAE-Cellulose Sephacryl S-200	2	
DEAE-Cellulose[16] IEF Collagen-Sepharose	3	C_1, C_2, C_3
Hydroxylapatite[17] Sephacryl S-200 L-Arg-Sepharose Red Dye Ligand DEAE-Cellulose SP-Sephadex	6	Class I & II (α, β, γ, δ, ϵ, ζ)
DEAE-Sephadex A50[18] Preparative PAGE[19]	2 6	CGN-A, CGN-B 1 – 6

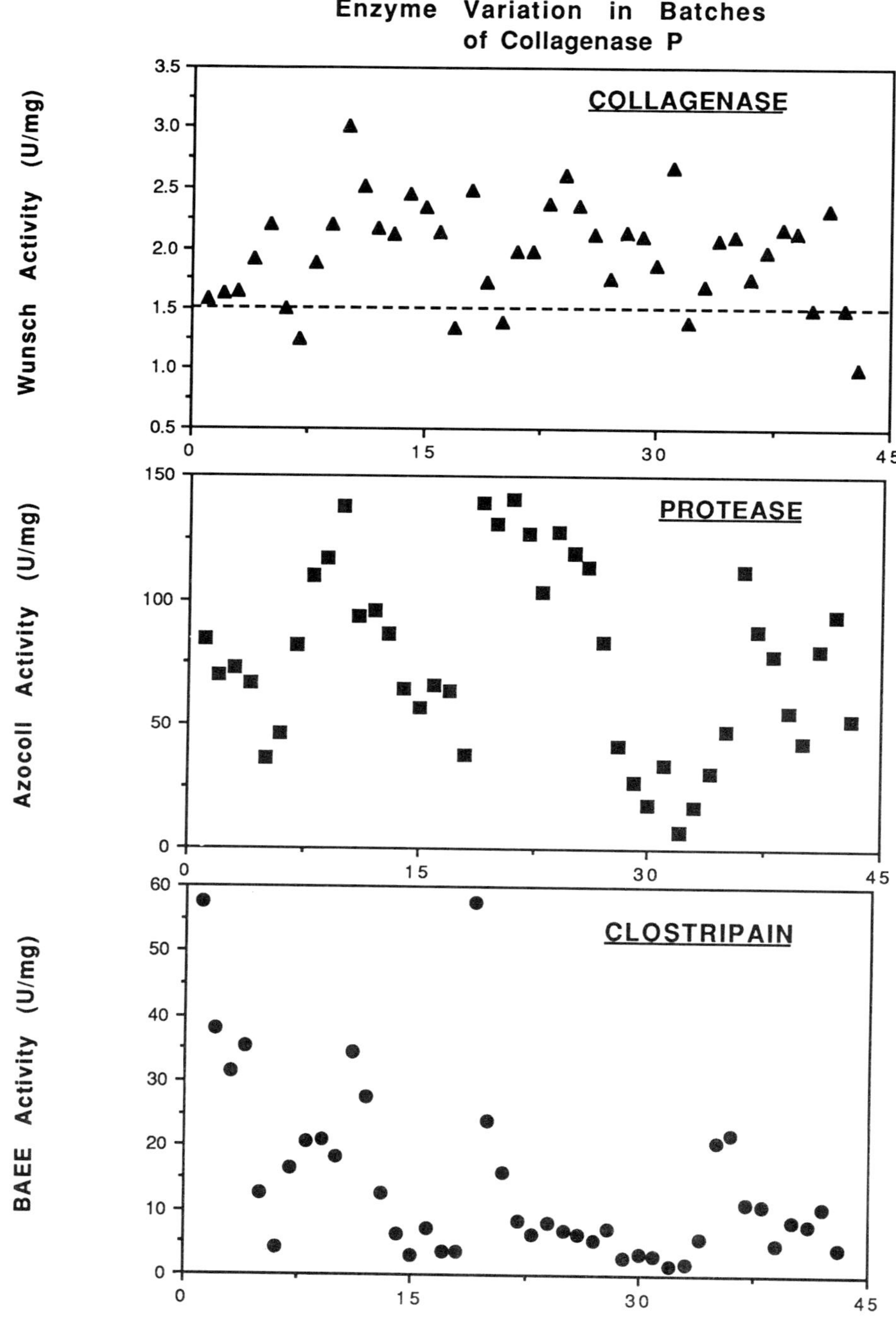

Fig. 4.2. Lot to lot variation in reported enzyme activities for Collagenase P (Boehringer Mannheim). Shown are Wunsch (▲), BAEE (●), and Azocoll (■) activities.

for each lot of Collagenase P which includes measured values for collagenase (Wunsch Units[22]), clostripain & trypsin (BAEE Units[23]), and protease (Azocoll Units[11]). Attempts to correlate enzymatic activities of crude collagenase with functional performance in pancreatic dissociation have not been successful. This may be attributed to the use of synthetic substrates for in vitro assays, which may not reflect in situ substrate specificities. However, biological or procedural noise may mask real differences due to collagenase variability. Therefore, in order to understand the effect of collagenase and its enzymatic constituents on pancreatic dissociation and islet liberation, other factors which affect the reproducibility of islet isolation must be identified.

OTHER FACTORS AFFECTING THE REPRODUCIBILITY OF ISLET ISOLATION

Investigators continue to modify their islet isolation procedures to optimize the yield of intact, functional islet mass. However, it is imperative to standardize the islet isolation procedure in order to properly evaluate new lots of collagenase. The goal of standardization is to have a reproducible procedure with one lot of collagenase so that contributions of biological variability to overall variability of the procedure can be estimated. If procedural factors contribute significantly to overall variability, neither biological parameters nor enzyme-related effects can be accurately assessed.

In the course of our evaluation of different collagenase lots for islet isolation, we have attempted to identify potential sources of procedural and donor variability which can be controlled. The influence of experimental noise can be minimized by attention to detail and controlled experimental design. Table 4.3 lists process-related factors potentially influencing islet yield, and suggests measures to minimize such variability.

DONOR PANCREATA

The effectiveness of different lots of collagenase varies with the species of the pancreas. Most lots of collagenase are effective in isolation of islets from rodent pancreas. As the same lots are applied to islet isolation from canine, porcine, and human pancreata, the percentage of "effective" lots decreases. Species-specific differences may be due to different types and amounts of peri-islet connective tissue, and the extent of direct endocrine to exocrine cell adhesion.[51]

Individual donor factors also influence islet recovery. For the purpose of collagenase evaluation, donor/organ selection criteria should be applied, if at all possible. For animal models such as the pig, selection of one specific strain helps to minimize biological noise. Animal age, size, feed and rearing conditions are also best kept constant. In our experience, the sex of the hog does not influence islet recovery. We have used both males (barrows) and unbred females (gilts) with similar results. We screen donor organs for attributes which might affect enzyme action or islet viability. Porcine pancreata which are visibly engorged with blood are excluded from analyses. We have observed retarded dissociation when using such tissues, possibly due to serum-based protease inhibitors which depress certain enzyme activities, or to serum proteins which may competitively inhibit collagenase enzymes. Donor factors may be beyond the control of the investigator when human pancreata are used for collagenase evaluation.

Variable pancreas size may also present a problem. In order to assess collagenase performance, it is necessary to standardize the enzyme-to-substrate ratio. It is probably not possible to determine this ratio in the strictest sense, since the enzyme substrate (intercellular connective tissue components) and the enzyme specific activities are ill-defined. A reasonable approach is to maintain a constant concentration of collagenase and limit the mass of the pancreas to a specific range. Our experiments, based upon the procedure of Ricordi et al,[29,41] use 667 mL of a 1.5 mg/mL solution of collagenase to dissociate porcine pancreata which weigh between 65 and 90 grams (splenic lobe only). Outliers are excluded from analysis.

Table 4.3. Critical process steps in islet isolation

Process	Factor	Impact on Tissue Dissociation/ Islet Purification	Comments / Solutions
Organ Procurement	Vascular flush	Solution may contain ingredients that alter the performance of dissociating enzymes. [24-29]	If vascular flush is required, use an inert solution such as Hanks balanced salt solution (BSS). BSS is used as a diluent for collagenase and does not alter dissociation activities.
	Warm ischemia time	Exocrine autolysis alters dissociating enzyme activities.[27]	Glands that experience greater than 15 minutes of warm ischemia should be disqualified from use.
	Blood content	Serum proteins inhibit dissociating enzymes (protease inhibitors), and may also serve as competing substrates of dissociating protease activities. Dissociation is retarded causing lower yields.	Glands that show evidence of gross blood congestion should be disqualified.
	Fat content	Excessive fat may retard the dissociation by clogging the dissociation circuit.	Remove excess fat from surface of pancreas.
Organ Perfusion	Quality of perfusion	High pressure may collapse or rupture duct resulting in poor perfusion. [30-32]	Initially perfuse with low pressure and visually confirm good tissue distension.
Tissue Dissociation	Amount and lot of enzyme	Variable results will occur if collagenase concentration or lot is changed. [1,4,29]	Maintain a constant volume and concentration of enzyme.
	Enzyme cofactors	Activities of pancreas dissociating enzymes require cofactors such as Ca^{++} and Zn^{++}. [1,33-35]	Ensure adequate cofactor concentrations in collagenase diluent.
	Enzyme stability	Certain lots of collagenase exhibit progressive loss of activity upon prolonged storage.	Store collagenase at or below -20°C, and avoid unnecessary freeze/thawing.
	Enzyme to substrate ratio	If enzyme to substrate ratio varies, kinetics of dissociation may be altered.	Do not exceed capacity of dissociating enzymes. Maintain tissue mass within allowable range.
Tissue Dissociation	Protein (Albumin , Serum, etc.) added to enzyme solution	Protein may compete as substrate for protease activity in dissociating enzymes.	Avoid addition of extraneous protein.
	Mechanical agitation	If too harsh, islets may be damaged; if not enough, dissociation may be prolonged. [1,29,36-41]	Porcine islets are fragile compared to canine or human islets. Avoid excessive agitation.
	Temperature	Enzyme activities are directly effected by temperature. [1,29,34,41-43]	Maintain constant temperature during tissue dissociation.
	Time (Duration)	The decision to stop dissociation is subjective. If this is early, islet cleavage is incomplete and embedded islets may not purify; if this is late, islet fragmentation may occur. Either case decreases the final yield.[1,4,29,40,41,44]	Screen new collagenase by intentional over digestion with intermittent sample evaluation to predict optimal dissociation time.
Purification	Cell lysis	Cell lysis yields extra cellular DNA which may induce tissue aggregation, impeding separation. [45]	Add DNase to the dissociation solution.
	Density of Gradient	If inappropriate densities are used, separation of endocrine and exocrine components may be sub-optimal. [29,45-50]	Confirm densities of gradient solutions with a densitometer prior to use. Do not change separation parameters without validation. Run test gradients when appropriate.
	Osmolarity of gradient	Density of tissue can be altered by the osmolarity of surrounding media. [47-49]	
	Centrifugation parameters	Centrifugal force and spin time must be optimal for peak separation. [29,46]	

Warm and cold ischemia times can also affect islet yield.[24,27] All attempts should be made to utilize pancreata which have similar ischemia times. Warm ischemia initiates exocrine autolysis and must be minimized. For example, we limit warm ischemia to less than 7 minutes, and cold ischemia to less than 40 minutes.

DISSOCIATION PROCEDURE

Although obvious, it bears stating that enzyme concentrations and formulations for dissociation should not fluctuate. Addition of protease inhibitors or proteins (such as trypsin inhibitor or 10% albumin) may have differential effects on different lots of collagenase, depending upon their composition. Additives such as these complicate comparison of collagenase lots and should be avoided. We have found it useful however, to include DNAse in the dissociation mixture at a concentration of 100 mg/mL. This prevents the clumping of dissociated exocrine cells and islets caused by release of free DNA.

Most pancreatic dissociations are performed by perfusing Clostridial collagenase via the pancreatic duct. A benefit of infusing the enzyme this way is preferential delivery of collagenase to the site of the desired substrate (not endocrine tissue). Consequently, initial tissue dissociation proceeds with reduced exposure of islets to Clostridial enzymes. Collagenase may be injected into the pancreatic duct at relatively high pressure (loading), or under controlled conditions of time and pressure. Initial high perfusion pressures may risk collapsing or rupturing some of the ducts, thereby reducing the thoroughness of ductal perfusion or changing the nature of the organ perfusion. Ductal perfusion is applied in three commonly used methods of pancreas dissociation: (1) collagenase loading followed by mechanical dissociation,[29,41] (2) continuous perfusion with modest mechanical tissue disruption,[52] and (3) monitored perfusion followed by mechanical dissociation.[53] In all cases, the risk of enzyme-mediated islet fragmentation increases with prolonged dissociation time. The investigator must decide when to terminate the tissue dissociation phase and initiate the islet purification phase. Different protocols for pancreas dissociation offer greater or lesser opportunity for process control; however, they all suffer from the subjectivity of dissociation endpoint determination. The controls discussed here are those we apply to the procedure described by Ricordi.[29,41]

Tissue perfusion must be performed in a reproducible manner. A standard volume of enzyme should be used for perfusion and uniform tissue distension should be confirmed by visual examination. To reduce variability in the rate of enzyme loss from the pancreas during initial phases of dissociation, we apply bulldog clamps to any 'leaks' encountered, as well as to the main pancreatic duct at completion of loading. In all of our studies, we began perfusion with low pressure, followed by a moderate increase in pressure to fully engorge the pancreas with enzyme.

The dissociation vessel and solution should be brought to the desired temperature at a controlled rate, and maintained as tightly as possible. For example, our experimental pancreas dissociations typically reach target temperature at 7-8 minutes, and are maintained at $37.2 \pm 0.2°C$. Many factors contribute to the time required to reach temperature, including pancreas mass and temperature, starting temperature of the perfusate, and time required to perfuse the pancreas and transfer it to the reaction vessel. Attention to timing at each step is required to facilitate reproducibility.

A reproducible and appropriate level of mechanical agitation is required during pancreatic dissociation. Since porcine islets are more friable than human islets,[36] mechanical agitation is not easily automated. Although the estimation is subjective, we attempt to maintain the same degree of agitation from one experiment to the next.

ISLET PURIFICATION

A great deal of scientific effort continues to be expended in optimizing recovery of islets from dissociated pancreatic tissue. This topic is addressed in greater detail in other chapters of this text. However, in the context of collagenase evaluation, variability of purification must be minimized. If the purification method is not generating reproducible yields, variability due to collagenase may not be recognized. Use of pre-Ficoll measurement abrogates the variability contributed by purification, but must be interpreted cautiously.

SAMPLE ANALYSIS

Islet yield is typically determined by staining a representative sample with diphenylthiocarbazone (DTZ) and examining it microscopically.[54] The total number of isolated islets is not an appropriate measure of yield due to islet size heterogeneity and the potential for islet fragmentation. An islet twice the diameter of another has eight times the endocrine biomass. Consequently, islets are quantitated in standardized volumetric units (Equivalent Islet Numbers: EIN). Islet equivalents relate to the number of 150 µm spherical islets that correspond to the equivalent mass of the sample in question. The EIN is therefore an indication of the total recovered endocrine biomass.[55] Expression of recovered endocrine biomass per mass of pancreas dissociated (EIN/g) enables yield comparison from one pancreas to the next.

The volume of sample examined must be sufficient to eliminate sampling error, since accurate determination of islet yield is central to the assessment of collagenase performance. The influence of sample size on sampling error is particularly evident when considering the influence of islet size on biomass. Islets larger than 250 µm are estimated to constitute only 15% of the total number of islets, but 60% of the total endocrine biomass of the pancreas.[56] Therefore, sample size must ensure a sample distribution which adequately represents in vivo islet size distribution. We have determined that a sample which contains a minimum of 200-250 islets is sufficient to minimize sampling error.

COLLAGENASE LOT SELECTION

As stated earlier, perhaps the single most significant source of error in the process of evaluating collagenase is the subjective decision of dissociation endpoint. This decision is made by the investigator, based upon visual examination of samples from the dissociation. However, there are no rules or guidelines on which to base this decision other than the investigator's experience. This is a critical determination since under-dissociation leads to sub-optimal islet cleavage from exocrine tissue, and over-dissociation extends islet exposure to dissociating enzymes, resulting in islet fragmentation and cellular damage. Either outcome is equally disappointing, and may preclude accurate assessment of collagenase performance. In an attempt to overcome this dilemma, we have developed a collagenase evaluation method that minimizes subjective analysis at this critical point in the dissociation procedure. Porcine pancreas is dissociated using a modified Ricordi procedure, with the exception that the tissue dissociation proceeds for up to 60 minutes. Samples are collected at 5 minute intervals and the size, number, and morphology of cleaved islets is determined in each sample. By correlating total mass of free islets with time, optimal dissociation time and yield can be projected.

Manual counting may not be practical using this method since samples are evaluated every 5 minutes. For this reason, we evaluate islets through imaging technology. Samples are stained by the zinc-avid fluorochrome N-(6-methoxy-8-quinolyl)-p-toluene sulfonamide (TSQ),[57] and gray scale images collected using a SIT black & white video camera mounted to an epi-fluorescence microscope. Typically, 24 images are collected per sample in order to minimize sampling error. Image analysis is automated by a command file written in Technical Control Language (TCL) through BDS-Image (Biological Detection Systems). Results are formatted to be consistent with EIN units. An additional benefit of using imaging technology is morphologic assessment of islet structural integrity. These parameters may also be monitored during the time course of dissociation.

Results from an evaluation of collagenase on porcine pancreas using this profile approach are presented in Figure 4.3. A 3-dimensional curve can be generated by comparing free islet size and time against number (Fig. 4.3A). In this example, two peaks of islet release are seen. These peaks are associated with relatively small islets

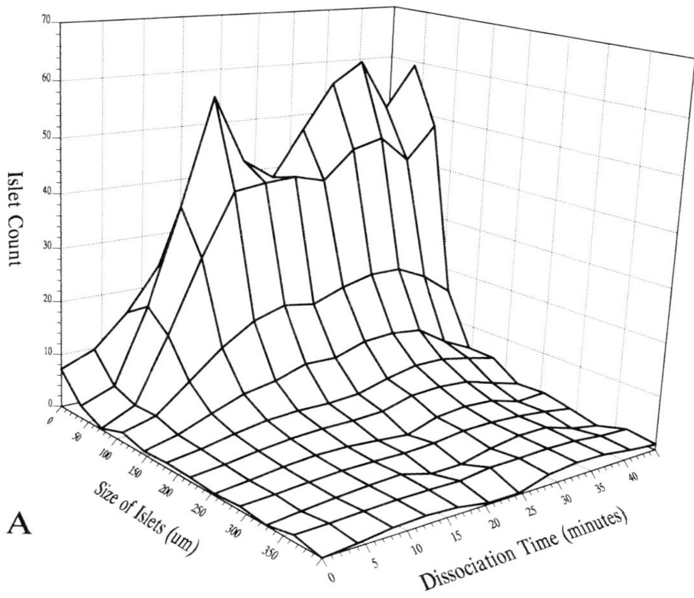

Fig. 4.3A

Fig. 4.3B

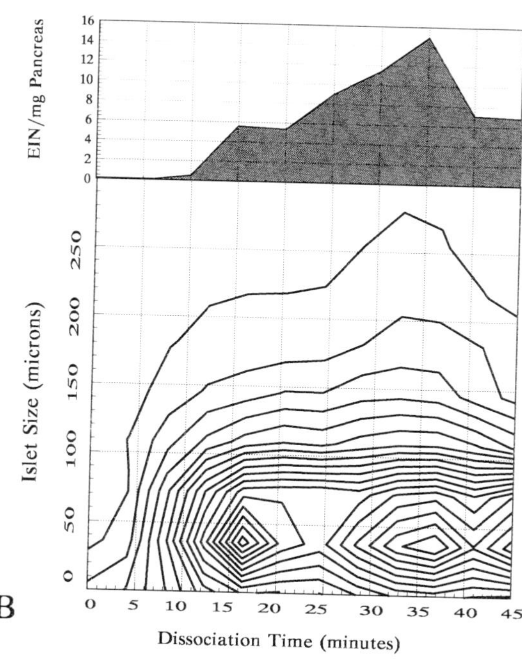

Fig. 4.3. Profile analysis of porcine pancreas dissociation in isometric display (A) and contour display (B). Maximum endocrine biomass yield is associated with the release of larger islets at 30 to 35 minutes and are demonstrated by the outer contour lines in the upper portion of the contour plot. The EIN results are shown above the contour plot (B).

(approx. 50 μm in diameter). However, it is difficult to ascertain the contribution of larger islets (>200 μm) to this curve. These same data are presented in a contour plot in Figure 4.3B. Again, islet size is plotted against dissociation time, although the scale of the ordinate (islet size) is reversed. Each contour represents increasing numbers of islets. The two peaks are seen as concentric accretions of contours in the lower third of the plot. There is a burst of large islets at 30 to 35 minutes as depicted by the outer contour lines. This activity immediately precedes the second peak. The shaded curve above represents the time course of EIN yield.

By plotting the kinetics of islet liberation during pancreatic dissociation, both optimal endpoint timing and pre-Ficoll EIN yield for a given lot of collagenase may be determined. In the example demonstrated in Figure 4.3, traditional methods for evaluating collagenase may have lead to an inappropriate termination of dissociation after the first release of islets (about 17 minutes). Peak endocrine biomass yield may have been missed, yielding inaccurate assessment of collagenase.

In six consecutive collagenase lot evaluations, profile analysis demonstrated similar dissociation kinetics and yields in duplicate studies. The profile approach yields consistent and reliable predictions of collagenase performance, and minimizes the risk of inaccurate collagenase assessment due to erroneous dissociation endpoint.

SUMMARY

Collagenase is recognized as the principal reagent for pancreatic dissociation. This crude mixture of bacterial enzymes varies from lot to lot in both composition and formulation. Such heterogeneity leads to irreproducible pancreatic dissociation and islet yields. Consequently, before investigators commit to the purchase of large amounts of any given lot, each must be pre-screened for functionality. However, evaluation of collagenase is hindered by other sources of variation. The pancreatic dissociation and islet isolation processes are fraught with biological and procedural noise which preclude accurate assessment of collagenase performance. In this chapter we described our efforts to control donor and procedural variables in order to minimize assay variability when evaluating collagenase. Despite attention to these experimental controls, subjective determination of dissociation endpoint remains a source of error. A new method for the evaluation of collagenase is reported, in which dissociation is allowed to proceed *ad finitum* and the kinetics of islet liberation are objectively determined. Analysis of tissue dissociation and islet liberation kinetics allows accurate estimation of the optimal dissociation endpoint, and minimizes the risks and costs of collagenase pre-screening.

ACKNOWLEDGMENTS

The authors wish to thank Bernice Ellis, Marilyn Smith, David Waters, Kathleen Wile and MaryJo Wright for their technical assistance. The expert assistance of Drs. Camillo Ricordi and Ray Rajotte is greatly appreciated.

REFERENCES

1. Gray DWR, Leow CK. Non-automated methods for islet isolation. In: Ricordi C, ed. Pancreatic islet cell transplantation. Austin: R.G. Landes Co. 1992;89

2. Hatton MWC, Berry LR, Krestynski F, Sweeney GD, Regoeczi E. The role of proteolytic enzymes derived from crude bacterial collagenase in the liberation of hepatocytes from rat liver. Identification of two cell-liberating mechanisms. Eur. J Biochem. 1983; 137: 311.

3. Kessler E, Yaron A. A novel aminopeptidase from Clostridium histolyticum. Biochim. Biophys. Res. Commun. 1973; 50:405.

4. Wolters GHJ, Vos-Scheperkeuter GH, van Deijnen JHM, van Schilfgaarde R. An analysis of the role of collagenase and protease in the enzymatic dissociation of the rat pancreas for islet isolation. Diabetologica 1992; 35:735.

5. Seifter S, Gallop PM. Collagenase from *Clostridium histolyticum*. Methods In Enzymol. 1961; 5: 659.

6. Seifter S, Harper E. Collagenases. Methods In Enzymol. 1970; 19:613.

7. Peterkofsky B. Bacterial Collagenase. Methods in Enzymol. 1982; 82:453.

8. Grant NH, Alburn HE. Studies on the collagenases of *Clostridium histolyticum*. Arch. Biochem & Biophys. 1959; 82:245.

9. Mandl I, Keller S, Manahan J. Multiplicity of *Clostridium histolyticum* collagenases. Biochemistry (Washington) 1964; 3(11):1737.

10. Yoshida E, Noda H. Isolation and characterization of collagenases I and II from Clostridium histolyticum. Biochim. Biophys. Acta 1965; 105:562.

11. Kono T. Purification and partial characterization of collagenolytic enzymes from Clostridium histolyticum. Biochemistry 1968; 7:1106.

12. Seifter S, Harper E. The Collagenases. Boyer PD, ed. The Enzymes, New York; Academic Press 1970; 3:649.

13. Takahashi S, Seifter S. New culture conditions for Clostirdium histolyticum leading to production of collagenase of high specific activity. J. of Appl. Bacteriol. 1972; 35:647.

14. Lwebuga-Mukasa JS, Harper E, Taylor P. Collagenase enzymes from Clostridium: characterization of individual enzymes Biochemistry 1976; 15:4736.

15. Oppenheim F, Franzblau C. A modified procedure for the purification of clostridial collagenase. Prep. Biochem. 1978; 8:387

16. Sugasawra R, Harper E. Purification and characterization of three forms of collagenase from *Clostridium histolyticum*. Biochemistry 1984; 23:5175.

17. Bond MD, Van Wart HE. Purification and separation of individual collagenases of Clostridium histolyticum using red dye ligand chromatography. Biochemistry 1984; 23:3077.

18. Hefley TJ. Utilization of FPLC-purified bacterial collagenase for the isolation of cells from bone. J. of Bone and Min. Res. 1987; 2:505.

19. Altieri P, Candiano G, Gineveri F, Ghiggeri GM. Purification of proteinase-free collagenase from commercial batches of the enzyme.Prep. Biochem. 1990; 20:137.

20. Van Wart HE, Steinbrink DR. Complementary substrate specificities of class I and class II collagenases from Clostridium histolyticum. Biochemistry 1985; 24:6520.

21. Scharp DW. Commentary. Cell Transplantation. 1993; 2:299.

22. Wunsch E, Heidrich HC. Zur quantitativen bestimmung der kollagenase. Z. Physiol. Chem. 1963; 333:149.

23. Mitchell WM, Harrington WF. Purification and properties of clostridiopeptidase B (Clostripain). J. Biol. Chem. 1968; 243:4683.

24. Kneteman NM, Warnock GL, Lakey JRT, Rajote RV, Pancreas procurement and preservation: impact on islet recovery and viability. In Ricordi C, ed. Pancreatic islet cell transplantation. Austin: R.G. Landes Co. 1992;72.

25. Yamaguchi T, Mullen Y, Watanabe Y et al. Isolation and function of islets from young adult pig pancreas, Transplant Proc 1992;24:1010.

26. Ohzato H, Gotoh M, Monden M et al. Intraductal injection of collagenase solution at the time of harvesting: A possible solution for preservation and collagenase digestion. Transplant Proc 1990; 22(2):782.

27. Ricordi C, Socci C, Davalli AM et al. Effect of pancreas retrieval procedure on islet isolation in the swine. Transplant Proc 1990; 22:442.

28. Zucker PF, Bloom AD, Strasser S, Alejandro R. Successful cold storage preservation of canine pancreas with UW-1 solution prior to islet isolation. Transplantation 1989; 48(1):168.

29. Ricordi C. The automated method for islet isolation. In Ricordi C, ed. Pancreatic islet cell transplantation. Austin: R.G. Landes Co. 1992;99.

30. Van Suylichem PT, Pasma A, Wolters GH, Van Schilfgaarde R. Microscopic aspects of the structure and collagen content of teh pancreas from the perspective of islet isolation. Transplant Proc 1987;19:3958.

31. Horaguchi A, Merrell RC. Preparation of viable islet cells from dogs by a new method. Diabetes 1981;30:455.

32. Rajotte RV, Warnock GL, Evans MG et al. Isolation of viable islets of Langerhans from collagenase-perfused canine and human pancreata. Transplant Proc 1987;19:918.

33. McShane P, Sutton R, Gray DWR, Morris PJ. Protease activity in pancreatic islet isolation by enzymatic digestion. Diabetes [Suppl 1] 1989;38:126.

34. Dono K, Gotoh M, Ohzato H et al. The role of calcium in collagenase digestion and preservation of islets. Transplant Proc. 1992; 24 (3):1000.

35. Bond, MD, VanWart HE. Characterization of the individual collagenases from clostridium histolyticum. Biochemistry 1984;23:3085.

36. Ricordi C, Socci C, Davalli AM et al. Isolation of the elusive pig islet. Surgery,1990;107:688.

37. Calafiore R, Calcinaro F, Basta G et al. A method for the massive separation of highly purified, adult porcine islets of Langerhans. Metabolism, 1990;39:175.

38. Hinshaw DB, Jolley WB, Knierim KH, Hinshaw DB. New non-enzymatic method for the isolation of functional pancreatic islets. Surg Forum 1981;32:381.

39. Warnock GL, Kneteman NM, Evans MG et al. Comparison of automated and manual methods for islet isolation. Can J Surg 1990;33:368.

40. Ricordi C, Lacy PE, Finke EH et al. An automated method for the isolation of human pancreatic islets. Diabetes 1988;37:413.

41. Ricordi C, Finke EH, Lacy PE. A method for the mass isolation of islets from the adult pig pancreas. Diabetes 1986;35:649.

42. Gray DWR, McShane P, Grant A, Morris PJ. A method for isolation of islets of Langerhans from the human pancreas. Diabetes 1984;33:1055.

43. Sutton R, Hammonds P, Hughes D et al. Isolation of islets from human pancreas using increased incubation temperatures and variable density gradients. Horm Metab Res [Suppl] 1989;25:35.

44. London NJ, Lake SP, Wilson J, Bassett D et al. A simple method for the release of islets by controlled collagenase digestion of the human pancreas. Transplantation 1990;49:1109.

45. Pretlow YG, Pretlow TP, Sedimentation of cells: An overview and discussion of artifacts. In : Pretlow TG, Pretlow TP, eds. Cell separation: methods and selected applications, Volume 1. San Diego: Academic Press, 1982:41.

46. Lacy PE, Kostianovsky M. Method for the isolation of intact islets of Langerhans from the rat pancreas. Diabetes 1967;16:35.

47. London NJM, James RFL, Bell PRF. Islet Purification. In Ricordi C, ed. Pancreatic islet cell transplantation. Austin: R.G. Landes Co. 1992;113

48. London NJM, Toomey P, Contractor H, Thirdborough ST, James RF, Bell PR. The effect of osmolality and glucose concentration on the purity of human islet isolates. Transplant Proc. 1992; 24(3):1002.

49. Hehmke B, Kohnert KD, Odselius R. The use of a new dextran medium for rapid isolation of functionally intact neonatal rat pancreatic islets. Diabetes Research 1986; 3:13.

50. Hering BJ, Muench KP, Schelz J, et al. The evaluation of neutral density separation utilizing Ficoll-sodium diatrizoate and Nycodenz and centrifugal elutriation in the purification of bovine and canine islet preparations. Hormone Metabol Res 1990;25[Suppl]:57.

51. van Deijnen JHM, Hulstaert CE, Wolters GHJ, van Schilfgaarde R. Significance of the peri-insular extracellular-matrix for islet isolation from the pancreas of rat, dog, pig and man. Cell Tissue Res.1992; 267(1):139.

52. Calafiore, R, Calcinaro F, Basta G, Pietropaolo M, Falorni A, Piermattie M, Brunetti P. A Method for the Massive Separation of Highly Purified, Adult Porcine Islets of Langerhans. Metabolism 1990; 39(2):175.

53. Ao Z, Lakey JR, Rajotte RV, Warnock GL. Collagenase digestion of canine pancreas by gentle automated dissociation in combination with ductal perfusion optimizes mass recovery of islets. Transplant Proc 1992; 24 (6):2787.

54. Latif ZA, Noel J, Alejandro R. A simple method of staining fresh and cultured islets. Transplantation. 1988; 45:827.

55. Ricordi C, Gray DW, Hering BJ, Kaufman DB, Warnock GL, Kneteman NM, Lake SP, London NJ, Socci C, Alejandro R, et al. Islet isolation assessment in man and large animals. Acta Diabetol Lat 1990; 27(3):185.

56. Bonner-Weir S. Anatomy of the Islet of Langerhans. In: the Endocrine Pancreas, Samols E, ed. The Endocrine Pancreas, New York; Raven Press, 1991:15.

57. Jindal RM, Taylor RP, Gray DWR, Esmeraldo R, Morris PJ. A new method for quantification of islets by measurement of zinc content. Diabetes 1992; 41:1056.

Islet Isolation from Rodent Pancreas

Part I

Gordon C. Weir

Jennifer Hollister

Alberto M. Davalli

Susan Bonner-Weir

The development of methods for isolating the islets of Langerhans has had an enormous impact upon diabetes research and provides a major step toward the goal of providing beta cell replacement therapy with islet transplantation for people with diabetes. The isolation of rodent islets has led the way for much of this progress. Rodents have become the most commonly used animals for experimental work on islets. Not only are they readily available and inexpensive, but the structure and function of their islets have marked similarities to what is known about human islets. Perhaps 90% of the work which forms the basis of our scientific understanding of islets come from work in mice and rats. In recent years the amount of work done with rodent islets has even increased because of the availability of valuable models of autoimmune diabetes, chemical diabetes, genetic forms of diabetes resembling NIDDM, and a variety of transgenic mice. Furthermore, mice and rats have been extraordinarily valuable for studies on islet transplantation.

DEVELOPMENT OF ISLET TRANSPLANTATION

The achievement of isolating the islets was impressive because these tiny micro-organs typically contain 1000-3000 cells and make up only about 1% of the volume of the pancreas. For many years virtually no biochemical studies on islets could be done except for histochemical observations. Some pioneers developed various ways to hand-dissect islets.[1] This proved easiest with the large islets of ob/ob mice,[2] but islets could also be obtained from normal mice.[1] Remarkable observations were made with as few as 1-3 islets. Pieces of pancreas were also used to study insulin secretion. Other workers explored the use of some species of fish, which have separate organs consisting of almost pure islet cells, that are usually adjacent to exocrine tissue.[3] These are called Brockmann bodies or principal islets, and in some species are more than one centimeter in diameter.

Pancreatic Islet Transplantation Volume I: Procurement of Pancreatic Islets, edited by Robert P. Lanza, MD, William L. Chick, MD; ©1994 R.G. Landes Company.

The major breakthrough in the isolation of rodent islets came when the enzyme collagenase was used to digest pancreatic tissue. It was found that with proper balance of digestion and agitation, intact islets could be separated from exocrine tissue and visualized with a dissecting microscope. The first use of this approach was reported in 1965 by Moskalewski, who isolated guinea pig islets.[4] The technique was then refined for use in rats by Lacy and Kostianovsky.[5] This technique was modified in countless ways by many laboratories, but the basic approach has remained the same. For many years there were problems with the consistency of the collagenase preparations, but this has not been a major issue in recent years. Initially the pancreas was distended by injecting the pancreatic duct with a buffer solution such as Hanks. Then the pancreas was minced and incubated in a collagenase containing solution. Some investigators have employed an arterial injection of neutral red to stain the islets for easier hand-picking.[6] More recently, most laboratories have been distending the pancreatic duct with a collagenase-containing buffer followed by a period of incubation and then agitation.[7] Further improvement came from gradient purification, using such materials as Ficoll-sodium diatrizoate, Nycodenz, Histopaque, or bovine serum albumin (BSA).[6] An automated digestion-filtration system has even been described, but this is not in wide use.[8]

Rodent pancreas is diffuse with more separation between lobules than the compact pancreata of larger species such as pig, dog, monkey and human. Rodent islets tend to be easier to isolate than islets from these larger species. The reasons for this are not known. Perhaps the diffuse nature of the pancreas allows easier digestion. Alternatively, the cells of rodent islets may be particularly adherent to each other so that their integrity is well maintained. There may be some special characteristic of the proteins around the islets that provides a useful susceptibility to the collagenase preparations. Some have thought that rodent islets must have a well defined capsule so that the outside layers might be digested away from the exocrine pancreas and a residual layer could hold the islet together. This may be true in some species, but in rats the capsule, when closely examined by electron microscopy, is very thin containing one layer of fibroblasts and collagen. Often there is no capsule between exocrine and islet cells. Furthermore, capsules are not found on isolated islets when studied by electron microscopy. Studies of collagenase preparations indicate that they contain a variety of other proteases which contribute to effective islet isolation. For isolation of primate islets pure collagenase preparations do not perform as well as those with various proteases.[9] The protease contaminants are probably also helpful for the isolation of rodent islets. A major factor behind the predictable success of isolating rodent islets must be the consistency of the pancreases and practice with the technique, as is expected when highly inbred strains of the same age are used on a frequent basis.

ISLET NUMBER, SIZE AND SHAPE IN RODENT PANCREATA

This is a frequently asked question with a complicated answer. If one assumes that a typical freshly isolated islet of 100-150 μm in diameter has an insulin content of 40 ng and the entire pancreas has an insulin content of 80 μg, there could be 2000 such islets. But this simplistic analysis does not take into account the considerable variability of islet size, nor the fact that continuous changes occur throughout the life of the animal.[10,11] A study by Lifson et al provides important insights into this issue.[12] A symmetrical distribution of islet diameter was described in normal 550 g rats, with a mean single islet diameter of 97 ± 4 (M ± SE) um and a median diameter of 83 ± 4 μm. The weight of the pancreases was about 1.8 g and estimated islet number was 3300/g of pancreas or about 6000 islets. The largest islets may be 800 μm in diameter, but these are rare; islets of 300 μm are few but not rare.[13,14] There have been question about whether the 800 μm islets are really one islet or several smaller islets that have merged. The development of these megaislets has not been studied, but they have a core of contiguous beta cells and a surrounding mantle.

The relationship between islet diameter and volume is an important consideration. The volume of an islet 800 μm in diameter would be the equivalent of about 500 islets with diameters of 100 μm. These numbers are not exact because islets are often not spherical, but instead are ovoid or in the case of very large islets, sometimes sausage-shaped. Most of the volume of the endocrine pancreas is accounted for by islets between 100 and 300 μm in diameter. Thus, even though the median islet diameter may be 83 μm, it has been estimated by Lifson et al that 72% of islet volume in a pancreas is accounted for by the largest 20% of the islet population, i.e., those with diameters of 140 μm or above.[12] All of the islets with diameters of 97 μm (the mean diameter) or below account for only 10% of the total islet volume. Thus, if there are 6000 islets, the smallest half of these (the median diameter being 83 μm) will only make up about 5% of the endocrine mass. There are questions about whether the very smallest islets have been accurately counted in these studies. Islets of 25 μm are described, but because beta cells have a diameter of only about 10 μm, these can only contain a few cells. Relatively few of these miniscule islets are seen with the immunostaining of sections, so they probably contribute very little to overall islet mass. These concepts are fundamental to predicting which islets will be retrieved during isolation. Most small islets will be unretrievable in the isolation process; some must be too small to identify, others are probably destroyed by enzymatic digestion. Many large islets are also lost, but their fate is not completely understood. Some are probably ruptured and digested, others can be seen attached to connective tissue, which usually makes them unretrievable. Large islets of over 225 μm may not be very useful for study and have limitations for transplantation because of anoxia of the beta cell cores (this phenomenon will be discussed later).

Expectations about islet yield are very dependent upon the size of the rodent because there is a good correlation between body weight and islet volume.[10,11] Laboratory rats tend to increase their weight until near the end of their life span and beta cell mass increases in parallel, except during the fetal and newborn period. Below 21 days of age the ratio of islet volume to body weight is higher, but afterwards is relatively stable. Presumably the insulin resistance of obesity and inactivity accounts for much of this increase in islet volume. Many laboratories use rats of 150-200 g for their islet isolations. Thus, if a 500 g rat has 6000 islets, these smaller rats should have about 2000. Of these 2000, 800 might be between 75-225 μm, a size we usually use for transplantation or other studies. Based upon studies in mice with similar looking isolated islets we estimate the mean isolated islet diameter to be about 160 μm.[15] On good days our laboratory can expect to isolate 500 islets per rat. Therefore, about 25% of the total number of islets may be isolated, but about 60% of the desirable larger islets might be obtained. Because they have a mean diameter of about 160 μm, they are larger than most of the islets in the pancreas. Furthermore, these relatively large isolated islets can be expected to contain about 40% of pancreatic islet volume. Not much is known about the efficiency of islet isolation from older large rats. Our limited experience suggests that the isolation procedures are not as effective in larger/older rats.

Islet volume and number has not been as carefully studied in mice, but the findings in rats generally hold true for mice. Bunnag found 421 ± 30 islets in one month old mice and 751 ± 47 islets in 14 month old mice.[16] The results of Parakal and Ali with a different method found about 25% fewer islets.[17] We typically use mice of 9-11 weeks of age weighing 25-30 g and obtain about 200-250 islets per mouse. Thus, our yield from mice as a percentage of islets in the pancreas seems to be better than from rats. Although isolated mouse islets have the same appearance and approximate size distribution as rats, it is our impression that there are fewer very large islets in mice than in rats. The ratio of islet volume to body weight is similar for mice and rats. For example, the islet volume for a 25 g mouse is about 1 mg and for a 250 g rat is about 6 mg.[15,16] Commonly used genetic models for obesity, insulin resistance and diabetes include ob/ob and db/db mice. At certain ages these mice are very hyperinsulinemic, and are found to have increased beta cell mass and larger islets.[2] They can be isolated with a conventional collagenase approach, but we are unaware of studies examining the efficiency of isolation.

INTEGRITY OF NON-BETA CELLS DURING ISLET ISOLATION

Morphometric studies of the rat pancreas indicate that the non-beta cells account for about 25% of the islet mass. In rodents these are found on the outer mantle of the islet and consist of alpha, delta, and PP cells, containing glucagon, somatostatin, and pancreatic polypeptide respectively. Isolated islets often have the same ratios of non-beta cell to total islet volume as the native pancreas,[17] but at times the proportion of non-beta cells can be reduced, presumably from over digestion. There are interesting questions about whether non-beta cells contribute to the insulin secretory capacity of islets.[18] Pipeleers et al[19] have found that transplanted purified beta cells function reasonably well. Recent studies of ours with rat and porcine islets indicate that non-beta cells can be lost during isolation for transplantation with little adverse impact upon the capacity of the grafts to secrete insulin.[20] Our impression is that the loss of non-beta cells is a bigger problem in the isolation of porcine islets than with rodent or human islets. Purposeful overdigestion might be useful as a strategy to obtain purified beta cells.

LIMITATIONS OF ISOLATED RODENT ISLETS

Even though isolated islets are extremely useful, they are not without their important limitations. Islets in vivo are richly vascularized, probably because of the high oxygen requirements of beta cells. For example, although islets make up only about 1% of pancreatic volume, they receive about 10% of the blood flow.[12] Following isolation, the center of islets may not receive enough oxygen. Careful studies by Dionne et al have shown that sufficient oxygen from a buffer can only penetrate about 75 μm into an islet.[21] This means that islets greater than 150 μm in diameter will have anoxia of their central beta cells. The larger the islet the more beta cell tissue will be vulnerable. This anoxia, when borderline, will lead to reduced glucose-induced insulin secretion and when severe will cause cell death. Studies of cultured islets reveal necrotic centers in large islets after several days. This important problem is often not taken into account when beta cell mass requirements for islet transplantation are considered.[22] When insulin secretion from freshly isolated islets is studied with static incubation, "basal" insulin secretory rates at a low glucose concentration are far higher than those from the well oxygenated islets of a perfused pancreas preparation.[23] A high rate of insulin release is also found with perifused isolated islets which should also have problems with anoxia. We assume that this high rate of insulin release is not from basal secretion, but represents leakage of insulin from anoxic beta cells.

Another important consideration is that the distribution of islet vasculature is highly specialized such that arterioles penetrate through an open "pore" in the outer mantle and break into a glomerular-like network of capillaries within the beta cell core, which then exit through the mantle before coalescing to form venules.[13] This pattern has important functional consequences because secreted insulin from the core is carried downstream to bathe the mantle cells, with a suppressive influence upon glucagon secretion. But the secretory products from the mantle would have a difficult time going upstream to reach the beta cell core.[18] When islets are isolated, this local portal system will be disrupted and other paracrine mechanisms will also be seriously disturbed. In addition, islets normally have a complex and functionally important sympathetic and parasympathetic neural innervation, which will also be disrupted. These disruptions may be at least part of the reason for why it is so difficult to study glucagon and somatostatin secretion from isolated islets. In spite of all of these changes, isolated islets can still be very useful for studies of insulin secretion, biochemistry, and electrophysiology, as long as the limitations are taken into account.

RAT ISLET ISOLATION METHOD AT JOSLIN

This is a modification of the method of Gotoh et al.[7] Collagenase (usually Boehringer Mannheim type P or Serva), 1.5-2.5 mg/ml, is dissolved in media M199, Hanks or RPMI 1640 without Calf Serum. The correct concentration should be determined for every lot of collagenase. About 6 mL of collagenase-containing solution should be made up for each rat. A 10 cc syringe with a dull 23 g needle is filled with 6 mL of collagenase solution. The needle is then attached to a 6 inch length of stiff PE 50 tubing, which is beveled at the end.

Donor rats between 180-220 g are most often used. They are overdosed with sodium amytal (100 mg/kg body weight) given intraperitoneally. The abdomen is opened to provide wide exposure of the pancreas. The pancreatic duct is tied off at its duodenal insertion taking care not to injure the surrounding pancreatic tissue. The bile duct is isolated near the point of branching toward the liver. Before canulation, fat is wiped from the duct area. A small incision is made in the duct with microdissecting scissors and the cannula is inserted to a point short of blocking the main duct of the dorsal lobe— some find a dissecting microscope to be helpful. The cannula is held in place by clamping it lightly with forceps and 6 mL of the collagenase solution is rapidly injected to fully distend the pancreas. The rat may then be sacrificed by cutting the diaphragm, heart or aorta.

The pancreas is then removed with careful dissection and placed on a piece of dental wax, whereupon fat and lymph tissue are removed. The pancreas is then placed in a 25 cm flask on ice until pancreata from the other rats are similarly processed. Up to two pancreata can be put into one flask. The pancreas-containing flasks are then placed into a water bath at 37°C for 15-25 min. The incubation time will vary with the lot of collagenase.

At the end of the incubation, 20 mL of media with newborn calf serum is added to the flask and the entire contents are poured into a sterile 50 mL Falcon tube on ice. After another 20 mL of media is added, the tubes are shaken vigorously for 5-10 seconds to disperse the tissue. To remove the collagenase, the islets are washed 3-4 times with 25-35 mL of media with 5-10% newborn calf serum using a clinical centrifuge. After the last wash, the pellet is resuspended in 20 mL of media and filtered through a 300-400 μm diameter wire mesh (Cellector) to remove the remaining undigested tissue, fat and lymph nodes. Add 5-10 mL more to each tube to collect any remaining islets and again filter through the mesh. The islets are then pelleted by spinning at 1200 rpm for 120 sec. As much media is removed as possible, with the help of turning the tubes upside-down on a paper towel. For the gradient separation procedure, the pellet is resuspended in 10 mL Histopaque 1077 (Sigma) and vortexed until the suspension is homogeneous. Ten milliliters media without serum is carefully overlaid on the Histopaque to maintain a sharp interface. The media is pipetted slowly down the side of the tube. The tubes are then spun for 20 minutes in a refrigerated centrifuge (10°C) at 2400 rpm (900 g) with very slow acceleration and no braking.

After centrifugation, the islets are collected from the interface with a disposable 10 mL serologic pipette. Unlike plastic materials, glass pipettes and all other glass surfaces must be siliconized. All of the islets are then placed in one or two 50 mL conical tubes. The islets are then washed three times to remove the Histopaque in the manner described above. After the final wash, the pellet is resuspended in 20-30 mL of media. Then 7-10 mL are added to 60 mm sterile culture dishes for hand-picking.

If necessary, the islets may be further purified by gravity sedimentation before use. The islets are resuspended in 25-35 mL media with neonatal calf serum and allowed to sit for at least 4 minutes on ice. The top 10 mL are then gently pipetted off and 10 mL of new media are added. The tube is inverted to redistribute the islets and then allowed to sediment for at least 4 minutes more. This process may be repeated for four to six times before the islets are hand-picked.

To hand-pick, a 10 μl pipette tip on any pipetteman can be used. For transplantation, we select only islets between 75 and 225 μm in diameter, which have a smooth surface and have a round or oval shape. We use a calibrated eyepiece micrometer. With overdigestion there are likely to be fewer small islets, with the proportion of large islets increasing. Also, the islets often have a ragged surface. With underdigestion there may be many small islets and fewer large islets. The conditions can be manipulated by either changing the concentration of collagenase or the time of digestion. The expected yield from 7-10 wk rats of 180-220 g is about 500 transplantable islets per pancreas.

For mouse islets the procedure differs only in scale, surgical approach and the digestion time. A 3 mL syringe with a 27 g needle bent 90 degrees is used. Once the pancreas is exposed, the end of the bile duct is clamped at its duodenal insertion with a small bulldog clamp and pulled taut. The bile duct is then isolated at the proximal end and the needle inserted. Then 2 mL of the collagenase solution is rapidly injected. The pancreata are digested for 3-4 min longer than those of rats. The rest of the isolation procedure is identical to that described for rats. The expected yield from a pancreas of a 9-11 wk mouse of 25-30 g is 200-250 islets, but can be less in some strains.

REFERENCES

1. Hellerstrom C. A method for the microdissection of intact pancreatic islets of mammals. Acta Endocr. (Kbh.) 1964; 45: 122-132.
2. Gapp DA, Leiter EH, Colemen DL, et al. Temporal changes in pancreatic islet composition in C57BL/6J-db/db (Diabetes) mice. Diabetologia 1983; 25:439-443.
3. Noe BD, Fletcher DJ, Bauer GE. Biosynthesis of Glucagon and Somatostatin In: Cooperstein SJ and Watkins D, eds. The Islets of Langerhans. New York: Academic Press, 1981; 189-221.
4. Moskalewski S. Isolation and culture of the islets of Langerhans of the guinea-pig. Gen Comp Endocr 1965; 5:342-353.
5. Lacy PE, Kostianovsky M. Method for the isolation of intact islets of Langerhans from the rat pancreas. Diabetes 1967;16:35-39.
6. Bretzel RG, Zekorn T, Hering BJ et al. Experimental Islet Transplantation in Small Animals. In: Ricordi C, ed. Pancreatic Islet Cell Transplantation. Austin: RG Landes, 1992:249-260.
7. Gotoh M, Maki T, Kiyoizumi T et al. An improved method for the isolation of mouse pancreatic islets. Transplantation 1985; 40:437.
8. Hering BJ, Milde K, Busam J et al. Oxygen bubbling enhanced collagenase digestion: A new approach to islet isolation. Proc Int Congress on Pancreatic and Islet Transplantation. Lyon, June 6-8, 1991.
9. Gray DWR, Leow CK. Non-automated methods for islet isolation. In: Ricordi C, ed. Pancreatic Islet Cell Transplantation. Austin: RG Landes, 1992: 89-98.
10. Hellman B, Petersson B, Hellerstrom C. The growth pattern of the endocrine pancreas in mammals. In The Structure and Metabolism of Pancreatic Islets Eds. Brolin S, Hellman B, Knudson. Pergamon Press, New York,1964: 45-61.
11. Hellerstrom C. Growth patterns of the pancreatic islets in animals. In: TheDiabetic Pancreas Eds. Volk BW, Wellman F. New York: Plenum, 1977: 61-97.
12. Lifson N, Lassa CV, Dixit PK. Relation between blood flow and morphology in the islet organ. Am J Physiol 1985; 249 (Endocrinol. Metab. 12): E43-E48.
13. Bonner-Weir S, Orci L. New perspectives on the microvasculature of the islets of Langerhans in the rat. Diabetes 1982; 31:883-889.
14. Jansson L , Hellerstrom C. Stimulation by glucose of the blood flow to the pancreatic islets of the rat. Diabetologia 1983; 25:89-94.
15. Montana E, Bonner-Weir S, Weir GC. Beta cell mass and growth after syngeneic islet cell transplantation in normal and streptozocin diabetic C57BL/6 mice. J Clin Invest 1993; 91:780-787.
16. Bunnag S. Postnatal neogenesis of islets of Langerhans in the mouse. Diabetes 1966; 15:480-491.

17. Parakkal RF, Ali MA. Regional differences in the distribution of the islets of Langerhans and of alpha and beta cells in the albino mouse. Rev. Can Biol 1961; 20: 781-788.

17a. Bonner-Weir DF, Trent DF, Weir GC. Partial pancreatecomy in the rat and subsequent defect in glucose-induced insulin secretion. J Clin Invest 1983; 71:1544-1553.

17b. Halban PA, Powers SL, George KL, Bonner-Weir SB. Spontaneous reassociation of dispersed adult rat pancreatic islet cells into aggregates with three-dimensional architecture typical of native islets. Diabetes 1987; 36:783-90.

18. Samols E, Weir G, Bonner-Weir S. Intraislet insulin-glucagon-somatostatin relationships. In: Lefebvre P ed. Handbook of Experimental Pharmacology GG/II. Berlin: Springer-Verlag,1983:133-173.

19. Pipeleers DG, Pipeleers-Marichal JC, Hannaert M, et al. Transplantation of purified islet cells in diabetic rats. Standardization of islet cell grafts. Diabetes 1991; 40:908-919.

20. Davalli AM, Ogawa Y, Scaglia L, et al. Function, mass, and replication of porcine and rat islets transplanted into diabetic nude mice. 1993, submitted

21. Dionne KE, Colton CK, and Yarmush ML. Effect of Hypoxia on Insulin Secretion by Isolated Rat and Canine Islets of Langerhans. Diabetes 1993; 42:12-21.

22. Weir GC, Bonner-Weir S, Leahy JL. Islet mass and function in diabetes and transplantation. Diabetes 1990; 39:401-405.

23. Weir GC, Leahy JL, Barras E. Braunstein LP. Characteristics of insulin and glucagon release from the perfused pancreas, intact isolated islets, and dispersed cells. Hormone Res. 1986; 24:62-72.

Islet Isolation from Rodent Pancreas

Part II

Francine Malaisse-Lagae

Willy J. Malaisse

The present account describes a method currently used for the isolation of islets from the pancreas of rats and other rodents.[1] This procedure involves the inflation of the pancreas, its dissection and further digestion, followed by the separation and eventual collection of isolated islets.

INFLATION OF THE PANCREAS

Rats

Fed rats (approximately 200 g body weight) are decapitated and bled. The peritoneal cavity is opened. The colon is gently freed and reclined downwards, so as to expose the duodenal part of the pancreas. The liver is then reclined upwards, allowing one to expose the biliary duct and its two main branches emerging from the liver. The duodenal extremity of the bile duct is occluded with a clamp, very close to the duodenum. An opening of the bile duct is performed close to the main branches of the biliary duct, and a plastic intravenous cannula (outer diameter 1.02 mm or less) is inserted a few millimeters in the bile duct, and secured in place with a ligature or a forceps. Through the catheter, fitted to a 10 mL syringe, 10 mL of Hanks solution are injected. This Hanks' solution consists of NaCl 137 mM; KCl 5.4 mM, $CaCl_2$ 1.3 mM; $MgSO_4$ 0.8 mM; Na_2HPO_4 0.3 mM; KH_2PO_4 0.4 mM. This solution is added with a saturated solution of $NaHCO_3$ to reach a pH of 7.4 when equilibrated in a stream of CO_2-O_2 (5-95, v/v). Since the main pancreatic ducts open in the biliary duct, the injected fluid fills the pancreatic ductular system in a retrograde way and causes its mechanical disruption.

Incidentally, the main duct draining the "dorsal pancreas", body, tail and upper part of the head, opens in the bile duct a few millimeters below the hepatic bifurcation.[2] Care should therefore be taken not to push the catheter too far. On the other hand, the main duct collecting the ventral pancreas, i.e., approximately the lower two thirds of the pancreatic head, opens in the biliary duct close to its duodenal extremity.[2] The clamp should therefore be placed very close to or on the duodenum.

Pancreatic Islet Transplantation Volume I: Procurement of Pancreatic Islets, edited by Robert P. Lanza, MD, William L. Chick, MD; ©1994 R.G. Landes Company.

OTHER RODENTS

The same procedure can also be applied to smaller rodents (mice, chinese hamsters, spiny mice), except that the volume of injected fluid is reduced to 2-3 mL. If canulation of the bile duct cannot be achieved, one can omit the step of pancreas inflation. The injection of Hanks' directly in the pancreas is, in our opinion, useless since it produces only an extraglandular edema, without disruption of the exocrine ductular system.

DISSECTION OF THE PANCREAS

Whether inflated or not, the pancreas is carefully dissected free from the extremity of stomach and from the duodenum. Its vascular connection (hilum) is cut, and the gland is transferred to a petri dish containing Hanks solution. It is then further dissected free from main vessels, ducts, and lymph nodes.

DIGESTION OF THE PANCREAS

Two or three glands are pooled in a beaker and minced into small pieces (1-2 mm size) with scissors. The minced tissue, corresponding to approximately 1 mL per rat pancreas, is transferred in a 10 mL test tube and mixed with 4 mg/mL of collagenase P (from Clostridium histolyticum; Boehringer-Mannheim). The tissue suspension is gently mixed by bubbling with a stream of O_2-CO_2 (95-5, v/v) for 12 to 14 min at 37°C. The tube is then closed with a rubber stopper and vigourously shaken by hand (200-250 strokes/min) for 1 to 2 min at 37°C. At this stage the tissue suspension should appear homogenous on visual inspection.

When using this method for the first time or applying it to a new species, it is advisable to check, under control of a dissecting microscope and at suitable time intervals, the extent of digestion. This allows the observation of the islets when they are still connected to small pancreatic ducts. It may also help in avoiding excessive digestion which may result in alteration of the islet integrity.

ISLET SEPARATION

The digested tissue is transferred and brought to a final volume close to 150 mL placed in a glass container. When the islets have sedimented at the bottom of the container (about 1 min), the supernatant solution is removed and replaced by an equal volume of Hanks solution. This procedure is repeated two to three times, in order to remove the bulk of the exocrine tissue, which sediments more slowly than the islets. One can, in addition, pass the tissue through a nylon mesh (400 µm) in order to remove items such as large ducts, remaining lymph nodes and clumps of acinar tissue.

The final digest, which is placed in about 50 mL of Hanks solution, is then used in aliquots of 2 or 3 mL dispersed in a petri dish already containing about 10 mL of Hanks solution for the collection of islets under a dissecting microscope (40 to 100 fold magnification). Whenever the collection is long, e.g. when large number of islets are to be collected by an untrained experimentator, it is advisable to place the main preparation on ice and/or to keep it under a gentle bubbling of O_2-CO_2.

When the islets are removed from hyperglycemic rats, the whole procedure from the inflation of the pancreas to the collection of islets can be performed in a Hanks solution enriched with D-glucose, in order to avoid the possible metabolic consequences (e.g. glycogenolysis) of glucose deprivation.

For preparation of islets under semi-sterile conditions, the washing of the islets and their further collection should be performed with sterile media and under a laminar flow hood.

ISLET COLLECTION

The usual yield of islets (100 µm or more in diameter) is in the range of 140 to 300 islets per rat pancreas.

Individual Picking

Islets can be collected with the aid of a glass loop. Such a loop is prepared from glass rods about 4 mm in diameter by heating on a flame, stretched and curved at the extremity. Each islet is transferred individually from the petri dish in a suitable collecting medium.

In order to avoid the sticking of islets to the vessels, it is recommended to use either non-adhesive plastic or siliconized glass, and to incorporate bovine serum albumin (1 to 5 mg/ml) in the collecting medium.

The islets that are collected one by one usually display a diameter of 100 µm or more. Individual variations in islet size are often far-from-negligible, especially considering that the islet volume is proportional to the cube of the islet diameter. Hence, when only 5 to 10 islets are placed in each collecting vial, e.g., for the purpose of secretion experiments, it might be desirable to assess, after incubation, the total amount of tissue present in each vial, by measuring insulin, protein and/or DNA content.

Batch Collection

When large numbers of islets are needed, another method of collection is preferred. A stretched siliconized Pasteur pipette is adapted to a rubber tube and the islets are collected by suction. For sterile sampling, a filter is inserted in the rubber tube. The islets are collected by groups of 10-30 and delivered in the appropriate collecting vessel. An obvious advantage of this procedure is the rapidity of islet collection. A disadvantage, however, consists in the necessity to discard, in a second step, the Hanks' solution which is aspirated together with the islets. A brief centrifugation can be performed for such a purpose.

This second procedure for the collection of large batches of islets increases the risk of contamination by dispersed acinar material. Repeated spontaneous sedimentation of the collected islets in Hanks solution may be helpful to remove such a contaminating material. Alternatively, the islets can be separated from the contaminating acinar cells by use of a 70 µm-mesh filter.

References

1. Malaisse-Lagae F, Malaisse WJ. Insulin release by pancreatic islets. In: Larner J, Pohl SL, eds. Methods in Diabetes Research. Vol 1. New York: Wiley and Sons, 1984: 147-152.
2. Orci L, Baetens D, Ravazzola M et al. Pancreatic polypeptide and glucagon: non-random distribution in pancreatic islets. Life Sciences 1976; 19:1811-16.

CHAPTER 6

PORCINE ISLET SEPARATION

Camillo Ricordi

One of the main problems conditioning the outcome of porcine islet separation is the ability to identify a reliable source of porcine pancreata that allows one to obtain consistent yields of islets with preserved function from each donor pancreas.

Since the introduction of the automated method for human islet transplantation in 1986,[1] many steps have been implemented to optimize this technique and to adapt it to the requirements of porcine islet isolation.[2-10] This represented a significant improvement over the originally described procedure for porcine islet isolation.[11]

DONOR SELECTION AND PANCREAS PROCUREMENT

Similarly to the human setting, donor selection can critically affect the outcome of porcine islet isolations, with the difference being that with pig pancreata many of the variables can be controlled and standardized. Strain, age, diet and weight are the main characteristics of the donor that can influence islet isolation outcome.

A classic example for strain and age related islet isolation outcome is in fact the pig, that was once considered a challenging species for islet isolation because of the marked fragility of the islets and their predisposition to fragmentation during the digestion process.[11] In our experience, the best selection for a successful islet isolation in swine is an older animal (possibly European large white) where we have observed that a consistently high number of islets could be obtained, may be because of the higher content in collagen matrix compared to younger donors.[2,3]

With respect to pancreas procurement, the gland is generally excised without perfusion, performing a total or segmental pancreatectomy, leaving the major vascular supply to the pancreas intact until the time of harvesting. At this time, when the gland is dissected and is ready to be removed, the vessels should be ligated on the donor side only, and divided. This allows blood outflow from the transected vessels from the organ. For pancreata obtained from a slaughterhouse the procedure can be significantly simpler. The porcine donor should be selected and made accessible to the procurement team as soon as possible after the animal is terminated (generally by gun shot to the head or electric discharge and bleeding). It is important to minimize the ischemia time and to place as soon as possible the excised pancreas in ice cold preservation solution (Eurocollins or UW).

ISLET ISOLATION EQUIPMENT AND SET UP

The entire procedure, (isolation and purification) can be performed in a standard tissue culture laboratory, equipped with at least one, possibly two, biological safety cabinets (class 100). Two refrigerated centrifuges are indicated for processing of the large volume of pancreatic tissue that become rapidly available during the dilution phase of the digestion process (e.g., IEC PR 7000, Fisher Scientific, Pittsburgh, PA, USA).

The isolation equipment can be set up in one of the safety cabinets, including a regulated water bath (Precision Stainless Steel Water Bath, model 182, Precision Scientific Inc., Chicago, IL, USA), a peristaltic pump (Masterflex Quick Load, model 7021-20, Cole Parmer Instrument Co., Chicago, IL, USA), a speed-drive system (Masterflex L/S Variable Speed-Drive System, Cole Parmer Instrument Co., Chicago, Illinois, USA), a temperature monitor (Mon-a-therm, model 6500, Vital Hospital Systems, Ballwin, MO, USA).

A double wrapped isolation pack, appositely prepared and sterilized is then opened under the hood. The isolation pack comprises:
- digestion chamber with o-ring,
- stainless steel screen,
- two temperature sensors,
- glass marbles,
- ring stand,
- three clamps (for chamber, tubing and cylinder),
- 100 mL graduated cylinder,
- small stainless steel tray,
- large stainless steel tray,
- two stainless steel tubing coils,
- surgical instruments including: large forceps, small curved clamps, large curved scissors, small curved scissors, and two mosquito hemostats.

The main component of the isolation procedure is a digestion chamber which retains the pancreas during a continuous digestion process (Fig. 6.1). Detailed designs of the chambers are available.[10]

The chamber can be made of any biocompatible material, provided it fulfills the necessary requirements of non-toxicity and sterilization. In laboratories at the beginning of their experience in islet isolation,

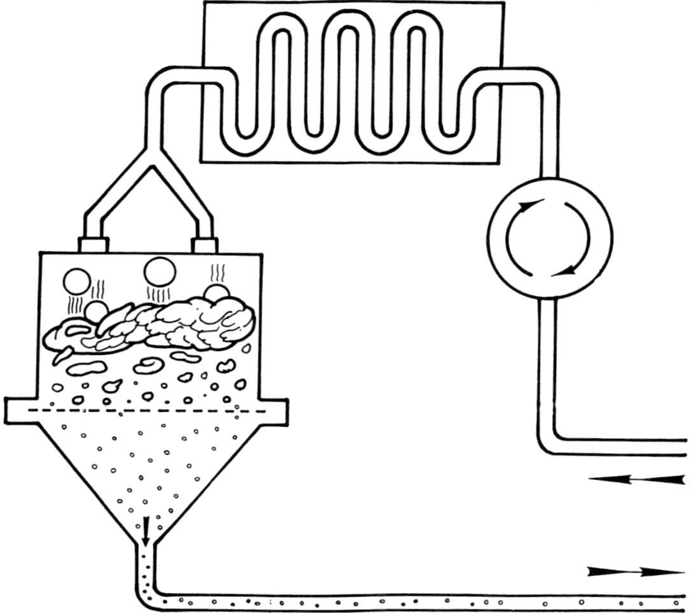

Fig. 6.1. The automated method (500 mL chamber): schematic representation of the isolation set-up. The pancreas is dispersed during a continuous digestion process. The continuous flow allows the islets that are progressively released to be saved from further digestion.

a transparent chamber (glass or plastic materials) may be preferable, to directly observe pancreatic tissue during the digestion process. However, a metal chamber will eventually be the first choice, i.e., stainless steel, for the ease of sterilization and durability compared to other materials. A compromise to be considered is a chamber with two directly opposed transparent windows to allow visualization of the chamber content. In all cases, possible changes in thermal conductivity across the chamber walls must be considered with any chosen material.

The stainless steel chamber that we use consists of a lower cylinder and an upper conical portion. Between these two main parts there is an o-ring, used as a sealing ring, and a removable stainless steel screen accurately positioned to completely cover the opening between the two components of the chamber. The function of the screen, with pore size of 320-500 μm, is to retain the pancreas into the lower portion of the chamber and to filter the tissue progressively digested during the isolation process. Furthermore, the lower cylinder contains 7 glass beads of 1 cm in diameter whose function is to prevent the pancreas from moving in unison with the chamber during the gentle shaking, therefore enhancing the dispersion of the pancreatic tissue within the chamber. Another consideration is the choice of chamber and marble material that can affect the dynamic of marbles' movement and consequently their interaction with the digesting gland, i.e., glass beads bounce less on a plastic compared to a stainless steel surface. Everyone has the innate pulsion to make "minor" changes to enhance or personalize the isolation procedure. For example, I have received the following comments: "We have some problems reproducing your procedure by the way we have chosen transparent plastic for the chamber to make it easier to follow the digestion and plastic beads instead of glass, since glass marbles have a predisposition to chip" or "We have built a 2 L chamber to better digest large porcine pancreata". These minor changes are indeed possible, but require appropriate modifications of the whole isolation procedure, including amount of

collagenase, temperature setting, shaking rate and amplitude, peristaltic pump rate and tubing size. All this assuming the donor selection and the collagenase blend were appropriate.

An important feature of the lower portion of the chamber is an opening in the lateral wall to connect a temperature transducer, that is connected to a monitor to determine intra-chamber temperature during the islet separation procedure. Additional openings may be applied to monitor other variables such as pH and pressure. The lower portion of the chamber also contains two inlet openings connected through a "Y" connector to a size 16 silicone tubing (Cole Parmer Instrument Co., Chicago, Illinois, USA). This tubing is connected to coils immersed in the 45°C water bath and then applied to the peristaltic pump (Fig.6.1). The outlet of the large chamber is connected to a larger (size 17) silicone tubing, to avoid increased pressure on the islets during the high flow collection phase of the separation procedure.

ISOLATION PROCEDURE

A large stainless steel tray is filled with sterile water and sterile ice (2 L of frozen sterile saline solution and 1 L of cold sterile saline solution). A smaller tray containing the pancreas and approximately 500 mL of cold Hanks with 10% fetal calf serum (FCS), is placed in the larger tray containing the iced saline solution. The pancreas is trimmed and weighed. We have obtained better results by processing only the splenic portion of adult pancreata of more than 90 g weight. In this case, the gland is divided at the level of the annular ring around the portal vein.

After duct cannulation, the Hanks solution is removed from the small tray and the large tray with iced saline is removed from the hood. The collagenase solution is injected in the duct using a disposable syringe (60 mL). Collagenase concentration (Boeringher Mannheim Biochemical, Type P, Indianapolis, IN, USA) is lot dependent and may even vary within the same lot in a time dependant fashion. We generally use 1-2 mg/mL in 350 mL of Hanks solution. The solution must be freshly prepared and it must be filtered (Nalgene Disposable Filterware, 500 mL, Nalge Company, Rochester, NY, USA; 0.8 and 0.2 µm pore size). An optimal temperature for the collagenase solution before injection is 28-32° C. This is important because injection of a cold collagenase solution would result in a temperature gradient between the inner portion of the gland and its surface. This differential temperature produces uneven collagenase activity on the different portions of the gland, resulting in a faster digestion of the superficial parenchyma, while the central portion of the gland remains relatively under-digested. During the preparation of the pancreas the chamber is kept at a temperature of 40-42° C by the recirculation of temperature controlled Hanks with 2% FCS. At the time of the intraductal collagenase infusion, the chamber is emptied and the temperature falls to 30-34° C.

An appropriate distension of the organ is critical to a successful islet isolation (as well as the quality and activities of the enzyme mixture that for reasons that are not apparent we still call collagenase).

At this time any remaining fat and/or connective tissue is removed from the pancreas (this may include ligation and resection of the tip of the splenic lobe). The gland is now loaded into the previously described stainless steel digestion chamber. The chamber is filled with the remaining collagenase solution contained in the small tray, the screen is placed, and the chamber is assembled.

Islets are separated from the exocrine during a continuous digestion process that lasts 30-60 minutes.[3] The content of the chamber is gently mixed by slow shaking that can be manual or by a controlled mechanical device, that standardizes the oscillation amplitude and rate during digestion. During the recirculation phase (flow rate 65-85 mL/min) the intra-chamber temperature is increased at a rate of 1-2°C/min by thermic exchange through the stainless steel coil immersed in the 45-50°C water bath until a temperature of 35-37°C is reached. The slow increase of intra-chamber temperature is necessary to allow the equilibrium between the surface and the inner gland portion dur-

ing digestion, therefore avoiding uneven enzymatic action.

Samples are first removed at 6 minutes and then every 2 minutes thereafter to monitor digestion. Even though experience generally allows one to clearly recognize islet tissue at the light microscopic level, it is recommended that one use dithizone (DTZ, Diphenylthiocarbazone, Sigma Chemical Co., St.Louis, MO, USA) for immediate detection of islet tissue.[12-14] DTZ solution is prepared adding 50 mg DTZ to 5 mL dimethyl sulfoxide (DMSO, Sigma Chemical Co., St.Louis, MO, USA), and diluting 1 mL of this solution with 20 mL of 2% FCS Hanks. A few drops of the freshly prepared and filtered (4-8 µm) final solution is added to the sample contained in a 35 mm petri dish with the result of a characteristic islet red stain given by the zinc contained in the insulin granules.[3] When a significant number of free islets is observed in a digestion sample (considering also the amount of tissue in the sample, the appearance of the islets and/or the PH of the solution), dilution and collection of the digested tissue is started. This is accomplished by aspiration of cold Hanks solution with 10% calf serum in the digestion circuit and collection of the digested tissue into a sterile 2 L flask. Gentle, slow motion shaking should be continued throughout the dilution phase and the coil should be removed from the water bath to interrupt the heating phase.

The digested tissue is first rapidly collected in the 2 L sterile flask pre-loaded with 1 liter of cold Hanks solution with 20% FCS. After the first liter of collection, the digested tissue can be directly loaded into 250 mL conical plastic bottles (250 mL centrifuge tubes, Corning Inc., Corning, New York, USA). The dilution phase lasts 20-50 minutes, until no islet tissue is detected in a sample. The digested tissue, containing the islets is then centrifuged (400 g for 4 minutes at 4°C) using the 250 mL conical plastic bottles. The pellet is collected into one or two bottles and resuspended in Hanks solution with 10% FCS. After an additional centrifugation and washing, the preparation is ready to be processed for purification with your favorite method. We generally use discontinuous gradients of Eurocollins-Ficoll using a COBE cell separator as described in the human islet isolation chapter.

DISCUSSION

Many problems still limit the availability of porcine islets for transplantation research. The main underestimated issue is the relevance of the source of porcine pancreata. Researchers can spend years trying to separate and transplant porcine islets from the wrong source with very frustrating results. We have recently described a method for rapid three-dimensional characterization of porcine pancreata before islet isolation[15] that could save significant energy and resources to screen the appropriate donors. If small and fragmented islets are present in the native porcine pancreas it will be very difficult to produce intact, large islets following the isolation procedure (even using the automated method). Another underestimated issue is how many porcine islets need to be transplanted to reverse diabetes, even in a nude mouse. We have previously reported that it was possible to reverse diabetes in a nude mouse with approximately 10 µL of porcine islets.[3,4] How many islet equivalent are 10 µL and how many 150 µm diameter porcine islets (flatter) are equivalent to one rat islet of 150 µm diameter (more spherical)? Moreover, how many porcine and how many rat islet equivalents correspond to 600 hand picked large rat islets, as they were traditionally selected before the introduction of islet isolation assessment "standards".[13,14] This will be a challenging task for an expert in islet mass related problems like Gordon Weir. Alternatively, you can take the 10 µL aliquot and count.

REFERENCES

1. Ricordi C, Lacy PE, Finke EH, Olack BJ, Scharp DW. Automated method for isolation of human pancreatic islets. Diabetes 37: 413-420, 1988.
2. Socci C, Ricordi C, Davalli A, et al. Selection of donors significantly improves pig islet isolation yield. Horm Metab Res (Suppl) 1990; 25:32-34.
3. Ricordi C, Socci C, Davalli A, Staudacher C, Baro P, Vertova A, Sassi I, Gavazzi F, Pozza G, Di Carlo V. Isolation of elusive pig islet. Surgery 1990; 107:688-694.
4. Ricordi C, Lacy PE. Renal subcapsular xenotransplantation of purified porcine islets. Transplantation 1987; 44: 721-723.
5. Ricordi C, Socci C, Davalli A, Baro P, Vertova A, Freschi M, Gavazzi F, Bertuzzi F, Di Carlo V, Pozza G. Effect of pancreas procurement on islet isolation in the swine. Transplantation Proceedings 1990; 22: 442-443.
6. Ricordi C, Socci C, Davalli A, Vertova A, Baro P, Sassi I, Braghi S, Giuzzi N, Pozza G, Di Carlo V. Application of the automated method to islet isolation in swine. Transplantation Proceedings 1990; 22: 784-785.
7. Ricordi C, Socci C, Davalli A, Staudacher C, Vertova A, Baro P, Freschi M, Gavazzi F, Bertuzzi F, Pozza G, Di Carlo V. Swine islet isolation and transplantation. Hormone and Metabolic Research 1990; 25:26-30.
8. Ricordi C. Automated method for islet isolation: A six year experience. Diabetes, Nutrition & Metabolism 1992; 5:59-62.
9. Ricordi C. Isolation of pancreatic islets for transplantation studies. Makowka, Cramer, Podesta (Eds.). Handbook of Animal Models in Transplantation, 1991. Los Angeles, California, Cedars-Sinai, May, 1992.
10. Ricordi C. The Automated method for islet isolation. Pancreatic Islet Cell Transplantation; 1892-1991: One Century of Transplantation for Diabetes. Ricordi C (Ed.). R.G. Landes Company, Austin, Medical Publisher, CRC Press (Distr.), May, 1992.
11. Ricordi C, Finke EH, Lacy PE. A method for the mass isolation of islets from the adult pig pancreas. Diabetes 1986; 35: 649-653.

12. Latif ZA, Noel J, Alejandro R. A simple method of staining fresh and cultured islets. Transplantation 1988; 45: 827-830.

13. Ricordi C. Qualitative and quantitative assessment of islet isolation in man and large mammals. Pancreas 1991; 6: 242-244.

14. Ricordi C, Gray D, Hering B, Kaufman D, Warnock G, Kneteman N, Lake S, London N, Socci C, Alejandro R, Zeng Y, Scharp D,Viviani G, Tzakis A, Bretzel R, Federlin K, Pozza G, James R, Rajotte R, Di Carlo V, Morris P, Sutherland D, Starzl T, Mintz D, Lacy P. Islet isolation assessment in man and large animals. Acta Diabetologica Latina 1990; 27: 185-195.

15. Fontes P, Rilo HLR, Bebhoo R, Alejandro R, and Ricordi C. A method for rapid characterization of porcine pancreata before islet isolation. In press, Transplantation Proceedings.

CHAPTER 7

Bovine Islet Isolation

Willem M. Kühtreiber

Robert P. Lanza

William L. Chick

Transplantation of islets of Langerhans is a promising therapy for treating patients with insulin dependent diabetes mellitus. A major problem, however, is that the supply of human donor material is extremely limited. Xenotransplantation, i.e., the use of non-human donor tissue, is a promising alternative. The large scale production of xenogeneic islet tissue would be most feasible with domesticated (farm) animals which already are available in large quantities, such as cows or pigs. Porcine islets are considered to be a particularly promising donor source because of the similarities between the amino acid sequences of porcine and human insulin (there is only a difference of 1 amino acid; for review see van Haeften[1]), and the relatively low levels of preformed human xeno-antibodies to pig tissues.[2]

The bovine pancreas is also a readily available and an inexpensive source of islets. Beef insulin differs from human insulin by 3 amino acids and therefore is slightly more immunogenic in humans than porcine insulin. Insulin-antibody complexes and insulin antibodies have been implicated in the development of lipoatrophy, insulin resistance and reduced glycemic control due to altered insulin pharmacokinetics.[1] Nevertheless, beef insulin has been used for the treatment of human diabetes since the early days of insulin therapy.

During the first 4 to 6 weeks of life, the neonatal bovine is considered to be monogastric and its islets respond to changes in blood glucose concentrations in much the same way as in other monogastric animals. However, at about 4 to 6 weeks after birth the rumen of the animals becomes functional and the animals become ruminants. The metabolism of the islets changes and they become less responsive to glucose and more responsive to short chain fatty acids that are absorbed through the rumen.[3] Indeed, Hering et al[4] have reported that bovine islets that were isolated from adult cows were unresponsive to glucose perifusions, whereas they did respond to a propionic acid challenge. These results confirm that free fatty acids represent major stimuli for insulin secretion in adult ruminants.

Given the glucose-unresponsiveness of adult islets, it has been questioned whether neonatal bovine islets would retain adequate glucose responsiveness in the long term and thus whether such islets could be successfully used for xenotransplantation in diabetic patients. In this chapter, we show the feasibility of large scale islet isolation from neonatal bovine pancreata and their long term culture in vitro. The islets maintain basal levels of insulin secretion that are comparable to levels from islets of monogastric species. Glucose responsiveness is shown to be maintained in long-term culture, and the islets are able to restore normoglycemia in vivo when transplanted into diabetic rats.

ISLET ISOLATION

Islets of neonatal pancreata were isolated by the method of Lacy and Kostianovsky[5] with some modifications. Pancreatic glands from male calves 1-10 days of age and weighing 20-40 kg were obtained from a local slaughter house. The calves were sacrificed and bled according to regular slaughter house procedures. A midline incision was made and the viscerae drawn forward to expose the pancreas. The pancreatic duct was transsected and cannulated in situ with a 14 gauge angiocath. Approximately 30 mL of an ice cold solution of UW-D (UW organ preservation solution variant D, see Sumimoto et al[6]) was then injected into the gland. The gland was then excised from the surrounding viscerae. Warm ischemia time was 10 to 40 minutes. Glands weighed on average 25 g before distension with UW. For a typical isolation, 5 to 7 glands were collected and transported to the laboratory in ice cold UW-D solution. In the laboratory the glands were distended via the pancreatic duct with a balanced salt solution containing crude collagenase. They were then digested by

gentle shaking in a flask. Once the glands began to disintegrate, the tissue was filtered through a screen and the larger pieces returned to the digestion flask for further treament with the collagenase solution. The filtrate was collected in ice cold culture medium, washed several times, and subsequently purified using discontinuous Ficoll gradients. Islets were recovered from the gradients, washed several times, and cultured in α-MEM based medium (see below) in 100 mm petri dishes.

The islet yield was 202,000 ± 113,000 EIN per pancreas or 8,800 ± 4,500 EIN per gram in the last seven consecutive bovine islet isolations performed in our laboratory (see Table 7.1). The average diameter was 101 ± 8 µm. It is not clear at this point why there is such a significant inter-isolation variation in the islet yields; part of this may reflect the variations in warm ischemia times that are inherent in the slaughter house situation.

An average yield of 8800 EIN per gram represents a significant improvement from values last reported by our group[7] (average 2,120 EIN per gram and average diameter of 80 µm) and also compares favorably to yields reported by others. Lacy et al[8] were able to isolate 20,000 islets per beef pancreas in a procedure that included the use of Velcro to retain partially digested collagen from pancreas that was distended, and chopped into large pieces. The number of EIN isolated per gland is unclear. Hering et al[4] isolated 2098 ± 292 islets per gram from

Table 7.1. Results of seven consecutive bovine islet isolations performed at BioHybrid Technologies Inc.

Isolation	vEIN	Diameter (µm)	EIN per pancreas (k)
B115	0.65	110	404
B114	0.74	96	279
B113	0.45	98	61
B112	0.55	98	120
B111	0.53	89	84
B110	0.61	102	233
B109	0.82	116	232
Average	0.6 ± 0.1	101 ± 8	202 ± 113

the duodenal part of the right pancreatic lobe of 12 to 18 month old cows with a single-endpoint technique and 2641 ± 292 islets per gram with the continuous digestion-filtration method. Giannarelli et al[9] report, 013 ± 313 EIN per gram using a sequential filtration method and density centrifugation with Histopaque.

Typical islet purity ranged from 90% to 95%. Bovine islets do not stain with dithizone and therefore it cannot be used to distinguish islets from exocrine tissue.[10] However, islets can readily be distinguished from exocrine tissue by standard phase contrast microscopy since the acinar tissue is heavily granulated. Figure 7.1 shows a bovine islet preparation before and after (a, b)

purification on the discontinuous ficoll gradient. The acinar tissue in Figure 7.1(a) appears much darker than the islets. The islet preparation in Figure 7.1(b) was estimated to be 94% pure. In case of doubt, islets can be distinguished from acinar tissue by means of the green light illumination technique of Finke et al.[11] With this technique the islets appear pink, while exocrine tissue, ducts and vessels appear green. After a successful isolation as in Figure 7.1(b), many islets have a fairly compact appearance and most of them round up and become even more compact after overnight culture.

To determine viability, islets were stained with a combination of Calcein-AM and Ethidium Bromide (Live/Dead Assay,

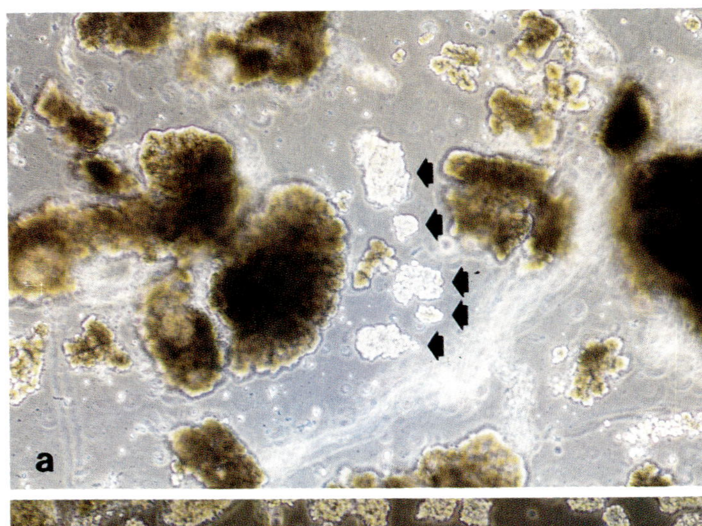

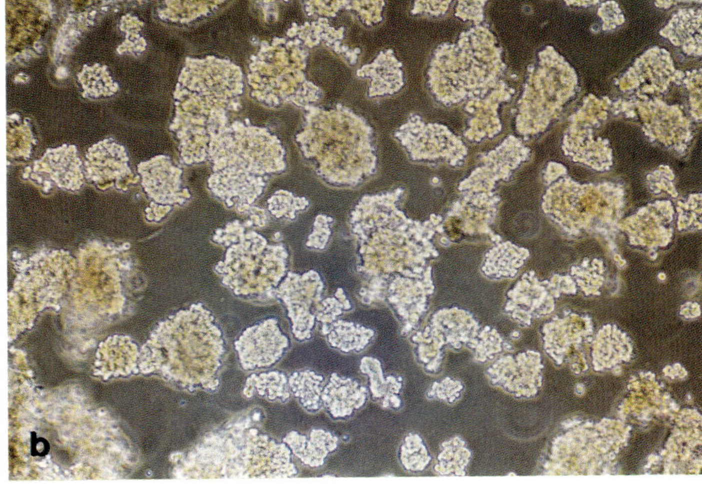

Fig. 7.1. Bovine islets can be distinguished easily from acinar tissue, since the latter is heavily granulated and appears much darker under phase contrast microscopy. This figure shows a bovine islet preparation before (a) and after (b) purification on a discontinuous ficoll gradient. This particular preparation was 94% pure after the ficoll gradient. The islets in (a) are indicated by arrow heads.

Molecular Probes Inc, Eugene, OR, USA) and viability was assessed by means of a fluorescence microscope equipped with FITC filter set. With this stain, living cells appear green whereas the nuclei of dead cells appear red. Typical islet-viability immediately after the completion of the isolation was 85 to 90%. This value typically rose to approximately 95% after overnight culture.

INSULIN SECRETION DURING LONG TERM CULTURE

To determine long term insulin secretion, islets were cultured in αMEM/HEPES containing 10% heat-inactivated horse serum with penicillin added. The medium was supplemented with glucose to a final concentration of 200 mg/dl. Alliquots of medium were harvested at periodic intervals and stored at -20°C for subsequent insulin analysis as previously described.[12]

Figure 7.2 shows the average insulin secretion of 19 different bovine islets preparations during long term culture of up to 9 months. The data indicate that neonatal bovine islets continue to secrete significant amounts of insulin over periods of several months, although there is a decrease from an average of approximately 250 µU/islet/day in the first month to approximately 120 µU/islet/day in the 9th month. This is similar to the pattern of insulin secretion from canine or human islets during long-term culture in our laboratory (unpublished data; see also Nielsen et al[13]). This gradual decline in insulin secretion may be related to cell death and a decline in the amount of insulin secreted per ß-cell.[14]

GLUCOSE RESPONSIVENESS

It is possible to distinguish three stages during bovine pancreas development (for references, see Bonner-Weir and Like ref 15). During the fetal stage, plasma glucose is low (10-30 mg/dL) and insulin secretion is stimulated by glucose and possibly fructose. Within 24 hrs after birth, blood fructose levels drop to zero, glucose levels are about 90 mg/dL and insulin secretion can be stimulated with short chain fatty acids as well as glucose. As the stomach develops and rumination becomes possible, plasma glucose falls

Fig. 7.2. Insulin secretion from bovine islets during long term culture in medium containing 200 mg/dl D-glucose. The medium was collected three times per week and assayed for insulin by RIA. Mean insulin secretion during each month of culture is shown. The numbers of different islet preparations is indicated above the error bar.

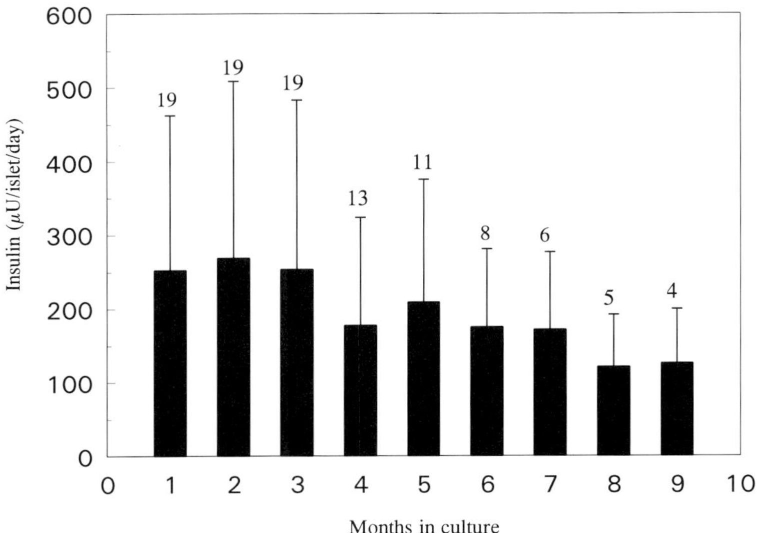

to 45-50 mg/dL and insulin secretion in response to glucose diminishes. This diminished sensitivity of adult bovine islets to glucose has raised concerns that these islets would respond less effectively to fluctuations in circulating blood glucose concentrations than islets of monogastric species. However, while this may be the case for adult bovine islets in situ, it was not clear whether isolated neonatal islets will also lose part of their sensitivity to glucose. Therefore, the acute responsiveness of isolated neonatal bovine islets to stimulatory levels of glucose was determined by means of glucose perifusion experiments after various periods of time in culture.

One day before the perifusion, the glucose concentration in the culture medium was lowered to 100 mg/dL. Approximately 8000 islets were used per perifusion. The islets were perifused at a rate of 0.5 mL/min at 37°C for 30 minutes with medium containing 100 mg/dL glucose, stepped up to 300 mg/dL glucose for 1 hr and then stepped back down to 100 mg/dL glucose for an additional 30 minutes. The secretion at 100 mg/dl was considered to be basal insulin secretion. Figure 7.3 shows the result of a typical perifusion experiment. In this case, the islets had been in culture for 40 days. There is a significant insulin secretory response to the glucose step from 100 to 300 mg/dL, with a delay of only 2 to 3 minutes. The insulin secretion then levels of to a lower plateau value that is maintained throughout the challenge period. Secretion then returns to basal values with a delay of about 15 minutes after stepping down from 300 to 100 mg/dL glucose. Table 7.2 shows an overview of perifusion experiments on bovine islet preparations that have been in long term culture.

It is clear that the islets remain glucose sensitive during the culture period. It must be stressed here that these islets are of neonatal origin. It is not clear whether islets

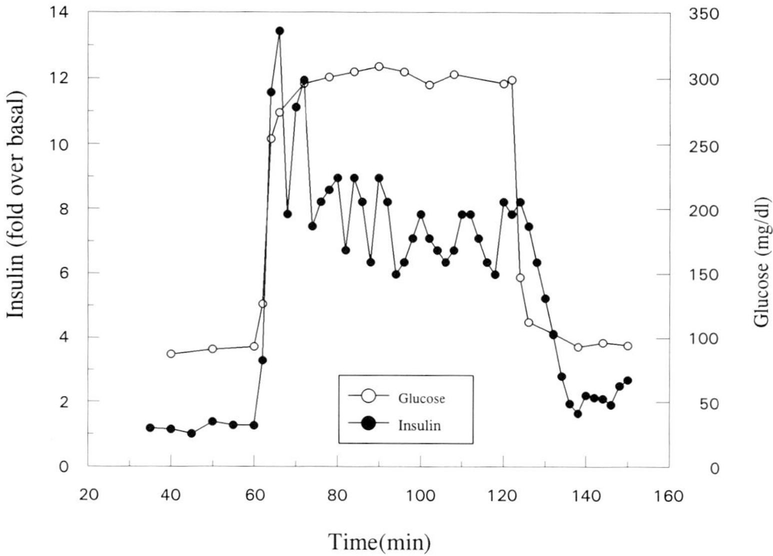

Fig. 7.3. Glucose stimulation of bovine islets after 40 days in culture. For details, see text. The open circles indicate the changes in glucose concentration, while the solid dots indicate the resulting alterations in insulin secretion.

Table 7.2. Glucose stimulation of insulin secretion during long-term culture of isolated bovine islets. Islets were removed from culture after the indicated number of days and perifused (see text for details)

Day in culture	Insulin peak (fold over basal)	Insulin plateau (fold over basal)
1	7.8	7.8
3	3.4	2.2
4	4.6	3.0
7	3.6	2.6
10	10.0	6.3
29	6.0	5.6
40	11.9	6.6
56	12.8	5.6
69	3.6	1.8
83	2.0	1.8
90	7.3	5.4
112	2.3	1.5
120	7.5	5.0
141	4.0	3.3
168	4.1	2.2
239	4.5	3.2

isolated from adult (ruminating) cows would show the same glucose sensitivity. In fact, data from the literature suggest that this is not the case. Hering et al[4] have shown that islets isolated from the duodenal portion of the right lobe of the adult beef pancreas fail to respond to a glucose challenge of 2.78 to 27.8 mM D-glucose, whereas they do respond with a two-fold increase in insulin secretion upon a propionic acid challenge from 0.05 mM to 0.5 mM.

Bonner-Weir and Like[15] have shown that there are two populations of islets in the bovine pancreas: large islets (100 to 1600 μm in diameter) and small islets (25 to 200 μm in diameter). The large islets appear well granulated from the 15th fetal week onward and remain well granulated throughout neonatal life and in the ruminating adult. In contrast, the small islets are depleted of most of their insulin shortly before birth, remain degranulated for 2 to 3 weeks post-partum, and regranulation is not completed until the calves are approximately six weeks of age. Although the relative contribution of these

two islet-populations to our bovine islet isolation yields is unknown, two lines of evidence suggest that the isolated islets are functionally competent. First, the evidence from our glucose perifusion challenges shows that bovine islets release substantial amounts of insulin in response to perifusion with 300 mg/dL glucose, even shortly after isolation. Second, the bovine islets can restore and maintain normoglycemia when transplanted into diabetic animals soon after isolation (see next section).

BOVINE ISLET TRANSPLANTS

Reports on the use of bovine islets in correcting hyperglycemia in diabetic recipients are very limited. Lacy et al[8] cultured beef islets for 3 days and then transplanted them into STZ-induced diabetic mice. The mice also received injections of anti-lymphocyte serum at the time of transplantation to delay rejection. The islets were able to maintain normoglycemia in the recipients for 9 days, after which hyperglycemia recurred. Hering et al[4] transplanted bovine islets be-

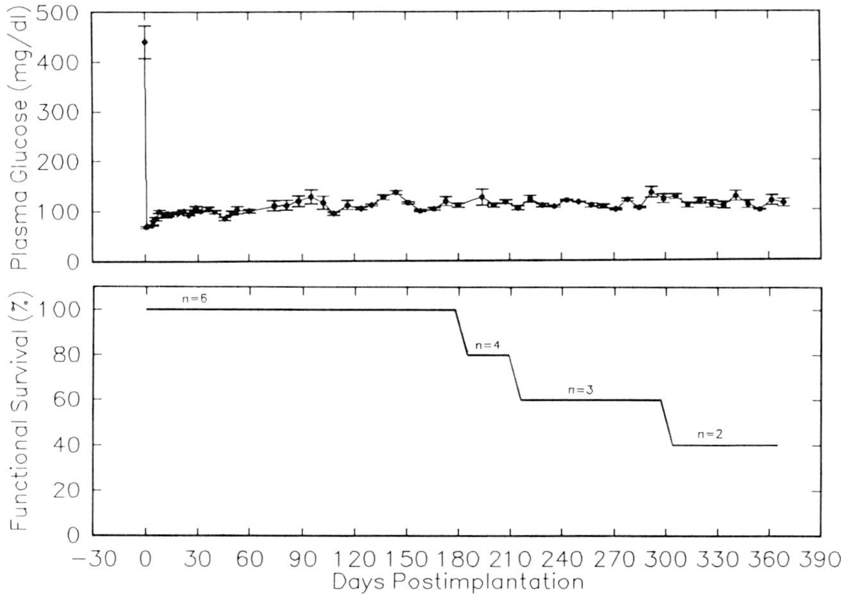

Fig. 7.4. Fasting plasma glucose levels (mean ± SEM) (upper) and functional survival rate (lower) of 6 diabetic rats that received intraperitoneal implants of encapsulated bovine islets. One implant recipient was killed with a functioning graft 88 days after implantation. (From Lanza et al; 1993; reproduced with permission).

neath the left renal capsule of STZ-induced diabetic male C57BC/6 mice. Normoglycemia was restored for 1 to 4 days and the islets rejected after 2 to 6 days.

Successful long term control of circulating blood glucose concentrations with immuno-isolated bovine islet xenografts in rats has been achieved by our laboratory and has been previously reported.[16-18] In these experiments, neonatal bovine islets were encapsulated in biohybrid diffusion chambers and implanted in streptozotocin induced diabetic rats. Islets (20,000 total per rat) were suspended in 1.2% (w/v) Pronova LVG sodium alginate (Protan, Drammen, Norway) at a concentration of 4-6 EIN/mm^3 and seeded into tubular permselective acrylic membrane chambers (nominal molecular weight cutoff 50-80 kD; W.R. Grace & Co.). The alginate was then gelled in 1.5% CaCl$_2$, the chambers washed in culture medium and the ends sealed. The chambers were introduced into the peritoneal cavity of 6 STZ-

induced diabetic Lewis rats (Charles River Laboratories, Wilmington, MA, USA) through a small midline incision. The grafts promptly normalized plasma glucose concentrations, with levels dropping from 468 ± 61 to 91 ± 10 mg/dl. Non-diabetic control rats maintained their blood glucose levels at 94 ± 3 mg/dl (see Fig. 7.4). All 6 grafts exhibited function for at least 6 months, with 2 grafts functioning for over 1 year. Islets that were retrieved from the animals showed varying degrees of viability. Figure 7.5 shows examples of islets retrieved after 200 days. The islets are clearly in good shape and well nucleated. Intravenous glucose tolerance tests on 3 rats with transplanted bovine islets resulted in K values (decline in glucose levels, %/min) of 3.3 ± 0.1, as compared to 3.3 ± 0.1 for normal and 0.9 ± 0.1 for untreated diabetic animals. These results clearly demonstrate that neonatal bovine islet-xenografts can restore normoglycemia in diabetic animals over extended periods of time.

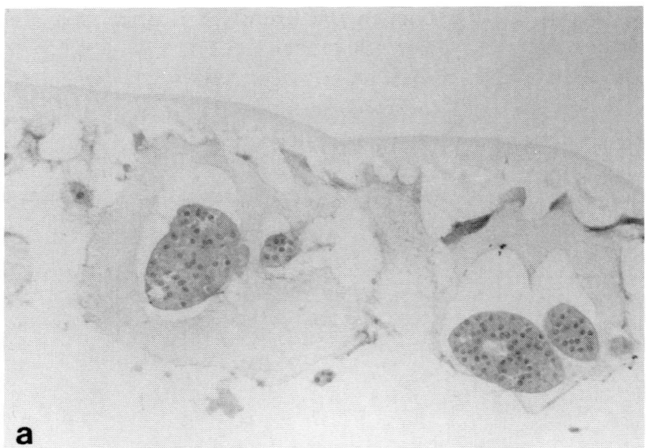

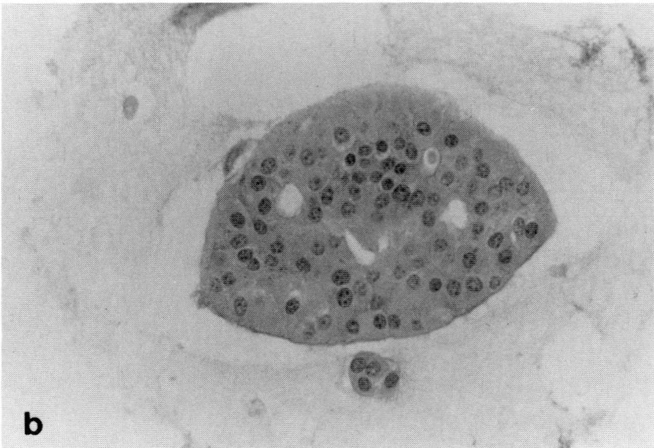

Fig. 7.5. Bovine islets from a biohybrid diffusion chamber retrieved from a rat after 200 days. (a) overview of a few islets near the acrylic permselective membrane. (b) Higher magnification of an islet. The islets are in good shape and well nucleated.

SUMMARY

We have shown the feasibility of large scale islet isolation from neonatal bovine pancreata. The islets could be maintained in long-term culture for periods exceeding 12 months. Throughout this period they continue to secrete insulin at levels comparable to those of monogastric species. Glucose responsiveness was shown to be maintained in long-term culture. Isolated bovine islets were also shown to restore normoglycemia in diabetic rats.

ACKNOWLEDGEMENTS

The authors thank Lisa Rock and Steven Carr for their expert technical assistance with the islet isolations and Kermit Borland and Sandy Sherman for their contributions to the long-term culture studies and perifusions.

REFERENCES

1. van Haeften TW. Clinical significance of insulin antibodies in insulin-treated diabetic patients. Diabetes Care 1989; 12: 641-648.

2. Kirkman RL. Of swine and men: organ physiology in different species. In: Hardy MA (ed.). *Xenograft 25 Amsterdam*. Elsevier, Amsterdam, New York, Oxford, 1989, 125.

3. Manns JG and Boda JM. Insulin release by acetate, propionate, butyrate, and glucose in lambs and adult sheep. Am J Physiol 1967;212: 747-55.

4. Hering BJ, Romann D, Clarius A et al. Xenogeneic Islet Preparation and Transplantation. Bovine islets of Langerhans. Potential source for transplantation? Diabetes 1989; 38 (suppl.1): 206-208.

5. Lacy PE and Kostianovsky M. A method for the isolation of intact islets of Langerhans from the rat pancreas. Diabetes 1967; 16: 35-39.

6. Sumimoto R, Jamieson NV, Wake K and Kamada N. 24-hour rat liver preservation using UW solution and some simplified variants. Transplantation 1989; 48: 1-5.

7. Borland K, Harvey J, Sherman S et al. Bovine pancreas as a source of islets for xenotransplantation. Transplantation Proceedings 1992; 24: 957-958.

8. Lacy PE, Lacy TE, Finke EH and Yasunami Y. An improved method for the isolation of islets from the beef pancreas. Diabetes 1982; 31 (Suppl. 4): 109-111.

9. Giannarelli R, Marchetti P, Villani G et al. Preparation of pure, viable porcine and bovine islets by a simple method. Abstract, Fourth International Congress on Pancreas and Islet Transplantation,1993, Amsterdam, The Netherlands, p. 78.

10. Latif ZA, Noel J and Alejandro R. A simple method for staining fresh and cultured islets. Transplantation 1988; 45: 827.

11. Finke EH, Lacy PE and Ono J. Use of reflected green light for specific identification of islets in vitro after collagenase isolation. Diabetes 1979; 28: 612 - 613.

12. Sullivan SJ, Maki T, Borland KM, Mahoney MD et al. Biohybrid artificial pancreas: long-term studies in diabetic pancreatectomized dogs. Science 1991; 252: 718-121.

13. Nielsen JH, Brunstedt J, Andersson A and Frimodt-Moller C. Preservation of beta cell function in adult human pancreatic islets for several months in vitro. Diabetologia 1979; 16: 97-100.

14. Leahy JL and Weir GC. Evolution of abnormal insulin secretory responses during 48-h in vivo hyperglycemia. Diabetes 1988; 37: 217 - 222.

15. Bonner-Weir S and Like AA. A dual population of islets of Langerhans in bovine pancreas. Cell Tissue Res 1980; 206: 157 - 170.

16. Lanza RP, Beyer AM, Staruk JE and Chick WL. Biohybrid artificial pancreas. Long-term function of discordant xenografts in streptozotocin diabetic rats. Transplantation 1993; 56: 1067-1072.

17. Lanza RP, Butler DH, Borland KM et al. Successful xenotransplantation of a diffusion-based biohybrid artificial pancreas: a study using canine, bovine and porcine islets. Transplant Proc 1992; 24: 669 - 671.

18. Lanza RP, Butler DH, Borland KM et al. Xenotransplantation of canine, bovine, and porcine islets in diabetic rats without immunosuppression. Proc Natl Acad Sci USA 1991; 88: 11100 - 11104.

CHAPTER 8

Islet Isolation from Canine Pancreas

Garth L. Warnock

Jonathan R.T. Lakey

Ziliang Ao

Ray V. Rajotte

Two decades have elapsed since procedures were initially developed to isolate and transplant islets of Langerhans in rodents.[1,2] Since then, islet isolation from rodent pancreas has become standardized and reproducible in many laboratories. However, the protocols are not suitable for islet isolation from large mammals and human subjects. Studies in large animal models provide more relevant preclinical prototypes for the procedure of islet separation. The canine pancreas provides an excellent model which simulates technical challenges anticipated with the more compact human pancreas. This provides an opportunity to refine the approach to clinical islet isolation, given the limited supply of cadaver adult human pancreas. Furthermore, the outbred canine population simulates the practical immune problems that can be anticipated with mass islet replacement in human subjects. The importance of this model in promoting advances in clinical islet transplantation is underscored by the observation that the best outcomes with human islet transplantation[3-7] have been demonstrated by those programs which have tested their islet isolation and transplantation procedures in the canine model.

In this chapter, investigations with the isolation of canine islets will be described from a perspective of literature accumulated from multiple research laboratories and from our own experience with this large mammal.

PANCREAS PROCUREMENT

As in all fields of islet cell isolation, success begins with careful pancreas procurement. The key is to avoid pancreatic warm ischemia and intraparenchymal hemorrhage into the pancreas during pancreatectomy. The dog is subjected to laparotomy and the entire pancreas is mobilized, care being taken to preserve all major vascular connections including veins and arteries. The structures can be readily skeletonized, leaving them intact until just before excision of the gland. Particular attention must be paid to avoiding compression of the gland parenchyma during retraction which causes

Pancreatic Islet Transplantation Volume I: Procurement of Pancreatic Islets, edited by Robert P. Lanza, MD, William L. Chick, MD; ©1994 R.G. Landes Company.

hematoma formation. Intraglandular hemorrhage will reduce the efficacy of subsequent collagenase digestion. Premature venous ligation also causes venous congestion, thereby reducing collagenase efficacy.

Both main branches of the pancreatic duct are cannulated in situ with a 20 cm length of PE90 (20 gauge) tubing. This should be completed at the conclusion of gland mobilization. Care must be taken to defer ligation of the pancreatic duct until immediately before gland excision. The entire gland is then excised, weighed, and chilled to 4°C by placing it on a cooling tray. The anterior surface of the left side of the gland is exposed at a point 5 cm from the tip of the gland. A cutdown is made at that site, sufficient to expose the pancreatic duct. A separate 20 gauge cannula is placed into the duct at that site. Each of the three cannulas is detailed in the Figure 8.1. Fifty milliliters of Hanks balanced salt solution (HBSS) containing collagenase at 4°C is injected into the catheter at each site of cannulation. This results in glandular distension. The pancreas is then transferred immediately for islet isolation.

Recent investigations suggest that appropriate selection of canine donors can maximize islet mass. Two factors which have independently been correlated to high islet mass are the size of the donor and the donor age. Islet separation can be optimized in those donors which exceed 20 kg of body weight and within the age range of 1 to 4 years.[8]

ISLET ISOLATION

Three key steps form the basis for adequate islet separation from the canine pancreas: (1) collagenase digestion of the fibrous connective tissue stroma; (2) gentle mechanical dissociation of islets from exocrine constituents; and (3) purification. Each of these components of the islet isolation process is detailed in the sections that follow.

COLLAGENASE DIGESTION

Although the optimal protocol to be followed has not been defined, two methods for collagenase digestion appear promising. The initial step is to deliver collagenase by injection through the pancreatic duct cannulae.[9,10] This gently distends the pancreas. Collagenase at this stage should be at 4°C. Multiple types of collagenase have been used with success.[9-14] We have used blends of different collagenase types containing more proteolytic activity.

A key is to deliver collagenase appropriately. This can be accomplished with a manual injection technique,[11] however, a perfusion technique that was initially described by Horaguchi and Merrell in 1981 appeared more promising,[9] and we have further developed perfusion of collagenase via the pancreatic ducts.[12] The technique of per-

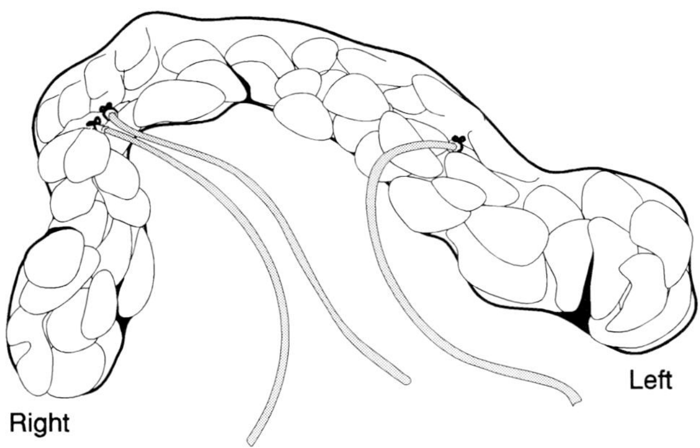

Fig. 8.1. Fully mobilized canine pancreas, demonstrating the triple cannulation technique with PE90 (20 gauge) cannulae. The cutdown in the left lobe ensures maximal delivery of collagenase to the distal left lobe, thereby improving digestion of the connective tissue stroma.

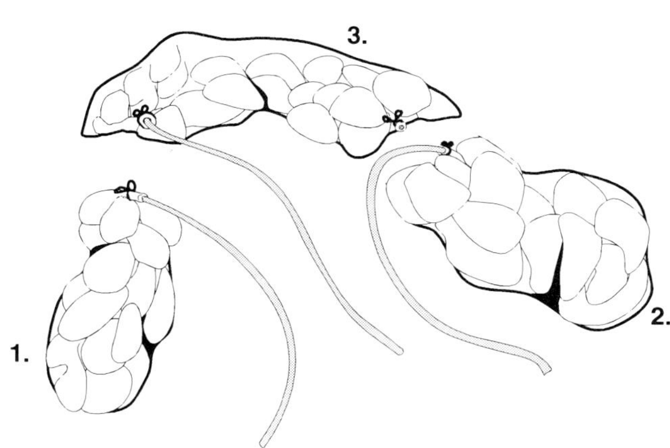

Fig. 8.2. Triple pancreas study that is used to select an appropriate dose of collagenase. The pancreas is divided into three segments, each of which is processed individually in the sequence shown. The study maximizes return of information on efficacy of the dose of any given lot of collagenase, while keeping variables of the type of pancreas constant.

fusion yields significantly better islet isolation results, at least for human pancreas.[15] Thus, each cannula in the pancreas is connected to a recirculating perfusion apparatus, permitting the warmed collagenase to be effectively delivered to the intrapancreatic, intralobular connective tissue.

The question is commonly posed as to how to select the appropriate dose of collagenase when the type has been chosen. The canine pancreas readily lends itself to a type of experiment in which more precise information can be collected on the dose of collagenase to be selected. As indicated in Figure 8.2, each of the three cannulated segments of pancreas can be separated from the adjoining gland. These are then processed individually, utilizing one of three concentrations of collagenase for each limb. The right limb is readily suited to initial evaluation, because it can be separated from the surgical specimen and the processing can

begin while segments two and three are left in situ with blood perfusion. Then segments two and three can be excised and processed in sequence with the alternate doses of collagenase. Each limb of the pancreas is kept separate and passed through all phases of the islet isolation protocol. Table 8.1 outlines the information which can be collected and then compared between the three doses. It should be noted, however, that quantitative data on the number of islets released per gram of pancreas cannot be directly compared, because of regional differences in the density of islets in each limb of the pancreas. However, valuable qualitative data can be collected, thus screening more rapidly for the appropriate dose. This type of experiment has the advantage that the variation expected between different pancreases can be minimized, thus providing more internal control over the conditions than comparing pancreata between different donors.

Table 8.1. Parameters for qualitative assessment of different doses of a given lot of collagenase in three segments from canine pancreas

- Duration of digestion required to yield free islets
- Size of islets
- Islet entrapment within exocrine tissue
- Islet morphology
- Number of islets per gram of pancreas
- Dissociation of exocrine tissue
- Purification of tissue on discontinuous density gradient

TISSUE DISSOCIATION

A variety of techniques has been described for mechanical dissociation of islets from the digested pancreas. These have included tissue chopping with counter-rotating blades,[16] tissue maceration with grinders,[17] gentle mechanical dissociation using teasing and trituration,[11,12] and automated dissociation.[18,19] A key principle to keep in mind, regardless of the dissociation process selected, is that the process be completed as gently as possible to avoid islet fragmentation. Manual teasing and trituration or automated dissociation techniques have been most popular. We currently use the manual technique when processing multiple lobes of the gland separately to select the appropriate dose of collagenase as detailed in the previous section. In this protocol, the cannulae in the gland are perfused at 300 mm Hg for 10 minutes initially with cold collagenase, then the collagenase is gradually warmed to 35°C over a 10 minute period. Visual inspection of the gland reveals the point at which it becomes mucoid (approximately 10-12 minutes after commencement of warming). The gland is then cooled by rapidly injecting 4°C

HBSS into the cannula and the segment is transferred to a beaker containing 4°C HBSS. Tissue forceps are used to gently dissociate the tissue, then it is passed sequentially through 14, 16, and 18 gauge needles three times each. At the conclusion of the 16 gauge trituration step, small aliquots of the tissue are stained with dithizone and inspected with the dissecting microscope to select the endpoint of additional trituration.

The automated protocol has been developed using a technique initially described by Ricordi and colleagues.[18] We currently use this protocol to separate mass quantities of islets for transplantation purposes. In this technique, collagenase perfusion is stopped when the temperature rises to 30-32°C and the pancreas is transferred to a digestion chamber. The digestion chamber is filled with collagenase at the same dose as the injected collagenase. Temperature is regulated to 37°C and the chamber is set into oscillation. Islets that are liberated in the chamber exit continuously with the effluent that flows from the superior port of the chamber. Aliquots of the effluent from the chamber are removed and inspected by micros-

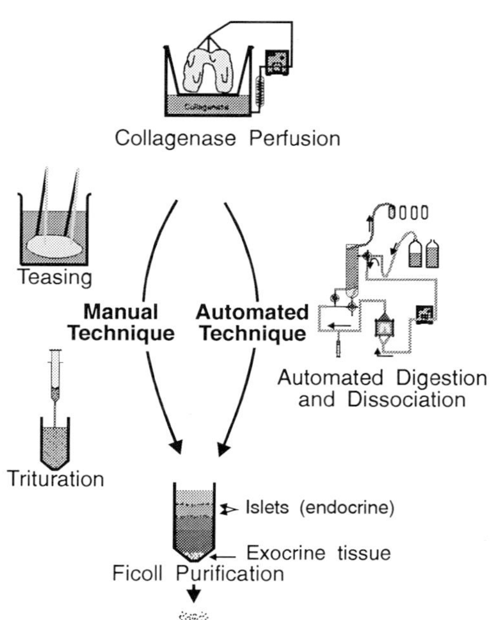

Fig. 8.3. Comparison of steps used in automated or manual islet isolation from canine pancreas. All pancreata were initially perfused with collagenase through three cannulas. They were then dissociated by manual (group 1, teasing and trituration) or automated (group 2, continuous digestion device) methods. Purification was completed with Ficoll gradients.

copy at 1-2 minute intervals. When most islets are judged to be free of attached exocrine tissue, the recirculating solution through the chamber is changed to plain HBSS containing 2% newborn calf serum and the effluent is collected and cooled quickly to 4°C.

In recent investigations in our laboratory we have had the opportunity to compare the manual and automated methods for canine islet isolation as outlined in Figure 8.3.[20] The type and dose of collagenase used in these experiments was held constant. The results are detailed in Table 8.2. In these studies, group 1 represented the standard manual technique for islet isolation. Group 2 represented initial attempts at islet separation using the automated protocol. There was a tendency to increased yields of islets when the automated protocol was used. However, variability amongst individual pancreata did not permit us to state that the results were significantly better with the automated technique. However, the use of more gentle shaking with the automated technique, as shown in group 3, permitted the recovery of significantly more islets compared with the manual method. A comparison of the islet size amongst these three groups is shown in Table 8.3. It can be seen that the advantage in group 3 was related to a greater size of islets. The mean diameter of islets isolated in group 3 was significantly higher than the counter parts in group 1. Thus, these data suggested that the use of an automated protocol must respect the need to maintain gentleness during the dissociation technique. An advantage of the automated protocol is that the digestion chamber augments the activity of collagenase originally delivered via the pancreatic duct by incubating the periphery of undigested pancreatic particles. Thus, the duration of exposure to collagenase at 37°C could be increased which may have freed more entrapped islets. In contrast, in the manual technique an abrupt endpoint to the digestion must be chosen and the gland subjected to further dissociation without maintaining activity of the collagenase. The quantity of collagenase solution needed to

Table 8.2. Islet yield and purity by different protocols

Group	Technique	n	Pancreas Weight (g)	Islet Purity (%)	Mean Islet Yield (± SE) Total (IE)*	IE/g
1	Manual	15	42.8 ± 1.5	89.3 ± 1.7	57,539 ± 7,066	1374 ± 171
2	Automated	26	43.8 ± 1.3	90.8 ± 1.3	93,511 ± 11,654	2236 ± 328
3	Automated with gentle shaking	13	49.5 ± 2.7	89.2 ± 1.2	120,256 ± 10,868	2515 ± 291[†]

* IE, islets equivalent to diameter 150 µm
† p < 0.002, compared with group 1, Mann-Whitney test

Table 8.3. Distribution of islet size

Group	n	Islet Size in µm (% of Total Islets) 51-99	100-149	150-199	200-249	>250	Mean Size Diameter (µm)
1	15	54.7 ± 2.3	35.2 ± 1.7	8.7 ± 1.2	1.3 ± 0.3	0.1 ± 0.1	103.4 ± 1.7
2	26	43.8 ± 2.0	40.6 ± 1.3	8.9 ± 1.2	2.1 ± 0.1	0.1 ± 0.1	107.6 ± 1.8
3	13	45.2 ± 2.6	38.4 ± 1.7	11.6 ± 1.3	4.2 ± 0.8	0.6 ± 0.4	113.3 ± 2.9*

* p < 0.005, compared with group 1

operate the automated system does exceed that needed for the perfusion and trituration method alone.

PURIFICATION

Initial attempts at purification of canine islets resulted in prohibitively low yields, possibly because of inadequate cleavage of free islets from the exocrine tissue. An alternative approach to this problem was to eliminate purification steps that resulted in a big loss of islets. Several investigators reported the use of unpurified canine islet-containing pancreatic microfragments to reverse diabetes in the late-1970s.[16,21,22] The use of impure pancreatic microfragments proved highly successful for investigation of dispersed pancreas transplantation in the dog. Transplantation into the spleen by direct puncture[21] or venous reflux[10] was highly successful, however, portal hypertension and disseminated intravascular coagulation resulted after intraportal embolization.[23] It was obvious that improved purification was needed to permit safe transplantation to the liver. Improvements of discontinuous density gradient purification techniques led to large scale high yield isolation of purified canine islets in 1982.[11] However, the quantity of islets separated from single donor pancreata still necessitated the use of multiple donors for a single recipient. In 1988, advances in collagenase digestion permitted sufficient highly purified islets to be isolated from a single donor pancreas to treat an individual recipient.[24]

The dissociated tissue (~15-25 mL) is weighed and resuspended at 4°C to a total volume of 120 mL in Medium 199 with 25 mM HEPES, 10% (v/v) fetal calf serum (FCS), and added 100 U/mL penicillin with 100 µg/mL streptomycin. Aliquots of 4 mL are removed to 50 mL tubes, suspended in 4.3 mL 5X Medium 199 and 16.7 mL Ficoll (density 1.125) and overlaid with 5 mL each of Ficoll with densities 1.085, 1.075, and 1.045. The desirable amount of tissue in the 50 mL gradients should not exceed 0.8 g. The tubes are centrifuged at 550x*g* for 25 minutes at 22°C. Tissue is collected from the interface at 1.045/1.075 and 1.075/1.085

layers, washed, recombined, weighed, and resuspended to a total volume in 30 mL of Medium 199 supplemented with 10% FCS and penicillin/streptomycin.

Ficoll solution should be prepared well in advance. It is mixed with distilled water to prepare a stock solution of density 1.125, from which all other densities are prepared. The solution is autoclaved at 110°C for 22 minutes, care being taken to remove the Ficoll immediately from the autoclave as soon as it has cooled. This avoids excessive polymerization of the Ficoll. It appears that a period of autoclaving is essential, since physicochemical properties of the Ficoll, including osmolarity and viscosity are changed, which may promote successful purification. Because the autoclave conditions are suboptimal for sterilization, the Ficoll should be sterile-filtered through a 0.22 µm filter in order to assure microbiologic sterility.

Other investigators have popularized the use of alternative gradient media for canine islet purification including Dextran[25] and Ficoll prepared with University of Wisconsin solution.[26] Ficoll has been used most widely, however, it is expensive. Dextran is a polysaccharide with a molecular weight of 72,000 which has been used clinically as a plasma substitute. Ficoll prepared with University of Wisconsin solution is reputed to have the advantage of reducing cell swelling, thereby enhancing separation of exocrine and endocrine particles.

We have recently investigated the efficacy of Dextran versus Ficoll in discontinuous density gradient purification of canine islets.[27] Digested canine pancreas was purified with discontinuous density gradients of Ficoll (n = 13) or Dextran (n = 7). For the Dextran group, 4 mL of tissue suspended in medium was placed in a 50 mL conical tube, pelleted, the supernatant removed, and the pellet vortexed with 12 mL Dextran stock solution (density 1.104). This was then overlaid with 5 mL stock solution, 5 mL Dextran at 1.085, and 10 mL of Dextran at density 1.075 and 1.041, respectively. Dextran gradients were centrifuged at 400 rpm for 4 minutes initially and 2000 rpm for 16 minutes thereafter. The purified islets were harvested from the interfaces of the upper layers and washed with Medium 199.

Comparison of islet yields from Ficoll or Dextran purification are presented in Table 8.4. Purity of the isolated islets was equivalent whether Ficoll or Dextran was used. The mean islet size was similar in both groups. Compared with the prepurification islet counts, 55.6% of the islets were recovered with Ficoll and 57.3% were recovered with Dextran.

For nine pancreases, the digest was split and purified with Ficoll or Dextran then the viability was determined in vitro by perifusion with glucose as shown in Figure 8.4. The basal insulin secretion (μU/islet/min) was 0.02 ± 0.007 for the Ficoll group and 0.04 ± 0.018 for the Dextran group. These increased after exposure to high glucose, a biphasic insulin release was observed, and all islets regulated insulin secretion back to basal. There was no difference in insulin secretion amongst the two groups.

Finally, islets isolated with Ficoll and with Dextran were autotransplanted into apancreatic recipients, as shown in Figure 8.5. Fasting normoglycemia (plasma glucose <150 mg/dL) was restored in both groups by 1 week, and this was well maintained during a follow-up of 2 months. Splenectomy at the conclusion of the follow-up induced prompt hyperglycemia which confirmed function of the islet autografts conclusively.

The results of this study have shown that Dextran has an equivalent efficacy for islet purification with similar isolation yields, purity, recovery, and viability. Considering the reduced cost, Dextran is an attractive alternative for large scale purification of canine islets.

Recent investigations have shown that purification of human islets can be achieved using the blood cell separation system developed by COBE BCT, Inc.[28] This offers the advantages of rapid purification of mass quantities of islets using discontinuous or continuous density gradients and a closed system which reduces the likelihood of bacterial contamination. Previous studies have reported use of the COBE system successfully for purification of canine islets[29] and we have reproduced these observations with Dextran or Ficoll.

ASSESSMENT OF ISLET MORPHOLOGY, SIZE, YIELD, AND PURITY

To assess islet size and numbers, the final islet suspension is thoroughly mixed, then 100 μL is removed x2 to separate tubes and incubated with dithizone.[30] Samples from the dithizone suspension are deposited on microscope slides and examined at microscopy. Two independent observers render separate counts for the two samples. The typical morphology of freshly-isolated canine islets stained with dithizone is shown in Figure 8.6. The islets tend to have an irregular morphology. Typical size distribution is between 50 and 350 μm diameter with mean islet diameters of 100–113 μm for an entire preparation (see Table 8.3). The diameter of each islet inspected at microscopy is measured with a graticule incorporated into the eyepiece of the microscope. The diameter is categorized within the size ranges of

---

Table 8.4. Profile of islet isolation with Ficoll versus Dextran

	Ficoll (n = 13)	Dextran (n = 7)
Islet purity (%)	89.2 ± 1.2	90.7 ± 1.5
*Pre-yield ([†]IE/g)	4523 ± 733	4207 ± 981
‡Post-yield (IE/g)	2515 ± 291	2411 ± 584
Islet recovery (%)	55.6%	57.3%
Mean islet size (μm)	113.3 ± 2.9	115.2 ± 5.3

*   Pre-purification
†   IE, number of islets equivalent to 150 μm in diameter
‡   Post-purification

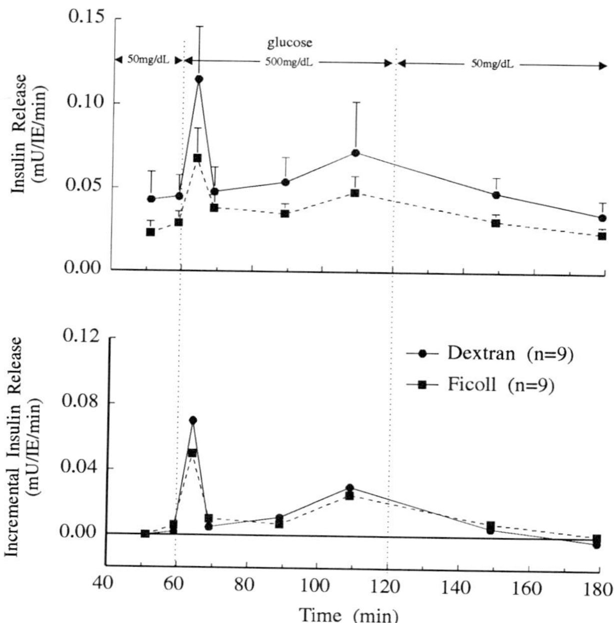

Fig. 8.4. Perifusate insulin release during challenge with glucose. Digests from nine canine pancreases were subjected to purification with discontinuous density gradients of Ficoll or Dextran, and the viability of each group of purified islets was compared.

Fig. 8.5. Daily fasting plasma glucose after autotransplantation of Dextran-purified (n = 6) or Ficoll-purified (n = 7) islets into the spleen of apancreatic dogs. Prompt onset of hyperglycemia occurred after splenectomy.

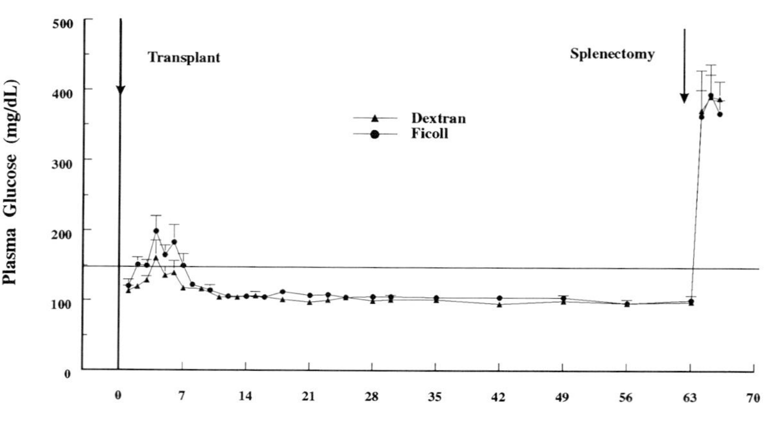

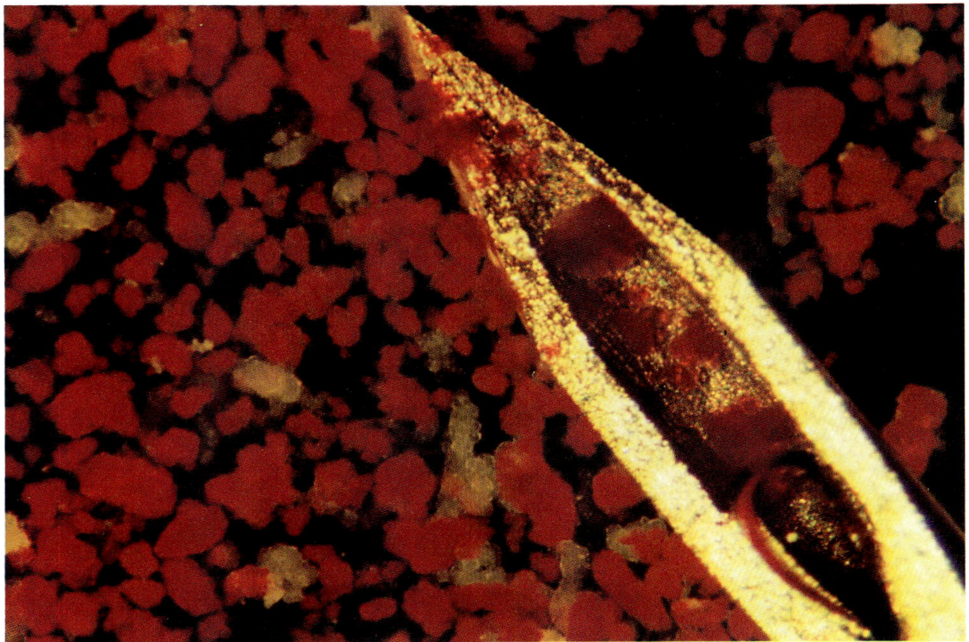

Fig. 8.6. Typical stereomicroscope appearance of highly-purified, freshly isolated canine islets. Included for reference to size is the tip of a 23 gauge needle, the internal bore of which has a diameter of 350 μm. Stained with dithizone.

60-99 μm, 100-149 μm, and in 50 μm increments thereafter to 400 μm and recorded on a count sheet. The number of islets in each size range is enumerated. To standardize the expression of islet quantity in numbers and volume, the crude islet counts in each size are converted to "islet equivalents". An islet equivalent is defined as an islet with a diameter of 150 μm. The number of equivalents in each size range is calculated from the product of crude islet counts and a conversion factor which corrects the size to a diameter equivalent to 150 μm. The final islet volume is determined from the product of the total equivalents and the volume constant for a sphere of 150 μ in diameter. Purity is estimated by comparing the relative proportions of dithizone-positive and dithizone-negative tissue seen on representative samples of the post-Ficoll pellet. Figure 8.7 is the detail sheet which we use to enumerate the findings during microscopic evaluation. This islet assessment system is based upon the guidelines that were set up at an International Workshop on Islet Isolation Assessment[31] in 1989.

Based upon morphometric studies performed on intact pancreas from dogs, a conservative estimate of the number of islets in a single pancreas is 500,000 islets.[32] However, current methods of islet isolation rarely achieve isolation of even 50% of this islet mass. Furthermore, it can be anticipated that some of the islets have reduced viability, or engraftment will be reduced following transplantation. Therefore, considerable additional progress is needed to optimize the mass isolation of islets from canine pancreas.

IN VITRO MAINTENANCE OF CANINE ISLETS AND QUALITY CONTROL ISSUES

For short-term (24 hour) maintenance of canine islets in vitro we use the following conditions. The islets are suspended free-floating in CMRL 1066 tissue culture medium containing 10% FCS and penicillin/streptomycin. They are dispensed, together with 10 mL of the culture medium, into 10 cm diameter petri dishes in groups of 5000 IE for incubation in a humidified atmosphere

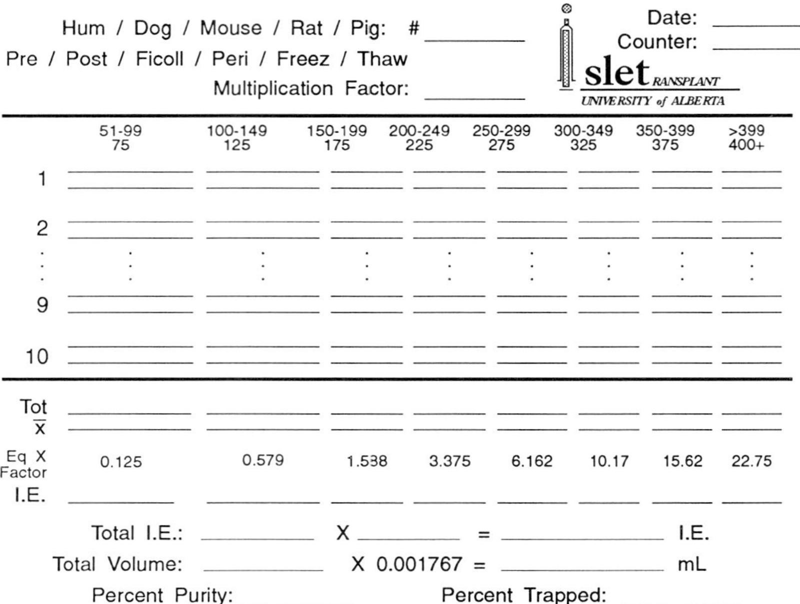

	51-99 75	100-149 125	150-199 175	200-249 225	250-299 275	300-349 325	350-399 375	>399 400+
1								
2								
:	:	:	:	:	:	:	:	:
9								
10								
Tot / $\bar{x}$								
Eq X Factor	0.125	0.579	1.538	3.375	6.162	10.17	15.62	22.75
I.E.								

Fig. 8.7. Protocol sheet for recording information on the size and quantity of islets isolated from canine pancreata

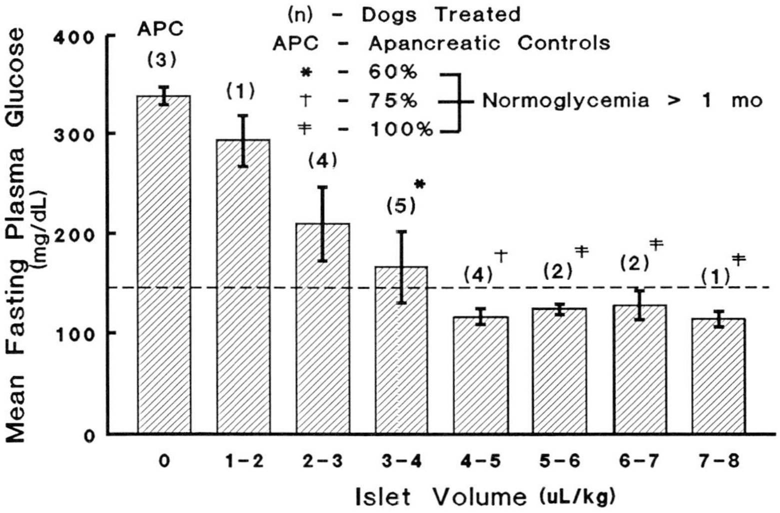

Fig. 8.8. Dose-response relationship of incremental volumes of highly purified autologous islets refluxed into the splenic vein of apancreatic recipients. Compared with apancreatic controls, there is a progressive reduction in plasma glucose levels as increasing quantities of islets are implanted. Consistent normoglycemia was observed during prolonged follow-up in dogs that received > 5 µL of islets per kilogram body weight (reproduced with permission from Warnock et al., In: Pancreatic Islet Cell Transplantation (Ricordi C, ed.), R.G. Landes Co. 261-278, 1992).

of 95% air/5% CO_2. For short-term culture, 37°C is acceptable and permits immediate assessment of islet viability with perifusion. For longer-term culture, 22°C is preferable, resulting in an improved islet recovery.[33]

One of the problems with in vitro short-term maintenance of canine islets is bacterial infection of the tissue. The principal contaminants appear to be gram-negative bacteria, coliforms, and pseudomonas species. Therefore, culture medium should contain penicillin/streptomycin or gentamicin. The principal risk points for colonization of canine islets with bacteria appear to be at five major stages. The first is contamination at the time of pancreatectomy. To minimize this, care should be taken to apply surgical drapes to the wound edges and to complete the pancreatectomy in as expedient a time as possible. The second major risk is colonization from improperly cleaned seals in the automated digestion system. It is preferable to remove all O-rings and seals and to autoclave these separately leaving adequate opportunity for sterilization of the tubing ports that conduct the collagenase and dilution medium. The third major risk is posed during the washing and recombining step. The centrifuge tubes are commonly placed into non-sterile cups in a centrifuge and then transferred back into the laminar flow hood. Care must be taken to avoid contamination with liquid which has accumulated on the outside of the tube during this stage. Similarly, the suction flasks which are used to evacuate supernatant from washed cells should be stored outside the cabinet and care taken to avoid reflux of aspirated supernatant from the suction tubing into the tube containing the graft. Finally, it should not be assumed that autoclaving of the Ficoll has achieved sterilization and this should be followed by filtration. Periodic microbiologic surveillance by sampling at multiple points during the procedure will help to enhance quality control by identifying the precise source at which the contaminants enter the system, especially when problems arise. Details on the microbiologic culture protocols follow those closely as reported in our earlier studies with human pancreata.[34,35]

VIABILITY TESTING

A key component of the islet isolation process is to ensure islet viability. Several indices of viability should be sought.

PERIFUSION

Perifusion studies are preferably completed on canine islets that have been subjected to a minimum of 24 hours in tissue culture at 37°C. This permits stabilization of basal insulin output. Groups of 250–300 islets are transferred to Millipore chambers and perifused with Kreb's Ringer Bicarbonate solution containing glucose during three consecutive periods of 1 hour each: initially with 50 mg/dL glucose, then with 500 mg/dL glucose, and finally with 50 mg/dL glucose. The effluent from the chamber is collected and subjected to radioimmunoassay for insulin.[36] Figure 8.4, detailed in the preceding section on purification, demonstrates a typical canine islet perifusion. Two samples should be collected during the 15 minutes of baseline period immediately before the glucose challenge. During the period of glucose challenge, samples at 5, 10, 30, and 45 minutes are collected. Finally, an attempt should be made to demonstrate a return to basal insulin release by collecting samples at 25 and 60 minutes following the cessation of glucose challenge. The minimum information that is presented should include the pattern of insulin release, and whether basal insulin secretion has been restored. Stimulation indices, which report the ratio of stimulated insulin output to the basal insulin release, are useful for descriptive data but should be reported in the context of the actual perifusion curves. The data in Figure 8.4 show that canine islets do respond to glucose challenge in vitro and that this response is characterized by a biphasic pattern of insulin release.

IN VIVO STUDIES

The ultimate test of viability is in a transplantation model. This can be accomplished with transplants of canine islet xenografts into mice,[37] autotransplantation, or allotransplantation. Autograft studies have

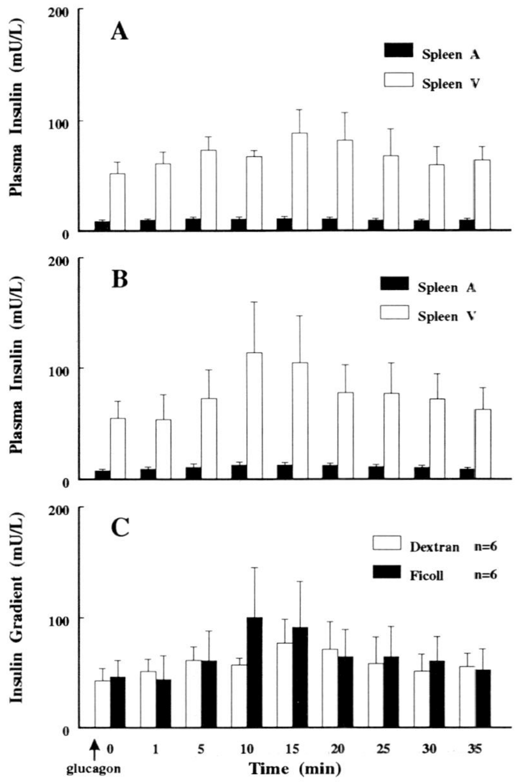

Fig. 8.9. Insulin levels in the splenic vein and femoral artery of apancreatic dogs that have received islets autografted into the spleen. In these studies, dogs in graph A have received Dextran-purified islets and dogs in graph B received Ficoll-purified islets. Graph C compares the veno-arterial insulin gradients of the two groups.

given the most detailed information on viability. Previous investigations have shown that purified islets can be transplanted into spleen,[12] liver,[13] and omental pouch[38] sites. However, it is critical to design the transplant so that objective evidence for function can be obtained. One way is to seek evidence that the islet grafts can induce euglycemia. In order to achieve euglycemia, the critical mass of islets must be provided. The dose response relationship after transplantation of carefully quantified volumes of islets has been investigated in studies from our laboratory.[12] When islets were implanted into the spleen by venous reflux or embolized to the liver via portal vein, consistent euglycemia was observed with graft volumes that exceeded 5 μL(2830 IE)/kg body weight (Fig. 8.8). Similar dose response studies have confirmed that this volume of autologous islets is also suit-

able for transplantation into the liver[13] and for islets that have been stored by cryopreservation.[39] In allograft studies, the critical mass of freshly-isolated or cultured islets that induced normoglycemia was 8 μL/kg body weight.[33,40] For the omental pouch site, an augmented volume of 10 μL/kg of autologous islets appears to be the critical threshold for consistent euglycemia.[38]

In the situation where euglycemia has not resulted, an alternative method of viability assay can be performed. In such circumstances, the recipient can be sustained with supplemental doses of daily insulin therapy. Then at the desired time, the venous effluent from the transplant site and blood from a systemic arterial source can be assayed simultaneously to determine evidence for insulin secretion. An in vivo challenge with glucose or glucagon can be used to seek evidence for responsiveness of the islets to an exogenous challenge. For example, Figure 8.9 demonstrates insulin output from intrasplenic islets that were purified using Dextran or Ficoll. The splenic vein and the femoral artery were cannulated. A bolus of intravenous glucagon (1 mg/20 kg) was administered, then assays were performed simultaneously from arterial and venous sites at 5 minute intervals throughout a 35 minute time. The use of glucagon has the advantage that the recipient does not necessarily need to be euglycemic at the time of assay.

SUMMARY

Isolation of canine islets has been performed in many laboratories with varying degrees of success. With attention to careful preparation and selection of donors and the use of either manual or automated techniques, mass separation of highly viable islets can be achieved. Automated protocols in combination with collagenase perfusion via the duct result in mass yields of islets. Purification with discontinuous density gradients of Ficoll or Dextran has equal efficacy. Following isolation of the islets, steps must be taken to ensure that their viability has been preserved. Although several laboratories have used the islet isolation procedures detailed in this chapter, all of the methods rarely lead to isolation of more than 50% of the islet mass estimated to be within the canine pancreas. The major obstacle to reproducible results is the lack of consistently effective lots of collagenase. There is a pressing need for improved collagenase to promote success in the canine model.

ACKNOWLEDGMENTS

This research was supported by grants from the Alberta Heritage Foundation for Medical Research, the Muttart Diabetes Research and Training Center, and the Medical Research Council of Canada. The authors are grateful to D. Bracewell, C. Lopushinsky, and H. Power, for technical help. We are grateful to C. Gardner for invaluable secretarial assistance.

REFERENCES

1. Moskalewski S. Isolation and culture of the islets of Langerhans of the guinea pig. Gen. Comp. Endocrinol. 5:342, 1965.
2. Ballinger WF, Lacy PE. Transplantation of intact pancreatic islets in rats. Surgery 72:175, 1972.
3. Tzakis AG, Ricordi C, Alejandro R, et al. Pancreatic islet transplantation after upper abdominal exenteration and liver replacement. Lancet 336:402, 1990.
4. Scharp DW, Lacy PE, Santiago JV. Results of our first nine intraportal islet allografts into type 1 (insulin-dependent) diabetic patients. Transplantation 51:76, 1991.
5. Warnock GL, Kneteman NM, Ryan EA, Rabinovitch A, Rajotte RV. Long-term follow-up after transplantation of insulin-producing pancreatic islets into patients with type 1 (insulin-dependent) diabetes mellitus. Diabetologia 35:89, 1992.
6. Socci C, Falqui L, Davalli AM, et al. Fresh human islet transplantation to replace pancreatic endocrine function in type 1 diabetic patient. Acta Diabetologia 28:155, 1991.
7. Gores PF, Najarian J, Stephanian E, et al. Insulin independence in type 1 diabetes after transplantation of unpurified islets from single donors with [15]-deoxyspergualin. Lancet 341:19, 1993.
8. Van Der Burg MPM, Guicherit OR, Frohlich N, et al. Assessment of islet isolation efficacy in dogs. In: Abstract Manual of the 4th International Congress on Pancreas and Islet Transplantation, (Amsterdam), #282, 1993 (abstract).
9. Horaguchi A, Merrell RC. Preparation of viable islet cells from dogs by a new method. Diabetes 30:455, 1981.
10. Warnock GL, Rajotte RV, Procyshyn AW. Normoglycemia after reflux ofislet- containing pancreatic fragments into the splenic vascular bed in dogs. Diabetes 32:452, 1983.
11. Noel J, Rabinovitch A, Olson G, et al. A method for large scale, high yield isolation of canine pancreatic islets of Langerhans. Metabolism 31:184, 1982.

12. Warnock GL, Rajotte RV. Critical mass of purified islets that induce normoglycemia after implantation into dogs. Diabetes 37:467, 1988.

13. Munn SR, Kaufman DB, Meloche RM, et al. Weight-corrected islet counts are predictive of outcome in the canine intrahepatic islet autograft model. Diab. Res. 9:121, 1988.

14. Lanza RP, Borland KM, Lodge P, et. al. Treatment of severely diabetic pancreatectomized dogs using a diffusion-based hybrid pancreas. Diabetes 41:886, 1992.

15. Warnock GL, Ellis D, Rajotte RV, Davidson I, Baekkeskov S, Egebjerg J. Studies of the isolation and viability of human islets of Langerhans. Transplantation 45:957, 1988.

16. Kretschmer CJ, Sutherland DE, Matas AJ, et al. The dispersed pancreas: transplantation without islet purification in totally pancreatectomized dogs. Diabetologia 13:495, 1977.

17. Alderson D, Kneteman NM, Olack BJ, Scharp DW. Isolation and quantification of canine islet tissue for transplantation. Transplantation 43:579, 1987.

18. Ricordi C, Lacy PE, Finke EH, et al. Automated method for isolation of human pancreatic islets. Diabetes 37:413, 1988.

19. Warnock GL, Kneteman NM, Evans MG, et al. Comparison of automated and manual methods for islet isolation. Can. J. Surg. 33:368, 1990.

20. Ao Z, Lakey JRT, Rajotte RV, Warnock GL. Collagenase digestion of canine pancreas by gentle automated dissociation in combination with ductal perfusion optimizes mass recovery of islets. Transplant. Proc. 24:2787, 1992.

21. Mirkovitch V, Campiche M. Successful intrasplenic autotransplantation of pancreatic tissue in totally pancreatectomized dogs. Transplantation 21:265, 1976.

22. Kolb E, Ruchert R, Largiader F. Intraportal and intrasplenic autotransplantation of pancreatic islets in the dogs. Eur. Surg. Res. 9:419, 1977.

23. Mehigan DG, Ball WR, Zuidema GD, et al. Disseminated intravascular coagulation and portal hypertension following pancreatic islet autotransplantation. Ann. Surg. 191:287, 1980.

24. Warnock GL, Cattral MS, Rajotte RV. Normoglycemia after implantation of purified islet cells in dogs. Can. J. Surg. 31:421, 1988.

25. Kaufman DB, Morel B, Field MJ, Munn SR, Sutherland DER. Purified canine islet autografts: Functional outcome as influenced by islet number and implantation site. Transplantation 50:385, 1990.

26. Van Der Burg MPM, Gooszen HG, Ploeg RJ, et al. Metabolic control after autotransplantation of highly purified canine pancreatic islets isolated in UW solution. Transplant. Proc. 23:785, 1991.

27. Ao Z, Matayoshi K, Yakimets WJ, Lakey JRT, Katyal D, Rajotte RV, Warnock GL. Comparison of Dextran and Ficoll density gradients for purification of canine islets. Transplant. Proc. 24:2788, 1992.

28. Lake SP, Bassett D, Larkins A, et al. Large-scale purification of human islets utilizing discontinuous albumin gradient on IBM 2991 cell separator. Diabetes 38 (Suppl.1):143, 1989.

29. Alejandro R, Strasser S, Zucker PF, Mintz DH. Isolation of pancreatic islets from dogs: semiautomated purification on albumin gradients. Transplantation 50:207, 1990.

30. Latif ZA, Noel J, Alejandro R. A simple method for staining fresh and cultured islets. Transplantation 45:827, 1988.

31. Ricordi C, Gray DWR, Hering BJ, et al. Islet isolation assessment in man and large animals. Acta Diabetol. Lat. 27:185, 1990.

32. Davis DJ, MacAulay MA, MacDonald AS, Estabrooks BL. Islets of Langerhans in dog pancreas. Transplantation 45:1099, 1988.

33. Warnock GL, Dabbs KD, Cattral MS, Rajotte RV. Improved survival of in vitro cultured canine islet allografts. Transplantation (in press).

34. Lakey JRT, Rajotte RV, Taylor GD, Kirkland T, Warnock GL. Microbial studies of a tissue bank of cryopreserved human islet cells. Transplant. Proc (in press).

35. Taylor GD, Kirkland T, Lakey J, Rajotte R, Warnock GL. Bacteremia due to transplantation of contaminated cryopreserved pancreatic islets. Cell Transplantation. IN PRESS.

36. Morgan CR, Lazarow A. Immunoassay of insulin: two antibody system. Diabetes 12:115, 1963.

37. Weber CJ, Zabinski S, Koschitzky, et al. Microencapsulated dog and rat islet xenografts into streptozotocin-diabetic and NOD mice. Horm. Metab. Res. (Suppl.25): 219-226, 1990.

38. Ao Z, Matayoshi K, Lakey JRT, Rajotte RV, Warnock GL. Survival and function of purified islets in the omental pouch site of outbred dogs. Transplantation 56:524, 1993.

39. Evans MG, Warnock GL, Kneteman NM, Rajotte RV. Reversal of diabetes by transplantation of pure cryopreserved islets. Transplantation 50:202, 1990.

40. Cattral MS, Warnock GL, Kneteman NM, Rajotte RV. Transplantation of purified single-donor canine islet allografts with cyclosporine. Transplantation 47:538, 1989.

CHAPTER 9

HUMAN ISLET SEPARATION

Camillo Ricordi

Benigno J. Digon, III

Daniel H. Mintz

Rodolfo Alejandro

Since the introduction of the automated method for human islet isolation and transplantation in 1986[1] many steps have been implemented to optimize the separation and purification of islets from the non-endocrine component of the pancreas that constitutes 98-99% of the gland.[2]

Since the human pancreas is generally retrieved from multiorgan cadaver donors, conditions such as the cause of death, status of the donor at the time of pancreas procurement, drug administration in the intensive care unit or in the operating room, and pre-existing donor conditions such as age, body composition and pathologic status of the pancreas are all variables that can influence the outcome of islet isolation. An appropriate and correct pancreas procurement is a critical factor for a successful isolation. We will attempt to give a precise and accurate description of our latest modification to the automated method. Presented is an overview of the islet isolation method followed by a brief yet concise protocol that we adhere to.

PANCREAS HARVESTING AND PROCUREMENT

Human pancreata can be obtained from multi-organ donors[3-5] after in situ perfusion of the abdominal aorta with 1500-2000 mL of University of Wisconsin solution (UW), and an additional 500-1000 mL of UW infused directly into the liver via the portal vein. Venous hypertension of the pancreas should be carefully avoided by venting the portal and/or splenic vein. Alternatively, the body and tail of the pancreas can be excised at the beginning of the procurement procedure and promptly perfused on the back table. The gland should then be immediately immersed in UW (600-800 mL per pancreas), placed in a sterile transport container and stored on ice until isolation. Eurocollins solution (Transplant Technology, Inc., Dallas, TX, USA) can be used for short-term cold preservation instead of UW, however, for longer storage periods (>2 hrs) we use UW. Regardless of the solution selected, the best purification results are generally obtained with less than 12 hours cold ischemia time. Saline solution should never be used as cold preservation solution, even for very short preservation periods.

Pancreatic Islet Transplantation Volume I: Procurement of Pancreatic Islets, edited by Robert P. Lanza, MD, William L. Chick, MD; ©1994 R.G. Landes Company.

ISLET ISOLATION EQUIPMENT AND SET UP

The procedure for islet isolation that we currently use is relatively simple and has been successfully reproduced in any animal model tested, i.e., dog, rabbit, sheep, swine, bovine, hamster, rat, mouse.

The entire procedure, (isolation and purification) can be performed in a standard tissue culture laboratory, equipped with at least one, possibly two biological safety cabinets (class 100), two refrigerated centrifuges with the capacity for 250 mL conical centrifuge tubes (e.g. IEC PR7000, Fisher Scientific, Pittsburgh, PA), and a COBE Blood Processing Centrifuge (COBE BCT, Inc., Lakewood, CO, USA 80215). For preparation of islets that will be eventually transplanted into a human recipient, a positive pressure, temperature regulated, laminar flow clean room is preferable to minimize the risk of contamination.

Details on the isolation equipment and set-up are available in the chapter on porcine islet isolation and will not be repeated here.

PANCREAS DISTENSION

The human pancreas is trimmed and divided at the neck. After ductal cannulation of both segments, the Hanks solution is removed from the small tray and the large tray with iced saline is removed from the hood. The collagenase solution is injected in the duct using a disposable syringe (60 mL syringe with Leur-Lok). Collagenase concentration (Boeringher Mannheim Biochemical, Type P, Indianapolis, IN, USA) has to be adjusted lot by lot and sometimes with time, even within the same lot. We generally use 2-3 mg/mL in 350 mL of Hanks solution with no antibiotic and no fetal calf serum (FCS). The solution must be freshly prepared and it must be filtered (Nalgene Disposable Filterware, 500 ml, Nalge Company, Rochester, New York; 0.8 and 0.2 μm pore size). Only immediately before injection, the temperature of the collagenase solution is raised to 28-32°C. Injection of a cold collagenase solution should be avoided, since it would result in a temperature gradient between the inner portion of the gland and its surface. This differential temperature would produce a different collagenase activity throughout the gland, resulting in a faster digestion of the superficial parenchyma compared to the central portion of the gland.

An appropriate distension of the organ is critical to a successful islet isolation. In the case of unsatisfactory intraductal distension, i.e., chronic pancreatitis pancreata, serial intraparenchymal collagenase injections using the same 60 mL syringe with a long needle, i.e., 18 gauge angiocatheter guide will increase the efficiency of the digestion. At this time any remaining fat and/or connective tissue is removed from the pancreas.

PANCREATIC DIGESTION AND ISLET SEPARATION (AUTOMATED METHOD)

The gland is then loaded into the previously described stainless steel digestion chamber kept at a temperature of 40-42°C by the recirculation of Hanks with 2% BCS through the waterbath heating, coil circuit. The chamber is filled with the remaining collagenase solution contained in the small tray, the screen is placed, and the chamber is assembled.

Islets are separated from the exocrine during a continuous digestion process that lasts 30-60 minutes. The content of the chamber is gently mixed by shaking that can be manual or by a controlled mechanical shaker, that standardizes the oscillation amplitude and rate during digestion (variable rate of 0-320 osc/min and fixed amplitude of 10 cm). During the recirculation phase (flow rate 65-85 mL/min) the intrachamber temperature is increased at a rate of 2°C/min by thermic exchange through the stainless steel coil immersed in the 45-50°C sterile water bath until a temperature of 37-38°C is reached. The slow increase of intrachamber temperature is necessary to allow the equilibrium between the surface and the inner gland portion during digestion, therefore avoiding uneven enzymatic action.

Samples are first removed at 8 minutes and then every 2 minutes thereafter to monitor digestion. Even though experienced observers can generally clearly recognize islet tissue at the light microscopic level, dithizone (DTZ, Diphenylthiocarbazone, Sigma Chemical CO., St.Louis, MO, USA) a vital stain of islet cells is vital for immediate identification of islet tissue.[6-9] A few drops of the freshly prepared and filtered (4-8 μm) final solution is added to the sample contained in a 35 mm petri dish which results in a characteristic red islet stain resulting from the chelating of dithizone to zinc in insulin granules. When a significant number of free islets is observed in a digestion sample (considering also the amount of tissue in the sample, the appearance of the islets and/or the pH of the solution), dilution and collection of the digested tissue is started. This is accomplished by aspiration of cold Hanks solution with 10% BCS and 1% Ab/AM (antibiotic/antimycotic) in the digestion circuit and collection of the digest into a sterile 2 L Ehrlenmeyer flask at a flow rate of 350 mL/ min. At this time, shaking should be continued (more vigorously for human adult pancreata and progressively more gentle for younger donors). During this dilution phase, the coil should be removed from the water bath to interrupt the heating phase.

The digested tissue is first rapidly collected in the 2 L sterile Erlenmeyer flask preloaded with 1 liter of cold Hanks solution with 20% BCS and 1% Ab/AM. After the first liter of collection, the digested tissue can be directly loaded into 250 mL conical plastic bottles (250 mL centrifuge tubes, Corning Inc., Corning, NY,USA). The dilution phase lasts 15-45 minutes, until no islet tissue is detected in a sample. The digested tissue, containing the islets is then centrifuged (400*g* for 4 minutes at 4°C) using the 250 mL conical plastic bottles. The pellet is collected into one or two bottles and resuspended in Hanks solution with 10% BCS and 1% Ab/AM. After an additional centrifugation and washing, the preparation is ready to be processed for purification using discontinuous Euro-Ficoll gradients on the COBE Blood Processor.[3]

In the following section, we present our brief yet concise modified protocol for islet isolation and purification.

HUMAN ISLET ISOLATION: MODIFIED AUTOMATED METHOD

BIOLOGICAL CABINET AND DIGESTION CHAMBER SET UP

1. The biological safety cabinet is thoroughly wiped with 70% ethanol and a sterile topper sponge.

2. It is of great importance to process the pancreas as sterilely and aseptically as possible, since all islet isolations are ultimately considered for human transplantation. Therefore, the operator must scrub with betadine and don surgical gloves and gown. A sterile half sheet is placed in the safety cabinet in order to cover the isolation area.

3. The outside wrap of the sterilized chamber package is opened and the sterile inside package is placed inside the safety cabinet. The package is opened and the wrap is removed from the hood.

4. The chamber is placed on a stand and a 100 mL graduated cylinder is attached to the lower clamp of the ring stand. The large tubing (size 17) and the short length of the small tubing (size 16) is threaded through the upper clamp and inserted inside the cylinder. The longer length of the small tubing is clamped off with a hemostat and put aside for the dilution phase.

5. The coil is brought outside the safety cabinet and immersed in the prewarmed sterile 45-50°C waterbath. The attached tubing, afferent to the chamber, is attached to the peristaltic pump.

6. A Monotherm temperature probe is attached to the chamber, the pump is started, and 600-700 mL of Hanks with 2% BCS and 1% Ab/AM is circulated through the system in order to warm the chamber to 40-42°C.

7. Once the fluid has completely filled the circuit, the pancreas is to be cleaned and distended.

PANCREAS CLEANING AND COLLAGENASE DISTENSION

1. 1 x 1L of cold sterile normal saline and 2 x 1L of crushed sterile frozen saline is added to the large stainless steel tray and approximately 500 mL of ice cold Hanks with 10% BCS and 2% Ab/AM is added to the small tray.

2. The pancreas is removed from the sterile transport container and immediately immersed in the small tray. A temperature reading is taken from the UW solution as well as a 5 mL sample for microbiological analysis.

3. The pancreas is dissected off any fat, connective tissue, and small bowel. Do not attempt to clean it too thoroughly since small tears and leaks could hinder the distension of the gland.

4. Collagenase is prepared at a concentration of 2-3 mg/mL and dissolved in 350 mL of room temperature Hanks solution with no Ab/AM and BCS. Once enzyme is in solution, it is sterile filtered through a 500 mL, 0.2 μm bottle filter system. After filtration, the bottle is tightly capped and placed in a waterbath at 45°C, until a temperature of 28-30°C is attained.

5. Once the pancreas is cleaned, it is weighed, and using a No. 10 blade scalpel, it is cut at the neck (just below the head). After ductal cannulation of both pancreatic segments with an 18G angiogatheter and tied in with 2-0 silk using a straight needle and a purse string stitch, the Hanks solution is removed from the small tray and the large tray with iced saline is removed from the hood.

PANCREATIC DISTENSION

1. Once the collagenase has reached 28-32°C, the pancreas is distended using a 60 cc Luer-Lok syringe. The head of the pancreas is distended first, followed by the tail segment. It is necessary to check for leaks and close them off with hemostats since an appropriate distension of the organ is critical to a successful islet isolation. In the case of an unsatisfactory intraductal distension, serial intraparenchymal collagenase distension using the same 60cc syringe with a long needle, i.e., 18 gauge angiocatheter guide will increase the efficiency of the digestion.

2. After the pancreas is distended, the recirculating fluid from the chamber system is discarded, and any remaining fat and/or connective tissue as well as the cannulas and suture material is removed from the gland. The distended pancreas is loaded into the chamber and filled with the remaining collagenase solution. The screen is placed, and the chamber is assembled.

3. The peristaltic pump flow rate is set to 65-85 mL/min and if needed, more Hanks is added to the system in order to prevent any air in the recirculation. Once no air in the system is observed, the chamber is gently mixed by shaking that can be manual or by a controlled mechanical shaker (variable rate of 0-320 osc/min and fixed amplitude).

4. The desired rate of heating is at a rate of 2°C/min. until a temperature of 37-38°C is reached. If a temperature greater than 38°C is obtained, the coil is removed from the waterbath and the temperature is allowed to decrease.

5. The length of digestion time varies, but in general, once the temperature has reached 37°C, the digestion is continued for around 20 minutes (for a total of approximately 30 minutes).

6. After 8 minutes of digestion, samples may be taken by vigorously shaking the chamber and collecting fluid with tissue from the large tubing (size 17) end. The sample is stained with a few drops of DTZ solution and observations are recorded. Normally, fat cells are seen first, followed by acinar and an occasional islet fragment. The digestion is considered complete once free large intact islets are observed and an increase is seen in the amount of tissue liberated from the chamber.

7. While the digestion is in progress, a sterile 2 L Erlenmeyer flask is placed in

the safety cabinet and 8 L of Hanks with 10% BCS and 1% Ab/AM is placed on ice near the hood. The longer length of the small tubing is placed into the flask and an additional 2 L Erlenmeyer flask with 1 L of ice cold Hanks with 20% BCS and 1% Ab/AAM is also placed in the cabinet. This serum is to inactivate the collagenase solution which is contained in the first liters of collection.

8. When the digestion is judged complete, the dilution phase is begun.

DILUTION PHASE

1. Several liters of Hanks with 10% BCS and 1% Ab/AM are continuously poured into a 2 L flask while the large tubing end is placed into the 2 L flask preloaded with Hanks with 20% BCS and 1% Ab/AM. All of the solution from the 100 mL cylinder is allowed to completely enter the circulation. The hemostat is unclamped from the adjacent tubing, and the small tubing from the 100 mL cylinder is clamped. This allows the Hanks with 10% BCS and 1% Ab/AM to circulate. At this time, the pump is turned up to provide a flow of 350 mL/min and the chamber is shaken vigorously. The coil is taken out of the waterbath to allow the chamber to be cooled. After the first liter of collection, the digest is directly loaded into sterile 250 mL conical sterile centrifuge bottles.

2. The digested tissue is centrifuged at $400g$ for 4 minutes at 4°C. The pellet is collected into one or two conical tubes, resuspended in Hanks with 10% BCS and 1% Ab/AM and stored on ice while the procedure is repeated until all of the collected fluid has been centrifuge.

3. Once all of the tissue has been collected and centrifuged, it is resuspended and evenly divided into as many 250 mL tubes as the number of gradients necessary to accommodate the volume of tissue obtained from the digestion. This number varies according to the size of the pancreas but should be chosen to allow from 15-20 mL of tissue per gradient. Also, once the tissue is combined, several samples of 100μl are taken, stained with DTZ, and evaluated. Comments on the condition of the acinar tissue and percentage of free islets are recorded.

4. The islets are then purified from the acinar tissue using discontinuous Euro-Ficoll gradients on a COBE Blood Processor.

PROCEDURE FOR THE SET UP AND OPERATION OF THE COBE 2991 IN THE SEPARATION OF ISLETS ON DISCONTINUOUS EURO-FICOLL GRADIENT

1. The COBE processor is positioned parallel to a biosafety (class 100) cabinet and the power is turned on. The plexiglass cover is opened by removing the weighted metal latch. The locking glass bowl cover, plexiglass cover and the underlying foam ring from the bowl area is removed.

2. The COBE centrifuge bag is placed in the bowl. This is done by carefully rolling the bag around the rotating seal and sliding it through the opening in the glass bowl cover. Care must be taken not to damage the rotating seal.

3. The bag is positioned over the four central posts in the bowl. The perimeter of the bag is tucked into the bowl so that the bag lies on the floor of the bowl, with the edge curving up the sides. The sampling port is positioned so that the stem lies flat, and parallel to the side of the bowl.

4. The plastic collar is placed around tubing at the center of the bag, below the rotating seal. The locking glass cover is lowered and locked in place. Take care not to catch any part of the bag in the slots at the edge of the bowl which holds the bowl cover. This could result in damage to the bag.

5. The sliding plexiglass cover is closed and the weighted metal latch is placed over the posts and the rotating seal. The rotating seal may require minor manipulation to position it to slide into the slot in the weight. Let the metal latch use its own weight to lock the cover and hold the rotating seal.

6. The tubing is placed into the valve slots on the COBE, using color codes to determine the position. The tubing is not loaded into the pinch valves, but merely held in place in the tubing guides. Each tube is clamped using hemostats.

7. The Masterflex pump is loaded with sterilized silicon tubing (size 16), and spiked to the green tubing from the COBE into the end of the silicon tubing. The other end of the tubing is placed into a sterile container (e.g. 50 mL tube, 250 mL tube, 100 mL bottle).

8. A 60 cc syringe is placed in a ring stand clamp. It should only be handled by the barrel of the syringe, as this will be used to load the suspended tissue into a 600 mL Transfer Bag. Remove the plunger and the tip cover. Place a COBE coupler/adapter onto the tip of the syringe. Spike the other end of the COBE coupler/adapter into a 600 mL Transfer Bag.

9. Prepare the solutions for the discontinuous gradients in the volumes listed below.

Bottom layer	Euroficoll	1.108	275 ml
Middle layer	Euroficoll	1.096	125 ml
Top layer	Euroficoll	1.037	100 ml
	Hanks BSS		50 ml

This is done by using the calculations below.

Volume	Density	Stock Volume	Eurocollins Volume	Calf Serum
100 ML	1.108	8.44/D-1.022	98-Stock Vol.	2 ML
100 ML	1.096	7.24/D-1.022	98-Stock Vol.	2 ML
100 ML	1.037	1.34/D-1.022	98-Stock Vol.	2 ML

Prepare the 275 mL for the bottom layer in a 250 mL tube. All others will fit in 100 mL bottles.

10. To prepare tissue for COBE separation, centrifuge tube at $400g$ for 4 min at 4°C. Decant supernatant and add ~50 mL of 1.108 Euroficoll solution. Resuspend tissue well using a sterile disposable pipet to break up any clumps. Add remaining 225 mL of 1.108 Euroficoll solution and mix well. Place on ice.

11. Euroficoll (1.108 w/tissue) is drained into a 600 mL Fenwal Transfer Bag via the set-up described in step 8. The filled Transfer Bag is attached to the red tubing and is hung with the green, yellow, purple and blue tubes clamped. The clamp on the red tube is released and the tissue is allowed to flow into the bag in the centrifuge bowl.

12. Once the tissue has entered the centrifuge bag, the red hose is clamped, the green and blue hoses are unclamped and the most dense of the Euroficoll layers (1.096) is pumped through the green tubing up to the junction. The green and blue tubings are then clamped.

13. The purple tube is then unclamped and the air in the centrifuge bag is removed by the following sequence of steps.
A. Hit the *Start/Spin* button and adjust the speed to 2000 rpm.
B. Allow the centrifuge to reach full speed, then push the *SuperOut* button and adjust the *SuperOut* rate to 100 ml/sec. The solution will be pushed up through the tubing towards the junction.
C. Press the *Hold* button when the solution reaches the junction, and clamp the purple tube.
D. Press the *Stop/Rest* button.

14. When the machine has stopped completely, press the *Start/Spin* button again and adjust the *SuperOut* rate to "0".

15. When the centrifuge has attained speed begin pumping the Euroficoll solutions of varying density at a rate of approximately 90 mL/min.
a) Pump in 125 mL of 1.096 Euroficoll on top of the 275 mL pellet layer which contains tissue and Euroficoll.
b) Pump in 100 mL of 1.037 Euroficoll on top of the 125 mL preceding layer.
c) Pump in 50 mL of Hanks Balanced Salt Solution until the fluid reaches midway down the tubing leading to the rotating seal.

16. Turn off the pump and clamp the green tubing. With the *SuperOut* adjusted to "0", push the *SuperOut* button and open any of the other three tubes (red, yellow or purple) to relieve the excess pressure, then reclamp the tubing and let spin for 3 min.

17. After 3 minutes collect the fractions through the yellow tubing. Unclamp the

yellow tubing and adjust the *SuperOut* rate up to about 175. Normally, 3 fractions are collected: the first has a volume of 100 mL, and fractions 2 and 3 are 125 mL each. Fraction 2 is referred to as the top and fraction 3 as the bottom. Between fractions the *SuperOut* rate is adjusted to "0" while the yellow tubing is moved to the next bottle (250 mL tube) to prevent spillage and tissue loss.

18. Once the fractions are collected the machine is stopped and a sample of the pellet is taken through the small port on the centrifuge bag, using a large (16 gauge) needle and syringe. The entire pellet may be collected by using a coupler and a 60 cc syringe.

19. Fractions 2 and 3 are filled with Hanks with 10% BCS and 1% Ab/AM and spun at $400g$ for 5 min at $4°C$, after which the tubes are rotated $180°$ and spun again (same speed, temp and time).

20. The supernatant is aspirated and resuspend and the pellets are resuspended in Hanks with 10% BCS and 1% Ab/AM for a second wash and spun at $400g$ for 4 min at $4°C$.

21. 100μL samples of the purified islets are taken and assessed for purity, counted, and converted to islet equivalents using DTZ staining.[5,6]

Discussion

Many "minor" factors can limit the outcome of human islet isolation. Yet the main variables seem to be the overall condition of the donor pancreata and the enzymatic activity of collagenase. These factors are still producing highly variable results in human islet isolation. The automated method has been used by most of the centers involved in clinical trials.[3,4,10-30]

However, there is still a lot of space for improvement in the islet isolation procedure (as well as in the results of clinical trials).

References

1. Ricordi C, Lacy PE, Finke EH, Olack BJ, Scharp DW. Automated method for isolation of human pancreatic islets. Diabetes, 37: 413-420, 1988.

2. The Automated Method for Islet Isolation. Pancreatic Islet Cell Transplantation; 1892-1991: One Century of Transplantation for Diabetes. Ricordi C (Ed). RG Landes Co, Austin, (Pub) CRC Press (Distr), May, 1992.

3. Ricordi C, Tzakis AG, Carroll PB, Zeng Y, Rilo HLR, Alejandro R, Shapiro R, Fung JJ, Demetris AJ, Mintz DH, Starzl TE. Human islet isolation and allotransplantation in 22 consecutive cases. Transplantation 53:407-414, 1992.

4. Tzakis AG, Ricordi C, Alejandro R, et al. Pancreatic islet transplantation after upper abdominal exenteration and liver replacement. Lancet, 336:402, 1990.

5. Ricordi C, Mazzeferro V, Casavilla A, Scotti C, Pinna A, Tzakis A, Starzl TE. Pancreas procurement from multiorgan donors for islet transplantation. Diab Nutr & Metab, 5:39-41, 1992.

6. Latif ZA, Noel J, Alejandro R. A simple method of staining fresh and cultured islets. Transplantation, 45:827-830, 1988.

7. Ricordi C. Qualitative and quantitative assessment of islet isolation in man and large mammals. Pancreas, 6:242-244, 1991.

8. Ricordi C, Gray D, Hering B, Kaufman D, Warnock G, Kneteman N, Lake S, London N, Socci C, Alejandro R, Zeng Y, Scharp D,Viviani G, Tzakis A, Bretzel R, Federlin K, Pozza G, James R, Rajotte R, Di Carlo V, Morris P, Sutherland D, Starzl T, Mintz D, Lacy P. Islet isolation assessment in man and large animals. Acta Diabetologica Latina, 27:185-195, 1990.

9. Ricordi C, Hering BJ, London NJM, Rajotte RV, Gray DWR, Sutherland DER, Socci C, Alejandro R, Carroll, PB, Bretzel RG, Scharp DW. Islet isolation assessment. Pancreatic Islet Cell Transplantation; 1892-1992: One Century of Transplantation for Diabetes. Ricordi C (Ed). RG Landes Co, Austin, (Pub) CRC Press (Distr), May, 1992.

10. Ricordi C, Carroll PB, Tzakis AG, Alejandro R, Zeng Y, Rilo HLR, Fontes PA, Shapiro R, Fung JJ, Starzl TE. Islet transplantation in diabetes: The Pittsburgh experience. Pancreatic Islet Cell Transplantation; 1892-1992: One Century of Transplantation for Diabetes. Ricordi C (Ed). RG Landes Co, Austin, (Pub), CRC Press (Distr), May, 1992.

11. Socci C, Falqui L, Davalli AM, Ricordi C, Maffi P, Secchi A, Di Carlo V, Pozza G. Substitution of the endocrine pancreatic function in IDDM patients by allotransplantation of fresh islets: The Milan experience. Pancreatic Islet Cell Transplantation; 1892-1992: One Century of Transplantation for Diabetes. Ricordi C (Ed). RG Landes Co, Austin, (Pub), CRC Press (Distr), May, 1992.

12. Alejandro R, Burke G, Shapiro ET, Strasser S, Nery J, Ricordi C, Esquenazi V, Miller J, Mintz DH. Long-term survival of intraportal islet allografts in Type I diabetes mellitus. Pancreatic Islet Cell Transplantation; 1892-1992: One Century of Transplantation for Diabetes. Ricordi C (Ed). RG Landes Co, Austin, (Pub), CRC Press (Distr), May, 1992.

13. Scharp DW, Lacy PE, Ricordi C, Boyle P, Santiago J, Cryer P, Gingerick R, Jaffe A, Anderson C, Flye W. Human islet transplantation in patients with Type I Diabetes. Transplant Proc 21: 2744-45, 1989.

14. Scharp D, Lacy P, Santiago J, McCullough C, Weide L, Boyle P, Falqui L, Marchetti P, Ricordi C, Gingerich R, Jaffe A, Cryer P, Hanto D, Anderson C, Flye M. Wayne. Results of our first nine intraportal islet allografts in Type 1, insulin dependent diabetic patients. Transplantation 51: 76-85, 1991.

15. Alejandro R, Tzakis A, Ricordi C, Zeng Y, Todo S, Mazzaferro Z, Mintz DH, Starzl TE. Combined liver-islet allotransplantation in man under FK506. Transplant Proc 23: 789-792, 1991.

16. Ricordi C, Tzakis A, Alejandro R, Zeng Y, Demetris AJ, Carroll P, Mintz DH, Starzl TE. Detection of pancreatic islet tissue following islet allotransplantation in man. Transplantation 52:1079-1080, 1991.

17. Ricordi C, Tzakis A, Carroll P, Zeng Y, Rilo HLR, Alejandro R, Shapiro R, Fung JJ, Mintz DH, Starzl TE. Human islet allotransplantation under FK-506. Transplant Proc 23:3207, 1991.

18. Socci C, Falqui L, Davalli AM, Ricordi C, Braghi S, Bertuzzi F, Maffi P, Secchi A, Gavazzi F, Freschi M, Magistretti P, Socci S, Vignali A, Di Carlo V, Pozza G. Fresh human islet transplantation to replace pancreatic endocrine function in Type I diabetic patients. Acta Diabetologia 28:151-157, 1991.

19. Ricordi C, Tzakis AG, Carroll PB, Zeng Y, Rilo HLR, Alejandro R, Shapiro R, Fung JJ, Demetris AJ, Bereiter DR, Mintz DH, Starzl TE. Human islet allotransplantation in 18 diabetic patients. Transplant Proc 24:961, 1992.

20. Ricordi C, Sever CE, Carroll PB, Tzakis AG, Zeng Y, Rilo HLR, Demetris AJ, Alejandro R, Starzl TE. Histologic findings of pancreatic islet tissue following intraportal human islet allotransplantation. Transplant Proc 24:976, 1992.

21. Socci C, Falqui L, Davalli AM, Ricordi C, Bertuzzi F, Braghi S, Maffi P, Secchi A, Gavazzi F, Freschi M, Magistretti P, Di Carlo V, Pozza G. Allotransplantation of fresh islets in four type I diabetic patients. Transplant Proc 24:965-966, 1992.

22. Alejandro R, Burke G, Shapiro ET, Strasser J, Nery J, Ricordi C, Esquenazi V, Miller J, Mintz DH.Intraportal islet allografts in Type I diabetes mellitus. Transplant Proc 24:959-960, 1992.

23. Sever CE, Demetris AJ, Tzakis A, Carroll P, Zeng Y, Fung JJ, Starzl TE, Ricordi C. Islet cell allotransplantation in diabetic patients - histologic findings in four adults simultaneously receiving kidney or liver transplants.Amer J Path 140:1255-1260, 1992.

24. Ricordi C, Tzakis A, Alejandro R, Zeng Y, Demetris AJ, Carroll P, Mintz DH, Starzl TE. Detection of intrahepatic human islets following combined liver-islet allotransplantation. Pancreas 7:507-509, 1992.

25. Carroll PB, Ricordi C, Shapiro R, Rilo HLR, Fontes PA, Scantlebury V, Irish W, Tzakis AG, Starzl TE. Frequency of kidney rejection in diabetic patients undergoing simultaneous kidney and pancreatic islet cell transplantation. Transplantation, 55:761-765, 1993.

26. Carroll PB, Ricordi C, Rilo HLR, Fontes PA, Tzakis AG, Shapiro R, Starzl TE. Intrahepatic human transplantation at the University of Pittsburgh: results in 25 consecutive cases. Transplant Proc, 24:3038-3039, 1992.

27. Carroll PB, Ricordi C, Fontes PA, Rilo HLR, Shapiro R, Starzl TE. Microbiological surveillance as part of human islet cell transplantation: results of the first 26 patients. Transplant Proc, 24:2798-2799, 1992.

28. Fontes PA, Ricordi C, Rilo HLR, Carroll PB, Tzakis AG, Selby R, Starzl TE. Human islet isolation and transplantation in chronic pancreatitis using the automated method. Transplant Proc, 24:2809, 1992.

29. Casavilla A, Ricordi C, Rilo HLR, Tzakis AG, Julian TB, Starzl TE. Laparoscopic approach for pancreatic islet transplantation. Transplant Proc, 24:2800, 1992.

30. Alejandro R, Burke G, Shapiro ET, Strasser S, Nery J, Ricordi C, Esquenazi V, Miller J, Mintz DH. Intraportal islet allografts in Type I diabetes mellitus - an update. Diab Nutr & Metab, 5:183-185, 1992.

CHAPTER 10

ISLET ISOLATION FROM THE FETAL PANCREAS

Thomas. E. Mandel

Maria Koulmanda

The fetal pancreas may be an excellent alternative source to adult pancreas of islets of Langerhans for transplantation. In contrast to adult islet cells, fetal islet cells have a large capacity for proliferation. The method of organ culture described in this chapter retains this proliferative capacity of the immature islets, in part by retaining intact the ducts and the islet precursor cells present in their walls, as well as maintaining the ability of the precursor cells to differentiate into functionally mature endocrine cells. Isolation of the islet and islet precursor tissue is achieved simply and relatively inexpensively. The method described has been extensively studied with fetal mouse and fetal pig pancreas and, to a lesser extent, also with fetal human tissue. Isografts and allografts of such immature organ cultured pancreata have been able to reverse streptozotocin-induced diabetes in mice, and xenografts of pig and human cultures have reversed drug-induced diabetes in athymic (nude) mice. Recently, these studies have been extended to test the survival of organ cultured fetal pig pancreas in NOD mice immunosuppressed with anti-T cell monoclonal antibodies to prevent rejection, and spontaneous diabetes in these animals has been reversed. The method described is compared with other techniques for islet isolation from immature islets described in the literature. We believe that the method that we have developed is more efficient and cheaper that these other methods, and may be applicable for the large scale production of xenogeneic immature islet tissue for possible clinical use. However, immature islets do not respond immediately to functional demands but this response develops with time in situ so that if the graft survives for a sufficient time in the host, it eventually develops appropriate function. The use of *fetal* islets in transplantation may be more appropriate *early* in diabetes, i.e., before structural diabetic complications have developed, where immediate graft function is not required and development of appropriate responses by the graft can occur over perhaps a prolonged period of time. In contrast, adult islet transplants and vascularized pancreas allografts may be more suitable for chronically diabetic patients that require immediate graft function.

Pancreatic Islet Transplantation Volume I: Procurement of Pancreatic Islets, edited by Robert P. Lanza, MD, William L. Chick, MD; ©1994 R.G. Landes Company.

INTRODUCTION

Transplantation of a pancreas, usually as a vascularized whole organ, offers suitable patients the opportunity of achieving long-lasting and perhaps even permanent normalization of metabolic control,[1] a state that cannot easily be attained and maintained constantly with insulin replacement by other means. However, patients considered for pancreas transplantation are usually those with Type I diabetes (insulin-dependent diabetes mellitus — IDDM) in end-stage renal failure in need of a kidney allograft, and at this stage of their disease they also generally have many other complications of chronic diabetes that cannot be reversed. Persistent excellent control of diabetes can reduce and, perhaps, if metabolic control is totally normalized, even prevent the development of the many serious complications that are the fate of many patients with IDDM. That good control can significantly reduce diabetic complications (e.g. nephropathy, retinopathy and neuropathy) was recently clearly shown in the DCCT trial, but even intensive control with parenteral insulin generally failed to maintain glycosylated hemoglobin levels within the normal range.[2]

The DCCT study clearly showed that tight control was highly beneficial but it is highly unlikely that most patients with IDDM will be able to maintain such levels of metabolic regulation continuously over many years. Pancreas transplantation can produce precise control but it is a major and relatively complex procedure that has many problems, not least being the need for continuing non-specific immunosuppression. Even if pancreas grafts are performed in pre-diabetic patients, the structural changes already present in their own kidneys are not reversed.[3] Pancreas transplantation is also made more complex by the need to cope with the copious secretions that are produced by the co-transplanted exocrine tissue although this problem has been largely but not totally overcome by urinary bladder drainage of the graft. Thus, if endocrine replacement in IDDM can be made simple, safe and effective it may have major long-term benefits.

A simple and potentially safe alternative to vascularized pancreas transplantation is the use of the isolated islets of Langerhans but there are still many problems with this approach. Even if all of these problems of non-specific immunosuppression and the need to transplant early and safely are solved, there is still the unresolved, and probably unresolvable, problem of the lack of suitable human donors. The most likely solution to this problem is the use of xenogeneic donors, or perhaps transplantation of genetically engineered autologous cells.

Many experimental studies mainly in rodent models have shown that isolated islet transplantation is effective and safe and, in certain circumstances, can also be successful as an allograft without the need for any immunosuppression. Isolation of the islets from the pancreas involves the elimination of the large excess of exocrine tissue, usually with collagenase digestion and some form of density gradient separation. The islets comprise only 1-2% of the entire pancreas and in their isolation and purification much islet tissue may be lost and large amounts of very expensive reagents (e.g. collagenase) used. Moreover, when adult islets are harvested the precursors of the islet cells, generally located in the ducts,[4] are also lost. Since the intra-islet endocrine cells are essentially non-replicating,[5] a potential pool of their precursors is thus also lost when the islets are isolated.

Experimental studies, mainly in rodents, have shown that very clean islets depleted of attached exocrine cells, lymphoid tissue and other non-endocrine elements are poorly immunogenic and in many rodent models of islet transplantation can be grafted into histo-incompatible recipients without the need for *any* immunosuppression. However, as islet purity is increased so islet yield is decreased. Thus, in the quest for cleaner and potentially less immunogenic islets from the adult pancreas a large amount of endocrine tissue is also usually lost. This problem compounds the shortage of suitable allogeneic cadaver pancreata for clinical transplantation, and islet isolation from the adult cadaveric pancreas for transplantation, at least at present, may be a poor use of an already scarce resource.

Indeed, the current results of islet allotransplantation in patients with typical autoimmune IDDM are still quite poor[8-12] and contrast sharply with the increasingly improving results of vascularized pancreas allotransplantation.[1,13] In contrast, the situation of islet transplantation in non-IDDM patients is rather different. Islet autografts in patients with total pancreatectomy for chronic pancreatitis[14] and, to a more limited extent, of allografts in patients that have had extensive abdominal resection for intra-abdominal tumors,[15] show that such grafts can indeed prevent surgically-induced diabetes. This suggests that it is possible to transplant isolated islets obtained from a single donor gland and produce insulin-independence, and further suggests that factors other than inadequate islet mass alone are responsible for the poor results of islet allografts in IDDM. However, a minimal islet mass, generally estimated as being between 4-6000 islets ("islet equivalents") per kg body weight, is required, and if this is achieved insulin independence may be attained. It is likely that if sufficient islets were to be transplanted they would function even in patients with IDDM, but the limited availability of allogeneic pancreata virtually precludes the usual cadaveric pancreas as a suitable source of tissue for islet transplantation on any large scale.

Xenogeneic pancreata may be an alternative source of islets. Such tissue is available in essentially unlimited amounts from suitable donor species such as pigs, but many predominantly immunologic problems remain with the use of such tissue, particularly from the "discordant" domestic species that could be considered for extensive clinical use where the presence of preformed natural antibody in the recipient may be a severe barrier to successful engraftment.

The use of immature pancreata, i.e., fetal or neonatal as a source of islets is a potentially attractive alternative option compared to the use of adult pancreata and has been tested extensively but so far predominantly in small animal experiments and to a more limited extent, in clinical trials.

Fetal islets have a number of potential advantages over adult islets but also some major disadvantages. Specifically, the major advantage of fetal islets is their capacity to proliferate[17] so that, potentially, a small graft of fetal tissue may generate a large and hopefully adequate mass of endocrine tissue after transplantation. This has been shown for islet isografts in mice where a small amount of organ-cultured tissue, representing less than one-half of the fetal gland, eventually grows to produce an islet mass that has an insulin content equal to that present in a normal adult mouse pancreas, and reverses diabetes fully with normalization of glycosylated hemoglobin levels.[17] In addition, the fetal pancreas appears to withstand relatively prolonged periods of ischemia and its harvesting can be easily accomplished under conditions where adult islets would be irreparably damaged. This makes the acquisition of the fetal glands logistically simple. Also, the fetal pancreas does not compete with adult pancreas as a source of tissue for transplantation. Disadvantages of the use of fetal islets are primarily due to their functional immaturity that prevents rapid physiologic function and long periods of time, weeks or even months in mice, may elapse before grafts of fetal islets function adequately. There are major ethical problems as well, particularly with the use of human fetal pancreata as this almost inevitably has to be from therapeutic abortions.

In this chapter, we describe a method of islet isolation that we have used over the past 15 years with fetal pancreata from mice, pigs and humans. The method is simple and relatively cheap and, although there are species-specific differences that determine the precise response of the fetal pancreas to various culture conditions, cultures of the fetal pancreas from all 3 species tested (mice, humans and pigs) behave in a fundamentally similar way. The experience that we have gained over a long period suggests that organ culture of the fetal pancreas may be a useful and reliable way of harvesting large amounts of islet tissue as well as the ductal tissue that contains islet precursor cells for transplantation. In addition, it is possible to modify the culture conditions readily so that *selective* survival of the endocrine cells with removal of potentially highly immunogenic non-endocrine cells is feasible. This may produce endocrine and endocrine-precursor tissue of reduced immunogenicity.

However, of probably more importance is the clear evidence that the capacity of the cultured tissue for proliferation and differentiation is retained. The growth of xenogeneic fetal human and fetal pig pancreas in athymic mice is also retained and transplants of quite small amounts of such tissue, each graft being equivalent to approximately one-half of a fetal mouse pancreas, can reverse streptozotocin-induced diabetes in such animals.[18-20] We have also shown that fetal pig pancreata can survive for prolonged periods (>5 months) in NOD mice that have been immunosuppressed with anti-T cell monoclonal antibodies[21] and we have now also reversed spontaneous autoimmune diabetes in NOD mice with such xenografts (Mandel and Koulmanda, unpublished data). Importantly, there is some evidence that in this model of pig islets transplanted to NOD mice the graft may also be resistant to recurrent disease.[22-25]

In addition to the method that we have developed, other methods of islet isolation from the fetal pancreas have been used by other investigators[26-37] and these will be described and contrasted to the organ culture technique we describe in detail herein.

ORGAN CULTURE OF FETAL PANCREAS

DONOR PREPARATION—ISOLATION OF THE PANCREAS FROM FETAL MICE

The mouse pancreas can be isolated from quite young fetuses but we generally use animals of 17-18 days gestation (the normal gestation for mice is 19-21 days, depending on the strain). Mice are mated so that pregnant animals of a defined gestational age are available. Mating is determined by examining the animal for the presence of a vaginal plug as an indication of mating and the morning on which a plug is detected is taken as day 0 of gestation. The presence of a vaginal plug only indicates that mating has occurred and is no guarantee of pregnancy but this can generally be established by inspec-

tion of the mated animal after 13 or 14 days. Late-gestation fetuses are used for preferance because they are quite large and easy to work with and their pancreas is readily identified and isolated. However, much younger fetuses can also be used and the pancreas can be easily identified even by 14 days gestation. We have even used mice of 12 days gestation, when the pancreas is present only as a mid-gut anlage and cannot be seen as a seperate organ but the duodenum containing the developing pancreatic buds can be readily identified. However, this very early fetal tissue is less effective as an isograft in reversing STZ-induced diabetes.[38]

The pregnant mice are killed by cervical dislocation or exposure to an overdose of CO_2 and placed on a cork dissecting board. The fur is washed with 70% ethanol and a long mid-line abdominal skin incision is made with scissors and the skin is reflected laterally and pinned out. The abdomen is opened via a long mid-line incision so that the intra-abdominal contents are exposed and the pregnant uterine horns clearly seen. The lower end of the uterus at the junction of the uterine horns is grasped with a pair of forceps, lifted up and cut away from the vagina, The uterine vessels and connective tissue and ovaries are cut away from the uterus and the isolated uterus is placed in a 9 cm diameter petri dish that contains 10-15 mL of PBS. The dissection of the fetuses and isolation of the pancreas is best performed in a laminar flow hood and frequent changes of instruments and the use of adequate quantities of sterile media and careful aseptic technique will usually eliminate contamination. It is unwise to rely on antibiotics in the culture media to maintain sterility.

The isolated uterus is grasped with a pair of small toothed forceps and the uterine horns are opened with a second pair so that the fetal sacs are exposed. Using a pair of small smooth curved forceps, each fetus is exposed, torn away from the placenta and placed into another petri dish. The fetuses can then be dissected at leisure. Generally, 10-12 fetuses are placed in each dish. The dishes can be kept at room temperature for some hours with no apparent loss of tissue viability, but if dissection is slow or there is likely to be a delay in isolating the pancreas, it is preferable to keep the tissue at 4°C until it is dissected, either in a cold room or on an ice slurry. We have found that fetal tissue is quite resistant to ischemic damage and will tolerate surprisingly long periods of ischemia even at room temperature.[39]

To remove the pancreas, each fetus is grasped gently with a pair of smooth curved forceps and held so that its abdomen is uppermost. The abdominal wall is then opened with a second pair of forceps and the abdominal contents everted and pulled away from the body. Generally this removes the intestines, stomach, spleen and liver *en block* and the organ cluster is placed into a separate petri dish. When 10-20 such clusters are collected they are further dissected under a dissecting microscope at low magnification (x3 to x5) using 26 gauge hypodermic needles mounted on 1 mL plastic syringe barrels. The pancreas is readily identified as an opaque white irregular mass that is clearly distinct from the dark red liver and the obvious intestine. The easiest way to locate the pancreas is to identify the stomach and follow its distal (pyloric) end to the duodenum. The spleen can be seen as an elongated thin strip of red tissue attached to the greater curvature of the stomach and the pancreas lying between the duodenum and the spleen. The gland can be quickly and easily isolated from the other adjacent organs with needles, cleared of any obvious attached tissue fragments and placed to one side in the dish. It is generally quickest to remove only the body and tail of the pancreas and we do not try to carefully dissect the head of the gland from the duodenum. The amount of tissue lost by not isolating the proximal part of the pancreas is generally well under one-half of the gland and its absence may have the added advantage that the developing pancreatic lymph nodes that are located in the mature pancreas near the proximal end of the pancreatic and bile ducts are not included in the tissue that is placed in organ culture. When all the pancreas pieces are free, they are set up in culture as described below.

DONOR PREPARATION—ISOLATION OF THE PANCREAS FROM FETAL PIGS

The method used is similar to that described above with the difference that more precise dissection is easy with the very much larger fetal pigs. The gestational age at term in pigs is around 114 days at which time in common domestic pig strains, e.g., Large white or Landrace, the fetuses measure about 22-26 cm crown-rump length. We generally use younger fetuses, preferably aged between 60-90 days when there is already quite well developed endocrine tissue present but the exocrine component is still poorly differentiated.

The fetal pigs may be obtained from a commercial slaughterhouse or, preferably, from animals killed specifically to obtain fetal tissue. In commercial slaughterhouse operations pigs are generally killed by stunning and exsanguination followed by scalding to remove body hair. This inevitably results in a period of 15-30 minutes of warm ischemia before the fetuses are removed. It is interesting, and perhaps even surprising, that in most instances viable pancreas is still present after this length of time but in some cases severe damage or even complete tissue death has occurred. The fact that viable fetal pancreas is often present under these conditions attests to the tolerance of fetal tissue to ischemic damage. Preferably, however, tissue that is as little exposed to ischemic damage as is possible is desirable and purpose-killed donors, or fetuses delivered by hysterotomy from anesthetized sows are the most certain to give consistently good islets. When the fetuses are removed from the uterus they are immediately placed in plastic bags and immersed in ice slurry to produce rapid body cooling and transported to the laboratory for dissection. The tissue will remain viable for many hours after rapid cooling.

Before the fetal pigs are dissected they are immersed in 70% ethanol for about 1 minute to sterilize the skin and placed on their right side on sterile towels in a laminar flow hood. The left (uppermost) body surface is then washed down with a stream of

70% ethanol and allowed to dry in the steam of sterile air in the laminar flow hood. The skin is removed from the left body wall by making an incision from the paravertebral mid-thoracic region anteriorly to about the mid-costal point, then distally to the hind leg and then dorsally towards the spine so that a large flap can be raised. This is reflected dorsally by dissecting it away from the underlying abdominal muscles. The muscle layer is exposed and using fresh instruments is excised so that the left lateral abdominal viscera are exposed. In order to get better exposure of the abdominal contents the left lower rib cage is also cut away and the left lung exposed. The stomach is retracted cranially and the pancreas can be seen lying with its tail and distal body attached to the spleen, greater curvature of the stomach and left kidney. In the fetal pig the pancreas has a very distinctive appearance and is readily identified. In young fetuses (approx 40-70 days gestation), the pancreas is an obviously glandular structure consisting of small white globules embedded in transparent jelly-like connective tissue. In more mature fetuses the mass of the gland is greater and the jelly-like connective tissue is no longer apparent.

To dissect the gland from the adjoining viscera it is necessary to detach it from the adjacent organs by grasping the tail of the gland with a pair of small forceps and carefully cutting the pancreas away from its attachments with iris scissors. The bulk of the head, body and tail of the pancreas can be easily mobilized but the proximal part of the head attached to the duodenum is difficult to remove cleanly and is best left behind. Usually, the splenic vessels are also removed with the gland but apart from these and some connective tissue there should be little if any other tissue removed. The detached pancreas is then placed in a fresh 9 cm petri dish for further dissection that takes place under a low magnification dissecting microscope.

Isolation of pancreatic pieces suitable for organ culture requires that the isolated gland first be cleared of as much irrelevant attached tissue as possible—principally the splenic vessels and obvious sheets of connective tissue. This is best performed initially with small sharp scissors under a dissecting microscope. The splenic vessels are easily identified and can be cut away from the superior margin of the gland and other obvious pieces of connective tissue can also be easily removed. The pancreas is then cut into approximately 0.5 cm^3 blocks that are diced into small (<1 mm^3) pieces with sterile 23 gauge needles mounted on 1mL syringe barrels. Much less tissue damage is produced with these than with scissors that produce more crush damage. If preferred, scalpel blades can be used to dice the gland. It is important to ensure that the fragments that are to be placed in culture are sufficiently small so that minimal tissue is lost through ischemic central necrosis in vitro (see below). During this dissection it is easy to remove tissue that is obviously not pancreas, e.g., large vessels, ducts and pieces with large amounts of connective tissue.

While the pancreas is quite resistant to ischemic damage it is preferable to maintain it as much as possible at a low temperature and we generally keep the petri dishes on an ice slurry when we are not actually working on them. The diced fragments are stored in PBS supplemented with 5-10% FCS until they are plated out on the culture plates.

DONOR PREPARATION—ISOLATION OF THE PANCREAS FROM HUMAN FETUSES

The principles for isolation of the human fetal pancreas are similar to those used for fetal pig tissue but there are some major and important differences. Firstly, it is not possible, and is indeed illegal, to obtain human fetal tissue primarily for therapeutic or experimental purposes in most Western countries. What tissue does become available must be obtained as a totally incidental consequence another procedure, i.e., a legally induced termination of a pregnancy. Termination of a pregnancy *in order to obtain tissue* is, in most countries, illegal. The maximum gestational age to which a legal termination is permissible is also a major limiting factor and varies from one country to another but is generally well below the age at which it is possible to maintain fetal viability ex utero.[40] Thus, in most countries where it is possible to perform legal terminations the upper age limit for this is generally around 20 weeks and conceivably this may decrease with advances in early neonatal care. In addition, while it is not legal to induce a termination in order to obtain tissue it is still necessary in most countries to have properly informed consent from the mother, and often also the father, for the use of fetal tissue for research purposes. Often the uses to which such tissue is put needs also to be clearly specified. In addition, the medical personnel involved in the care of the mother and in performing the termination must not be involved in the research project and the dissection of the fetus must not be performed by them. There must be a clear dissociation of interest between the teams involved the management of the mother and the subsequent use of the tissue, as is, incidentally, also the case in the use of any post-natal donor tissue.

The manner in which a termination is performed is also an important factor in determining the viability of the pancreas. In many instances for mid-trimester terminations, i.e., from about 12-20 weeks gestation prostaglandin-induced premature labor is used and in many and perhaps most such cases there is a long period of warm ischemia before the fetus is delivered. In such cases the fetus has often died in utero and the tissue is already autolysed. We have found that in most such cases the tissue is dead and fails to produce sustained insulin secretion in vitro.[41] When a mid-trimester termination is performed by other methods, e.g., by dilatation and vacuum extraction or by hysterotomy there is a much shorter period of warm ischemia and indeed there may be evidence of spontaneous fetal activity, e.g., heart beat or spontaneous muscle movement. All such activity must cease and the fetus be in permanent cardiac arrest, i.e. dead before any procedure can be performed on it. However, when tissue is obtained from such fetuses there is consistently good insulin production over a period of some weeks in organ culture with rising insulin levels in media aliquots.[41,42]

Once these criteria have been fulfilled and fetal tissue becomes available the pancreas can be isolated. It is generally advisable that the fetal organs be removed as part of a general autopsy but the method of performing this is modified so that it is performed *immediately,* fetal death is established and with the use of strictly sterile techniques. The abdominal viscera are removed, placed in sterile medium, examined for any abnormalities and the pancreas is then isolated. It is dissected away from the attached organs and cleared of adherent obviously non-pancreatic tissue, and then diced into small pieces (<1mm^3), as for fetal pig tissue.

One frequent difference between fetal human and fetal pig pancreas is that with the former the precise duration of ischemia may not be known and the amount of damage that the tissue has suffered may be such that it is not worthwhile using it. Ischemic damage can be roughly gauged by inspection of the tissue and by its feel when it is being dissected. If a piece of liver is available it can be a good guide to the viability of the other organs. Fresh liver is uniformly dark in color and soft but firm to touch. If there is obvious mottling and particularly if the liver is very friable it is likely that it has undergone severe ischemic damage and under these circumstances it is probably unwise to proceed further with organ dissection. If liver is not available the pancreas can give similar clues, not so much from its color but rather from its consistency when it is being processed. A fresh viable pancreas is firm and when it is being cut into small fragments for culture the pieces are discrete; in contrast when severe damage has occurred the pancreas fragments and dissociates readily.

PREPARATION OF DISHES FOR ORGAN CULTURE

We use the same method we originally described in 1978 for the culture of fetal mouse thymus[43] for organ culture of fetal islets from all of the 3 species studied. The principle of the method is that the tissue fragments are maintained at a gas-medium interface so that there is excellent gas exchange, with a ready uptake of nutrients and disposal of metabolic wastes by diffusion into the underlying medium. We have also used this method for the maintenance of other fetal tissues, including lymph nodes and spleen, but it is not possible to predict how any particular organ will behave in terms of its survival and differentiation nor what variations will be encountered with different species. However, with fetal pancreata from the mouse, human and pig the common factor is that there is selective survival of the ductal and endocrine tissue while the poorly differentiated exocrine elements either do not develop or, more likely, are selectively killed. The reason for this differential survival is not fully understood but is most likely due to an absence of factors necessary for survival of the exocrine cells and it has been suggested that corticosteroids are one such component that allows exocrine cells to survive.[44] In any case, since the aim of the method is the selective elimination of non-endocrine cells with retention of the endocrine cells and their precursors, the precise reasons for the selective loss of the irrelevant cells, though interesting is of less immediate concern.

The limiting factor for tissue survival in organ culture is the size of the pieces explanted as this determines the degree of oxygenation available to cells farthest removed from their surface. Total immersion of tissue pieces in media greatly limits oxygenation with consequent ischemic necrosis of the more deeply placed cells. The benefit of having the entire tissue pieces exposed in the gas phase is that there is much better oxygenation with a resultant decrease in the central ischemic necrosis that is a major feature of methods that use immersion culture. Generally, with fetal pancreas a viable cell layer about 10-20 cells deep, i.e., about 100-150 μm) is present when the tissue is maintained in the gas phase in 10% CO_2/ 90% air but this is greatly reduced when the entire tissue piece is fully immersed. Thus, in the gas phase method much larger pieces of tissue survive and the process of dispersing the pancreas is simplified and accelerated because larger fragments can be viably maintained. As detailed below, the size of the fragments initially plated out can be

futher enlarged by increasing the ambient O_2 concentration but this can result in O_2 toxicity.

This organ culture method is also easy to modify with respect to ambient gas concentration, medium type and additives. A potential problem with the method is that the tissue pieces are generally too large for intravenous embolization, e.g., for intraportal transplantation, but this is not really a serious problem since the need for such transplantation is not obligatory. On the other hand, the tissue pieces harvested are large enough to be easy to handle and do not require the use of methods to increase their total size, e.g., by placing them in plasma clots for renal subcapsular transplantation. On the other hand, the pieces are still small enough so that they survive after transplantation by diffusion of nutrients from the graft bed vasculture during the time it takes to establish an adequate ingrowth of host vessels. This does of course imply that the graft bed is well vascularized as in, for example, the renal subcapsular space, at least in rodents.

The petri dishes we routinely use are 9 cm diameter plastic tissue culture plates (e.g. Steritech #23484, 14 x 90 mm plastic gamma irradiated, Steritech Pty Ltd, Dandenong, Victoria 3175, Australia) but other brands of similar tissue culture grade dishes are equally suitable. This specific size is also not mandatory but is convenient since the gelatin foam rafts that act as a primary support are well suited for this dish size. The dishes are filled with about 15 mL of medium and this is changed routinely twice a week, but more often if serial measurements, for example, of insulin secretion are required. Each dish can be used for 15-20 1 mm^3 organ fragments. With this amount of tissue it is unlikely that medium depletion will occur even if less frequent changes are made.

The primary support for the tissue fragments that maintain them in the gas phase is a block of surgical gelatin foam. It is important to use a gelatin foam that is not soluble in aqueous media and the brand that we have found to be ideal is "Gelfoam-7"

(Absorbable gelatin sponge, USP. Size 12 [20 x 60 x 7mm] Upjohn Co., Kalamazoo, Michigan, USA). These gelatin sponges are sterile and individually packed in sealed bags in packets of four. Despite their cost they are ideal for this use as they have a coarse pore size that allows for free diffusion of macromolecules and are very hydrophilic so that they adsorb the culture medium readily. The sponges are insoluble and, unless there is bacterial contamination or the presence of very mature exocrine pancreas when they rapidly dissolve because of the release of proteolytic enzymes, they will remain intact for at least 3 weeks in vitro.

However, the softness and large pore size of the gelatin foam means that the tissue fragments cannot be placed directly on to the surface of the sponge and an intermediate support is necessary. This is most easily provided by using sterile strips of an inert material such as Millipore filter strips. Approximately 5 mm x 20 mm strips are cut from sheets or circles of 0.45 μm pore size Millipore (#HVLP 04700 filters) and boiled in distilled water to wash out any residual detergent, sterilized by autoclaving and stored in 70% ethanol or in the autoclave bags. The surface of the strips is smooth and there is no actual ingrowth of cell processes into their substance so that the tissue fragments can be very readily stripped off the filters with no discernable damage to the tissue. In addition, the white opaque surface of the millipore makes examination of the attached tissue simple as the tissue fragments can be easily seen against the background. It is important to wash the strips well in media or other aqueous solvents since traces of detergent may be present that are toxic to tissues with prolonged contact. We routinely boil the millipore strips in distilled water as this not only promotes their sterility but also effectively washes out any residual traces of detergent.

Other gas-phase organ culture systems have been described using the same principles. Variants include the use of other supports, e.g., Nuclepore, or the use of a stainless steel mesh as the primary support instead of gelatin foam. Indeed, even simple flota-

tion of strips may be successful but at the risk of these sinking and resulting in total immersion of the tissue. Stainless steel mesh supports are useful because they are much cheaper than commercial gelatin foam and can be reused, but the cost of cleaning them and the need to have a more precise medium level so that the mesh is exactly level with the medium surface makes this support less convenient than Gelfoam. Especially designed organ culture dishes are also available but are of less value because of their cost and the constraints that they impose on the amount of tissue that can be processed per dish.

MEDIA

We have systematically only tested three media (TCM199, Dulbecco's Modified Eagles Medium [DMEM] and RPMI1640) with fetal mouse pancreas. When the insulin secretion by, and the extractable insulin content of 17 day fetal CBA pancreata were compared in these media there was little consistent difference between RPMI1640 and DMEM, but less insulin production was noted when TCM199 was used.[45] However, since RPMI1640 has a "non-physiological" glucose content—2 gm/L (approx 11 mM)—and DMEM has a more physiological glucose content of 1gm/L (5.5 mM), we routinely use the latter. We have indeed shown that with fetal mouse pancreas at least, exposure to a constantly hyperglycemic environment can result in sustained abnormal function when the tissue is subsequently transplanted into a diabetic recipient.[46] Perhaps the "set-point" for insulin secretion by the immature fetal beta cells is altered by constant exposure to a supraphysiologic glucose content. That this may indeed be the case was supported by studies of Brown et al who showed that uncultured fetal rat pancreas isografts in diabetic rats performed less well than if they had first been transplanted into a euglycemic primary host and *subsequently* grafted into a diabetic recipient, i.e., they showed that functional development of the fetal islets was influenced by the ambient glucose concentration.[47,48] Similar aberrations in insulin secretion are sometimes seen in infants born of diabetic mothers.

Fetal calf serum (FCS) supplementation is also used routinely and we have not found major problems with either FCS batch variation or concentration within quite broad limits[46]—generally we use 5-10% FCS. Since FCS is expensive and there may be occasional batch variation (although we have not found this to be a problem), there is no reason to use more FCS than necessary. Other sera supplements may also be used and systematic studies have been performed with fetal pig pancreas by Sandler et al who showed that human serum (HS) appeared to be better than FCS and that pig serum appeared to disrupt pig islets.[49] The gas phase we use routinely is 10% CO_2 in air at an ambient temperature of 37-37.5°C with maximum humidity as this prevents evaporation of the media. Under these conditions—referred to as "conventional culture" or "CC"—there is excellent survival of fetal mouse,[18,38,39,45,46] human[41,50] and pig pancreatas[51] for prolonged periods—generally 2-3 weeks or even longer—with routine media changes twice weekly, although this is probably unneccesary as the volume of medium is large for to the amount of tissue present and nutrient depletion is unlikely.

GAS CONCENTRATIONS—THE EFFECT OF ALTERING O_2 CONCENTRATION

There are two quite separate effects of O_2, the obligatory need for this gas to maintain viability and the totally distinct effect of O_2 toxicity, presumably because of the effects of the formation of highly reactive O radicals. These toxic effects of O_2 are differentially expressed on the various cells of the fetal pancreas and seem also to be species dependent. Thus, selective exposure to O_2 can have beneficial effects on the cultured tissue and O_2 can be used to modify the cellular composition of the cultured organ pieces.

We have routinely used a mixture of 10% CO_2 in air with media buffered with HCO_3^- to maintain a pH of about 7.2. However, with this relatively low O_2 content there is a large amount of central necrosis in the tissue pieces of the size we generally use and a surviving rim of about 10-20 cell diam-

eters is present with a sharp demarcation between viable and dead tissue. This demarcation line becomes apparent within the first 1-2 days of culture and thereafter the surviving rim of viable tissue remains essentially static in depth while the central necrotic core gradually shrinks as the dead cells fragment and are removed. There are frequent mitoses present in islet and ductal cells and particularly with pig fetal pancreas there are frequently pyknotic cells seen amongst the interstitial cells. It is interesting that there is such a sharp demarcation line between the peripheral viable and central dead tissue with little evidence of an intermediate zone of damaged cells, at least as detected by light microscopy. With increasing time in culture the central necrotic zone is gradually absorbed and the total volume of the cultured fragments decreases. The duration of survival of the tissue pieces in vitro depends to a large extent on the species used. Generally, viable tissue can be obtained for many weeks with all the species studied but there is a gradual loss of cells with time and we have found that 2-3 weeks is a reasonable limit beyond which there is increasing tissue loss. This is more apparent with fetal pig islets than with fetal human or fetal mouse tissue.

Clearly, hypoxia is a limiting factor in determining the size of organ pieces that can be maintained in culture. In an attempt to improve oxygenation we have increased the O_2 concentration to 90% with 10%CO_2. With this O_2 concentration there is no central necrosis present when 1 mm³ pieces are used and these larger tissue fragments can be maintained in culture for varying periods. However, there are marked species differences in the ability of the tissue to withstand exposure to such high O_2 concentrations. Fetal mouse islet cells appear able to survive for at least 2-3 weeks under such conditions but the non-endocrine cells, specifically fibroblasts, macrophages, dendritic cells and probably endothelial cells, are all selectively killed after some time in this gas phase.

The gas phase variation produces marked effects on the appearance of the cultured tissue. When fetal mouse pancreas fragments are examined under a dissecting microscope conventionally-cultured fragments are discoid in shape with a marked outgrowth of cells from the explant, but when cultures are maintained in 90% O_2 they become quite spherical without the outgrowth from their edge. Indeed, it is possible to predict with some accuracy the fate of such "immuno-modified" fetal mouse cultures when they are tested as allografts in non-immunosuppressed mice on their pretransplant appearance, with the spherical pieces generally being far less immunogenic, presumably as a result of the more complete elimination of immunogenic "passenger leukocytes." The duration of tolerance to 90% O_2 is limited and after some time (14-21 days in mice) the endocrine cells also start to die—the maximum survival of fetal mouse pancreas seems to be about 4-5 weeks. However, we have found that allografts of fetal mouse pancreata seem to need about 21 days exposure to 90% O_2 to be sufficiently depleted of immunogenic cells so that they will usually survive in MHC-mismatched allogeneic recipients without need for any immunosuppression.[52,53]

In contrast to fetal mouse pancreata we have found that human fetal pancreata are very much more sensitive to O_2 toxicity and the islet and all other cells are rapidly killed usually within a few days of culture.[54] Fetal pig pancreas appears to be intermediate in its sensitivity to O_2 toxicity between mouse and human fetal pancreas with the endocrine and ductal cells showing excellent survival for some days while the non-endocrine cells are rapidly killed—usually within 24-48 hours. Histologic examination of fetal pig pancreas after 48-72 hours in 90% O_2 shows that the islet and ductal cells are intact with many in mitosis whereas the non-endocrine and non-ductal cells are pyknotic. An interesting appearance is seen in such organ cultured pieces where the entire tissue fragment is intact wihout evidence of central necrosis but with marked pyknosis of interstitial cells adjacent to viable endocrine and ductal and presumably endocrine-precursor cells, many of which are dividing. Thus, with fetal pig pancreas there seems to be a highly selective difference in the susceptibility of the various

cell types present in the fetal pancreas to withstand exposure to high concentrations of O_2. This may be of major benefit both in eliminating potentially highly immunogenic non-endocrine cells ("passenger leukocytes") as well as enabling the dissection of the fetal pancreas to be rapid and easy as quite large pieces of tissue can be used. However, there is O_2 toxicity for *all* cells with increasing duration of exposure and we generally see death of all cells in fetal pig pancreas after 5-7 days in 90% O_2. Thus there is a strict limit to the duration of exposure of the tissue to such high concentrations of O_2.

We are presently studying the effects of somewhat reduced O_2 concentrations (50%) to see whether the benefit of adequate oxygenation can be retained while its toxic effects are reduced. We have some evidence that reducing the O_2 concentration to 50% can help achieve this aim. Since O_2 toxicity is presumably mediated by highly reactive superoxide radicals we are also studying the effects of adding to the culture media superoxide scavengers such as superoxide dysmutase and catalase. Our data suggest that these enzymes may be beneficial in reducing O_2 toxicity while allowing adequate oxygenation to facilitate the selective survival of endocrine cells and their precursors but we have not as yet defined the optimal conditions. Ideally, it would be beneficial to use the maximum amount of O_2 to maintain viability of the endocrine cells while allowing selective cell death to occur to those cells that are irrelevant, and possibly even harmful, for a graft. As a compromise we are currently using an initial brief exposure (2-3 days) of fetal pig pancreas to 90% O_2 to improve overall viability by reducing or even eliminating central necrosis and then transferring the cultures to "conventional" conditions for some days as this allows the reduced tissue volume, now composed principally of islet and ductal cells, to survive well for a much longer period.

The result of these procedures is also the production of tissue pieces that are small enough to survive the initial post-transplantation ischemia in vivo while they are reliant on diffusion of O_2 and nutrients from the adjacent vasculature in the graft bed before the implants become vascularized by ingrowth of host vessels that will then provide adequate oxygenation and nutrition. The tissue fragments produced by the method we use are too large for intravenous embolization and must be placed into a very well vascularized site. Probably the best such site, at least in rodents, is the renal subcapsular space where the grafted fragments are placed directly onto a dense capillary bed in an organ that has a very high blood flow. Whether the renal subcapsular site is as good in large animals is uncertain but there are data that suggest that grafts can survive in this location in primates and perhaps also in dogs.

Thus, the use of selective gas concentrations may enable the culture conditions to be modulated so that there is maximum survival of the endocrine cells and, most importantly, also of their precursors, while at the same time eliminating from the tissue as much as possible any irrelevant tissue. It is also essential with fetal islet tissue to retain its capacity for proliferation so that this can be utilized after transplantation to increase the bulk of the graft to a functionally adequate amount. In contrast to grafts of adult islets that are essentially non-replicating, the prime advantage of fetal islets lies in their capacity for continuing proliferation, either from the islet cells themselves or perhaps more likely from duct-wall precursors that are co-isolated with the fetal islets. In any case there is ample evidence that whatever the precise source of islet cells the fetal grafts do show continuing growth and differentiation, a potential that must be retained if fetal islets are to be transplanted.

A COMPARISON OF OTHER METHODS OF FETAL ISLET ISOLATION

A number of groups have also used fetal pancreata as a source of islet cells for transplantation. In general, the methods used by others rely on varying degrees of tissue dispersion so that either a cell suspension or major disruption of the gland into very small cell aggregates is produced. To the best of our knowledge there has not been a strict quantitative comparison of the various methods to determine which is the optimal with regard to islet yield.

Ideally, if islet transplantation could be performed without a need for immunosuppression, it could have much wider potential application and this has been repeatedly demonstrated in rodent models of diabetes. Therefore a major aim of islet isolation has been to reduce immunogenicity and most methods have been designed to optimize this, usually at the expense of islet cell yield.

However, yield cannot be ignored, if only from cost considerations, and if immunogenicity can be reduced while high islet yield is retained, this would constitute the ideal situation.

One method that clearly is very effective in eliminating immunogenic cells was developed by Simeonovic et al[32] and is described in detail in reference 55. This method relies on an initial digestion of the fetal pancreas with collagenase to produce a partial digest that is then placed in tissue culture to produce "proislets". This method has been used with success by Simeonovic and her colleagues with both murine and porcine fetal pancreas. In their method the fetal mouse pancreas is removed from 17 day gestation animals and is carefully cleared of attached mesentery before being cut into 3 pieces and placed in collagenase solution where digestion occurs for a few minutes. The partial digest is then placed in tissue culture using RPMI 1640 medium for 4 days at 37°C. During this time the acinar tissue degenerates while the endocrine cells and their precursors remain viable and form variably sized clusters referred to as "proislets". Similar methods are used for fetal pig pancreas. The "proislets" appear to consist of clean islet-like tissue with a sizeable component of precursor cells. Following transplantation into suitable recipients the proislets undergo further differentiation and proliferation and can reverse diabetes in a range of models. When compared with uncultured fetal pancreas as allografts, the proislets are clearly much less immunogenic.[56] Thus, this method is effective and clearly can be readily adapted for large scale use.

While we have not made a direct comparison of the efficiency of proislets and organ-cultured fetal pancreas to reverse diabetes, we believe that our organ culture method may be more efficient since much less donor tissue is required and reversal of diabetes occurs sooner than with proislets. For example, Simeonovic et al generally use 4-8 donor equivalents of islets for an allo or isograft[57] and between 1/2 (in spontaneously diabetic NOD mice) and 1/20 (in streptozotocin-diabetic CBA mice) of a fetal pig pancreas to produce proislets for a xenograft to achieve euglycemia in mice.[57-59] In contrast, with organ cultured tissue prepared as described above, <1/2 of a fetal mouse pancreas and as little as 1% or less of a fetal pig pancreas can achieve the same end and often in less time. This suggests that there are much larger losses of tissue in the preparation of proislets than in the preparation of organ cultured fragments. In addition, the proislets are much smaller and for renal subcapsular transplantation are generally placed into a plasma clot for ease of handling. This is rather more demanding than the manipulation of the organ cultured fragments that can be handled directly and may also contribute to post-transplantation loss of tissue due to ischemic damage before vascularization develops. An advantage of the proislets, however, is that they are probably small enough to embolize intravenously.

Digestion of fetal or neonatal pancreas can also be used to prepare a single cell suspension or a mass of small cell aggregates that can be plated out onto the surface of appropriate petri dishes. When these cell suspensions are placed in culture, nests of islet cells grow out from the underlayer of attached cells and these free-floating or loosely attached cell aggregates can be harvested as quite clean populations of endocrine cells. This method or variants of it have been used by Hegre et al[34-37] and Korsgren, Sandler et al[26-31] to prepare islet tissue from rodents and pigs, and in the case of the Swedish group also recently for clinical use in a small series of patients with IDDM.[60-64] In each case a clean preparation of islet tissue that is capable of continued growth is

generated but again, as for the preparation of proislets, there appear to be major losses of tissue, either in its initial digestion from the fetal pancreas or subsequently during tissue culture. Thus, for their clinical trials many fetal pigs, sometimes pooled from a number of litters were required to prepare enough tissue for transplantation into a single patient and even with this there appeared to be no clinical benefit, although both sustained porcine C-peptide production and in at least one instance histological evidence of graft survival was noted.

A suggested major advantage of the preparation of islets or proislets from digests of fetal pancreata is that there is a selective loss of immunogenic contaminating cells that results in tissue of much reduced immunogenicity. Simeonovic and Lafferty have indeed compared fresh fetal pancreas and proislets as allografts and clearly demonstrated that the proislets are much less immunogenic.[56] However, the results that we have had with allografts of organ cultured fetal mouse pancreas and indeed with similarly-treated fetal pig pancreas suggest that a similar reduction in immunogenicity can be achieved with the organ culture methods using 90% O_2 exposure.

In the studies in Sweden where islet cell-like clusters (ICC) were used there also appear to be major cell losses although it is likely that well-defined endocrine tissue was prepared. The Swedish group developed their method for preparation of ICC initially using rat fetal pancreata.[65] The method relies on collagenase digestion to produce a cell dispersion that is plated out into dishes containing tissue culture media. After a few days in vitro, fibroblasts attach to the surface of the dish and ICC consisting of endocrine cells, and presumably their precursors, grow out of the attached monolayer and form loosely attached or free-floating nests of cells that are the ICC.

When this method was adapted for human fetal pancreata[27,28,30,31] the authors found, as have we and others,[41,42] that only a proportion (<50%) of specimens from prostaglandin-induced abortions produced viable ICC. Initially using their standard methods each pancreas yielded between 100–200 ICC that were up to 400 μm in diameter.[27] Although these ICC had at least some immunohistologically differentiated beta cells they failed to respond to physiologic stimuli in vitro by increasing insulin secretion. As in previous studies with the fetal pancreas of large mammals that have a long gestation period, there was a long delay in the development of a normal response of the beta cells to glucose-induced insulin release[66,67] whereas the pancreas of small mammals that have a short gestational development will mature functionally in vitro.[68]

In subsequent studies the Swedish group attempted to increase the efficiency of their method by the addition of various supplements to the culture media. For example, addition of human serum (HS) increased the yield of ICC about 7-fold compared to FCS but the cell number per ICC was reduced by about 50%.[27] ICC development was also enhanced when the media were supplemented with amniotic fluid.[31] Addition of 10mM nicotinamide further increased ICC yield by 40% and the insulin content by 50% but there was no alteration in stimulated insulin release.[28] There also appeared to be no increase in the amount of DNA per ICC. This suggested that the addition of nicotinamide was useful in increasing the absolute number of ICC and their insulin content but without either increasing the size of the cell clusters or their capacity to secrete insulin in response to pharmacological stimuli. Addition of growth hormone as a supplement was also beneficial in increasing insulin production.[32]

Another feature of note is the variation in the types of cells present in the ICC. When rat fetal pancreas was grown in this way, there were many beta cells whereas these cells represented only a minority in the ICC that developed from the human fetal pancreas. As in the culture of human fetal pancreas, fetal pig pancreas showed variable growth depending on the serum supplementation used. When FCS was used, there was a marked outgrowth of fibroblasts whereas with human serum (HS) fibroblasts were less evident and ICCs developed more rapidly and

in a 2-3-fold greater number.[27] Interestingly, the ICC growth was apparently complete by days 4-5 after the initial plating. Quantitative estimates from entire litters suggested that only about 10^5 ICC were produced *per litter*.[27]

Thus, there appeared to be major cell losses in the preparation of ICC although this may have been due, in part at least, to ischemic damage of the pancreas before it was processed for culture. Indeed, when this method was used to prepare ICC very many fetuses were required to generate sufficient islets for each recipient and up to 5 pregnant pigs were needed to produce sufficient tissue for a clinical transplant, and even this was not adequate to reverse diabetes. However, it should be emphasized that graft losses after transplantation due to rejection or failure of engraftment may have been responsible for the absence of an effective graft mass. Nevertheless, the costs and effort required to process such large amounts of donor tissue would be prohibitive for large-scale application and means of generating sufficient tissue at a reasonable cost and with relatively simple methods are essential. The primary benefit of the organ culture method that we described above is that it is simple and efficient while, at the same time, producing grafts of excellent viability and reduced immunogenicity.

CONCLUSION

Fetal pancreata may well be a highly attractive source of islets for transplantation, particularly if xenogeneic tissue from suitable domestic species can be used. There are clearly a great many unsolved problems still present before the use of such grafts can be contemplated, but one problem where advances have been made is in the efficient isolation of the endocrine cells. For this to be optimally effective there should be a high recovery of the appropriate cells, retention of their precursors that can produce new cells after transplantation, and elimination of irrelevant and potentially harmful cells from the fetal tissue. Many prerequisites will need to be satisfied before these aims can be achieved and, because of the many variables much experimentation is still required. At present it is not at all clear which of the methods that have been described is best, but we would like to suggest that the method that we have developed and describe in detail herein may have significant advantages in terms of cost and efficiency without sacrificing the potential benefit of reducing immunogenicity. For experimental studies in small animals where tissue availability is not a major concern probably any of the methods described are adequate, but for clinical application where large amounts of tissue may be required, costs and efficiency are of major importance. We believe that the method that we have developed may fulfil many of the requirements for tissue preparation for potential clinical use.

Acknowlegments

The studies reported in this chapter that were performed in the Transplantation Unit at the Walter and Eliza Hall Institute were supported by the National Health and Medical Research Council of Australia, and by grants from J.B. Were and Sons, The Perpetual Trustees and Executors Association of Australia, Hoechst Diabetes Research Fund, Australia, and by various grants from the Juvenile Diabetes Foundation, International. Many graduate students, post-doctoral fellows and technicians were involved and are acknowledged in the references cited.

References

1. Robertson RP. Pancreas transplantation in humans with diabetes mellitus. Diabetes 40: 1085-1089, 1991.
2. The diabetes control and complications trial research group. The effect of intensive treatment of diabetes on the development and progression of long-term complications in insulin-dependent diabetes mellitus. N Engl J Med 329: 977-986, 1993.
3. Fioretto P, Mauer SM, Bilous RW, Goetz FC, Sutherland DER, Steffes MW. Effects of pancreas transplantation on glomerular structure in insulin-dependent diabetic patients with their own kidneys. Lancet 342: 1193-1196, 1993.
4. Dudek RW, Lawrence IE. Morphologic study of cultured pancreatic fetal islets during maturation of the insulin-secretion mechanism. Diabetes 29: 15-21, 1980.
5. Hellerstrom C, Swenne I. Growth pattern of pancreatic islets in animals. eds Volk BW, Arquilla ER. "The Diabetic Pancreas" 2nd edn. NY Plenum Medical Book Co, 1985; pp. 53-79.
6. Bretzel RG, Hering BJ, Stroeder D, Zekorn T, Federlin KF. Experimental islet transplantation in small animals. in "Pancreatic islet cell transplantation" (ed Ricordi C) pp 249-260, RG Landes Co, Austin TX 1992.
7. London NJM, James RFL, Bell PRF. Islet purification, in "Pancreatic islet cell transplantation" (ed Ricordi C) pp 113-123, RG Landes Co, Austin TX 1992.
8. Warnock GL, Ryan EA, Kneteman NM, Rajotte RV. Transplantation of pancreatic islet cells into type I diabetic humans: the University of Alberta experience. in "Pancreatic islet cell transplantation" (ed Ricordi C) pp 400-409, RG Landes Co, Austin TX 1992.
9. Alejandro R, Burke G, Shapiro ET, Strasser S, Nery J, Ricordi C, Esquenazi V, Miller J, Mintz DH. Long-term survival of intraportal islet allografts in Type I diabetes mellitus. in "Pancreatic islet cell transplantation" (ed Ricordi C) pp 410-413, RG Landes Co, Austin TX 1992.
10. Socci C, Falqui L, Davalli AM, Ricordi C, Maffi P, Secchi A, Di Carlo V, Pozza G. Substitution of the endocrine pancreatic function in IDDM patients: the Milan experience. in "Pancreatic islet cell transplantation" (ed Ricordi C) pp 414-422, RG Landes Co, Austin TX 1992.
11. Gores PF, Najarian JS, Sutherland DER. Clinical islet allotransplantation: the University of Minnesota experience. in "Pancreatic islet cell transplantation" (ed Ricordi C) pp 423-433, RG Landes Co, Austin TX 1992
12. London NJM, James RFL, Robertson GM, Chadwick D, Feehlay J, Burden F, Bolia A, Bell PRF. Human islet transplantation: the Leicester experience. in "Pancreatic islet cell transplantation" (ed Ricordi C) pp 454-461, RG Landes Co, Austin TX 1992.

13. Sutherland DER. Report from the international pancreas transplant registry. Diabetologia 1991; 34 (suppl 1) S28.

14. Farey AC, Sutherland DER. Islet autotransplantation. in "Pancreatic islet cell transplantation" (ed Ricordi C) pp 291-312, RG Landes Co, Austin TX 1992.

15. Ricordi C, Carroll PB, Tzakis A, Alejandro R, Zeng Y, Rilo HLR, Fontes PAC, Shapiro R, Fung JJ, Starzl TE. Islet transplantation in diabetes: the Pittsburgh experience. in "Pancreatic islet cell transplantation" (ed Ricordi C) pp 448-453, RG Landes Co, Austin TX 1992.

16. Tuch BE, Simpson AM. Experimental fetal islet transplantation. in "Pancreatic islet cell transplantation" (ed Ricordi C) pp 279-290, RG Landes Co, Austin TX 1992.

17. Mandel TE The fetal pancreas: a valuable source of tissue for islet transplantation? Clin Transplant 4: 87-92, 1990.

18. Mandel TE, Koulmanda M. Effect of culture conditions on fetal mouse pancreas in vitro and after transplantation in syngeneic and allogeneic recipients. Diabetes 34: 1082-1087, 1985.

19. Mandel TE, Collier SA, Hoffman L, et al. Isotransplantation of fetal mouse pancreas in experimental diabetes: effect of gestational age and organ culture. Lab Invest 47: 477-483, 1982.

20. Mandel TE Fetal islet transplantation in diabetic mice: a model for human islet transplants. eds Peterson CM, Jovanovic-Peterson L, Formby B. "Fetal Islet Transplantation. Implications for Diabetes"; pp 165-184, Springer-Verlag, NY, 1988.

21. Mandel TE, Koulmanda M. Effect of immunosuppression with anti-T cell mAbs on the survival of organ-cultured fetal pig xenografts in NOD mice. Transplant Proc. (in press).

22. Mandel TE, Koulmanda M, Loudovaris T, Bacelj A. Xenografts of fetal pig islets in NOD mice; recurrence of disease and rejection of allografts precedes xenograft rejection in anti-CD4 treated mice. ed. E Shafrir, "Lessons from Animal Diabetes III", pp 120-125, 1990.

23. Mandel TE, Koulmanda M, Loudovaris T, Bacelj A. Islet grafts in NOD mice: a comparison of iso, allo, and xenografts. Transplant Proc 21: 3813-3814, 1989.

24. Mandel TE, Koulmanda M, Bacelj A. Fetal pancreas transplantation in non-obese diabetic (NOD) mice: a comparison of iso, allo, and xenografts. Horm Metab Res. Suppl 25: 166, 1990.

25. Mandel TE, Koulmanda M, Loudovaris T. Xenografts of organ cultured fetal pig pancreas in NOD mice: a comparison with allografts and isografts in transiently immunosuppressed mice. Transplant Proc 22: 816-817, 1990.

26. Korsgren O, Sandler S, Jansson L et al. Effects of culture conditions on formation and hormone content of fetal porcine islet like cell clusters. Diabetes 38 (suppl 1): 209-212, 1989.

27. Sandler S, Andersson A, Korsgren O, Tollemar J, Petersson B, Groth C-G, Hellerstrom C.. Tissue culture of human fetal pancreas. Effects of nicotinamide on insulin production and formation of islet like cell clusters. Diabetes 38 (suppl 1): 168-171, 1989.

28. Sandler S, Andersson A, Schnell A, Mellgren A, Tollemar J, Borg H, Groth C-G, Hellerstrom C. Tissue culture of human pancreas: development and function of B-cells in vitro and transplantation of explants to nude mice. Diabetes 34: 1113-1119, 1985.

29. Korsgren O, Sandler S, Schnell Landstrom A, Jannsson L, Andersson A. Large scale production of fetal porcine isletlike cell clusters. Transplantation 45: 509-514, 1988.

30. Sandler S, Andersson A, Schnell A, Landstrom A, Tollemar J, Borg H, Petersson B, Groth C-G, Hellerstrom C. Effects of amniotic fluid on the development of human fetal pancreatic b-cells in tissue culture. Transplant Proc 18: 57-59, 1986.

31. Sandler S, Andersson A, Korsgren O, Tollemar J, Petersson B, Groth C-G, Hellerstrom C. Tissue culture of human fetal pancreas: growth hormone stimulates the formation and insulin production of islet-like cell clusters. J Clin Endocrinol Metab 65: 1154-1158, 1987.

32. Simeonovic CJ, Lafferty KJ. The isolation and transplantation of foetal mouse proislets. Aust J Exp Biol Med Sci 60: 383-390, 1982.

33. Mullen Y, Watt PC, Stein E. Proliferation of porcine fetal islets in vitro and in vivo. Implications in development of an artificial pancreas. Diab Nutr Metab 5 (suppl 1) 79-82, 1992.

34. Hegre OD, Wells LJ, Lazarow A. Response of beta cells to different levels of glucose. Fetal pancreases grown in organ culture and subsequently transplanted to maternal hosts. Diabetes 22: 906-915, 1970.

35. Hegre OD, McEvoy RC, Bachelder V, Lazarow A. Organ culture of fetal rat pancreas: quantitative analysis by linear scanning of islet and other tissue components. In Vitro 7: 366-376, 1972.

36. Hegre OD, McEvoy RC, Bachelder V, Lazarow A. Fetal rat pancreas: differentiation of the islet cell component in vivo and in vitro. Diabetes 22: 577-583, 1973.

37. Hegre OD, Marshall S, Schulte BA, Hickey GE, Williams F, Sorenson RL, Serie JR. Nonenzymatic in vitro isolation of perinatal islets of Langerhans. In Vitro 19: 611-620, 1983.

38. Mandel TE, Collier SA, Hoffman L, pyke KW, Carter WM, Koulmanda M Isotransplantation of fetal mouse pancreas in experimental diabetes: effect of gestational age and organ culture. Lab Invest 47: 477-483, 1982.

39. Mandel TE, Koulmanda M. Effect of ischemia and temperature on fetal mouse pancreas: Insulin production in vitro and function following isotransplantation. Diabetes 33: 376-382, 1984.

40. Allen MC, Donohue PK, Dusman AE. The limit of viability — neonatal outcome of infants born at 22 to 25 weeks' gestation. N Engl J Med 329: 1597-1601, 1993.

41. Mandel TE, Georgiou HM. Insulin secretion by fetal human pancreatic islets of Langerhans in prolonged organ culture. Diabetes 32: 233-237, 1983.

42. Lim SM, Heng KK, Lim NK, Seah ML, Wee A, Li SQ, Soh P, Rauff A, Vengadasalam D. An in vitro assessment of human fetal pancreatic islets of Langerhans in culture. Ann Acad Med Singapore 20: 465-471, 1991.

43. Mandel TE, Kennedy MM. The differentiation of murine thymocytes in vitro and in vivo. Immunology 35: 317-331, 1978.

44. McEvoy RC, Hegre OD. Foetal rat pancreas in organ culture: effects of media supplementation with various steroid hormones on the acinar and islet components. Differentiation 6: 105-111, 1976.

45. Collier S, Mandel TE, Hoffman L, Caruso G. Organ culture of fetal mouse pancreas: the effect of various culture conditions on insulin secretion. Diabetes 30: 804-812, 1981.

46. Collier SA, Mandel TE, Carter WM. Detrimental effect of high medium glucose concentration on subsequent endocrine function of transplanted organ cultured foetal mouse pancreatic islets. Aust J Exp Biol Med Sci 60: 437-445, 1982.

47. Brown J, Heininger D, Kuret J, Mullen Y. Islet cells grow after transplantation of fetal pancreas and control of diabetes. Diabetes 30: 9-13, 1981.

48. Mullen Y, Clark WR, Molnar IG, Brown J. Complete reversal of experimental diabetes mellitus in rats by a single fetal pancreas. Science 195: 68-70, 1977.

49. Sandler S, Andersson A, Schnell Landstrom A, Tollemar J, Borg H, Petersson B, Groth C-G, Hellerstrom C. Tissue culture of human fetal pancreas. Effects of human serum on development and endocrine function of isletlike cell clusters. Diabetes 36: 1401-1407, 1987.

50. Hoffman L, Mandel TE, Carter WM, et al. Insulin secretion by foetal human pancreas in organ culture. Diabetologia 23; 426-430, 1982.

51. Thompson SC, Mandel TE. Fetal pig pancreas: Preparation and assessment of tissue for transplantation, its in vivo development and function in athymic mice. Transplantation 49: 571-581, 1990.

52. Collier SA, Mandel TE. Reduction of the immunogenicity of fetal mouse pancreas allografts by organ culture in 90% O_2. Transplantation 36: 233-237, 1983.

53. Collier SA, Mandel TE, Carter WM. Effect of duration of organ culture and gestational age on the function of fetal pancreas grafts. Transplant Proc 16: 1052-1054, 1984.

54. Mandel TE, Hoffman L, Collier SA, Carter WM, Koulmanda M. Organ culture of fetal mouse and fetal human pancreatic islets for allografting. Diabetes 31 (suppl 4) 39-47, 1982.

55. Simeonovic CJ, Teittinen KUS, Brown DJ, Wilson JD. Preparation and transplantation of fetal proislets. in in "Pancreatic islet cell transplantation" (ed Ricordi C) pp 238-248, RG Landes Co, Austin TX 1992.

56. Simeonovic CJ, Lafferty KJ. Immunogenicity of mouse fetal pancreas. A comparison. Transplantation 45: 824-827, 1988.

57. Simeonovic CJ, Ceredig R, Wilson JD. Effect of GK1.5 monoclonal antibody dosage on survival of pig proislet xenografts in CD4+ T cell-depleted mice. Transplantation ; 49: 849.

58. Simeonovic CJ, Wilson JD, Ceredig R. Antibody induced rejection of pig proislet xenografts in CD4+ T cell-depleted diabetic mice. Transplantation 1990; 50: 657.

59. Simeonovic CJ, Wilson JD. Xenotransplantation of fetal pig proislets in anti-CD4-treated diabetic NOD/Lt mice. Transplant Proc. 1992 24: 2287-2288, 1992.

60. Groth CG, Korsgren O, Andersson A, Hellerstrom C, Bjoersdorff A, Tibell A, Tollemar J, Bolinder J, Ostman J, Kumagai M, et al. Evidence of xenograft function in a diabetic patient grafted with porcine fetal pancreas. Transplant Proc. 24: 972-973, 1992.

61. Kumagai-Braesch M, Groth CG, Korsgren O, Andersson A, Hellerstrom C, Bjoersdorff A, Tibell A, Tollemar J, Bolinder J, Ostman J, et al. Immune response of diabetic patients against transplanted porcine fetal islet cells. Transplant Proc. 24: 679-680, 1992.

62. Andersson A, Groth CG, Korsgren O, Tibell A, Tollemar J, Kumagai M, Moller E, Bolinder J, Ostman J, Bjoersdorff A, et al. Transplantation of porcine fetal islet-like cell clusters to three diabetic patients. Transplant Proc. 24: 677-678, 1992.

63. Korsgren O, Groth CG, Andersson A, Hellerstrom C, Tibell A, Tollemar J, Bolinder J, Ostman J, Kumagai M, Moller E, et al.Transplantation of porcine fetal pancreas to a diabetic patient. Transplant Proc. 24: 352-353, 1992.

64. Groth CG, Andersson A, Korsgren O, Tibell A, Tollemar J, Kumagai-Braesch M, Moller E, Bolinder J, Ostman J, Bjoersdorff A, et al Transplantation of porcine fetal islet-like cell clusters into eight diabetic patients. Transplant Proc. 25: 970, 1993.

65. Hellerstrom C, Lewis NJ, Borg H, Johnson R, Freinkel N. Method for large scale isolation of pancreatic islets by tissue culture of fetal rat pancreas. Diabetes 28: 769-776, 1979.

66. Tuch BE, Jones A, Turtle JR. Maturation of the response of human fetal pancreatic explants to glucose. Diabetologia 28: 28-31, 1984.

67. Hullett DA, Falany JL, Love RB, Burlingham WJ, Pan M, Sollinger HW. Human fetal pancreas — a potential source for transplantation. Transplantation 43: 18-22, 1987.

68. Freinkel N, Lewis NJ, Johnson R, Swenne I, Bone A, Hellerstrom C. Differential effects of age versus glycemic stimulation on the maturation of insulin stimulus-secretion coupling during culture of fetal rat islets. Diabetes 33: 1028-1038, 1984.

CHAPTER 11

PROCUREMENT OF FISH ISLETS

James R. Wright, Jr.

Most of the literature pertaining to experimental islet xenotransplantation consists of studies in which rat islets have been transplanted into mice.[1] The severity of concordant islet xenograft rejection in rat-to-mouse models is quite mild relative to that seen with other species combinations. As a result, it is extremely difficult to extrapolate from the results of rat-to-mouse islet xenotransplantation studies. Therefore, it is necessary to develop and standardize alternative islet xenograft models that are more aggressively rejected than rat islets transplanted into mice.

We have recently develop a model using teleost fish as islet donors that allows us to perform islet xenograft studies across a wide phylogenetic barrier.[2-5] The islet tissue, called principal islets or Brockmann bodies (BBs), in certain teleost fish is anatomically distinct from their pancreatic exocrine tissue and can easily be identified macroscopically. If a suitable teleost species (see below) is readily available, using fish as islet donors offers a major cost advantage relative to mammalian donors because islet isolation procedures are not necessary to generate islet tissue; the BBs can simply be harvested with a scalpel and forceps. Not only are BBs simple and economical to harvest, they are also remarkably similar to mammalian islets.[2,6]

SELECTION OF APPROPRIATE DONOR SPECIES

The ideal donor species should meet seven criteria.[7] First, it should be readily available or easily bred. Second, it should be large enough to work with easily. Third, the species should have one or more discrete BBs composed of relatively pure endocrine tissue. Fourth, the BBs must be able to tolerate culture at 37°C without undergoing necrosis, degranulation, or loss of function. Fifth, the species should maintain fasting plasma glucose levels in a mammalian range. Sixth, insulin secretion must be glucose dependent. And seventh, the BBs must be able to maintain long-term normoglycemia after transplantation into diabetic nude mice.

This last criterion is an absolute prerequisite to xenograft studies in non-immunocompromised mice. BBs from most teleost species do not function at mammalian body temperatures;[2,8-10] however, insulin leaching from non-viable BB grafts can give the appearance of function for several days after transplantation.[2] In the absence of studies demonstrating long-term graft function after transplantation into diabetic nude mice, it would be

---

impossible to interpret the results of xenotransplantation studies in immunocompetent mice. Specifically, it would be difficult to know whether graft failure was due to technical problems, non-function secondary to the effects of higher mammalian body temperatures, or xenograft rejection.

To date, convincing long-term function of BB grafts has only been demonstrated using two species of tropical fish, *Osphronemus gourami*, i.e., the giant gourami[11,12] (Fig. 11.1A) and *Oreochromis nilotica*, i.e., tilapia[3] (Fig. 11.1B). Undoubtedly, other tropical fish species would make suitable donors for xenograft studies, but additional studies will be required to identify these species. For the purpose of this chapter, we will focus on the latter species because it is the model used in our laboratory.

TILAPIA

Tilapia are members of the family Cichlidae, i.e., cichlids, the second largest family of perciform fish. Classification of tilapia is complicated because there is not uniform agreement on systematology and taxonomy.[13] In fact, our donor species has been placed into two different genera depending upon which classification system is used. The prevailing convention at this time is that the scientific name *Tilapia nilotica* (Linnaeus) has been replaced by *Oreochromis nilotica*; this re-classification is behavioral, rather than morphologic, and is based on the fish's peculiar manner of breeding, i.e., oral incubation or "mouthbrooding". However, the common name remains tilapia.

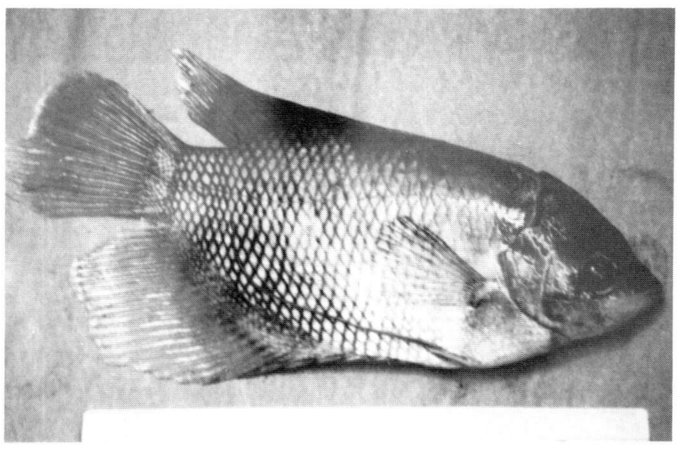

Fig. 11.1A. Osphronemus gourami (compliments of Prof. J. Schrezenmeir).

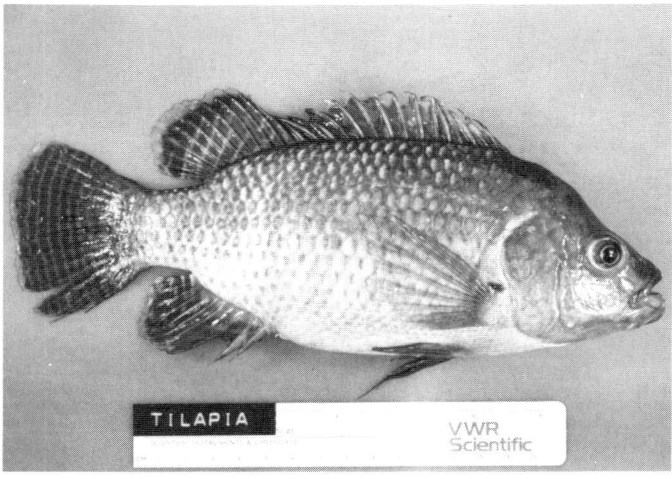

Fig. 11.1B. Tilapia (Oreochromis nilotica).

Tilapia nilotica are omnivorous freshwater fish that are native to Africa and the Middle East, but have been introduced around much of the world by fish farmers.[14,15] They breed easily and grow rapidly, attaining a maximum size of about 75 cm and a weight of about 3 kg. Tilapia flesh is a delicious, mild white meat.

Tilapia usually have 2-6 BBs which are composed of relatively pure endocrine tissue (Fig. 11.2A) and an abundance of beta cells (Fig. 11.2B). Like mammalian islets, tilapia BBs are composed of four endocrine cell types (Figs. 11.3A-C) with the beta cells tending to be centrally located. Tilapia BBs will tolerate mammalian body temperature in vitro and in vivo and will function well after transplantation. The mean fasting plasma glucose levels (+ S.E.M.) of tilapia is 75.4 + 3.0 mg/dL (n = 140).[2]

INTRODUCTION TO METHODS

The methods described and illustrated in this chapter are those used in our laboratory to harvest and culture BBs from tilapia. These methods are equally applicable to harvesting and culturing BBs from Osphronemus gourami. The latter model was developed by Professor Jürgen Schrezenmeir of Mainz, Germany who was the first to harvest, culture, and transplant BBs successfully. The major differences between our methods and those of Schrezenmeir will be reviewed briefly near the end of the chapter. Methods

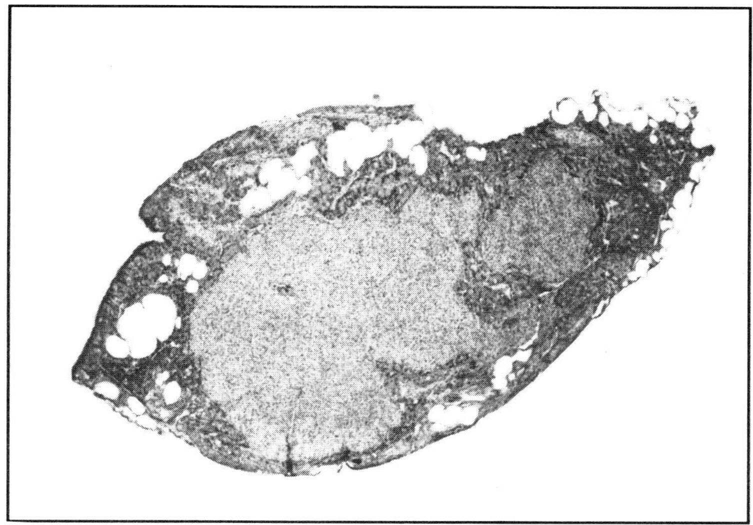

Fig. 11.2A. Histologic section showing one of several BBs from a tilapia. Note that the BB is composed of a central core of relatively pure endocrine tissue surrounded by a capsule containing exocrine and connective tissue (H&E; original magnification, 40x).

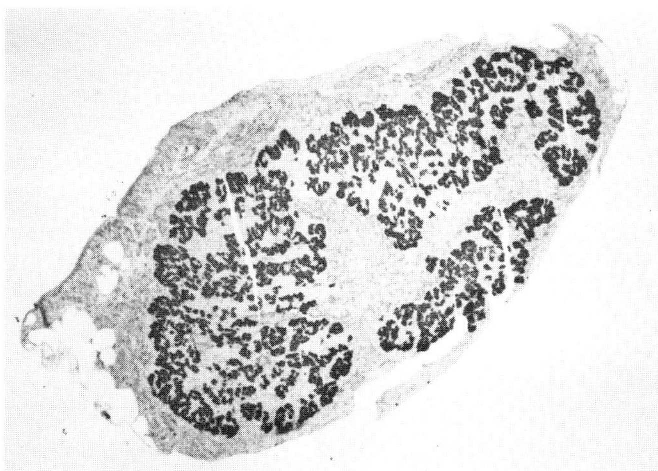

Fig. 11.2B. Section of tilapia BB stained for insulin by immunoperoxidase showing darkly stained beta cells surrounded by a mantle of unstained non-beta cells (original magnification, 40x).

Both Fig. 11.2A and Fig. 11.2B are reproduced with permission from: Wright,Jr., JR. Experimental transplantation using prinicpal islets of teleost fish (Brockmann bodies). In C Ricordi, ed. 1892-1992. One Century of Transplantation for Diabetes. Pancreatic Islet Cell Transplantation, Austin: RG Landes Co., 1992, pp. 336-51.

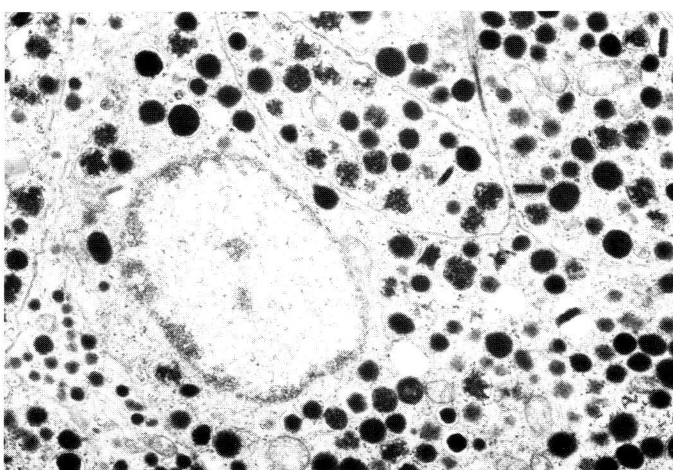

Fig. 11.3A. Electron micrograph showing a beta cell containing insulin granules (12,500x).

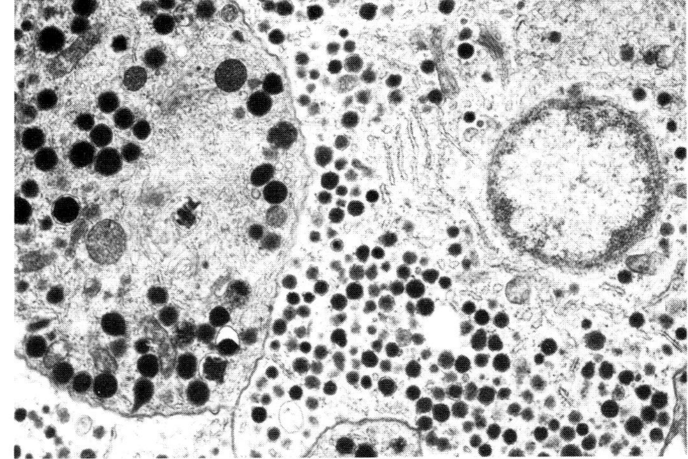

Fig. 11.3B. Electron micrograph showing an alpha cell (glucagon) on the left and a PP cell (pancreatic polypeptide) on the right (12,500x).

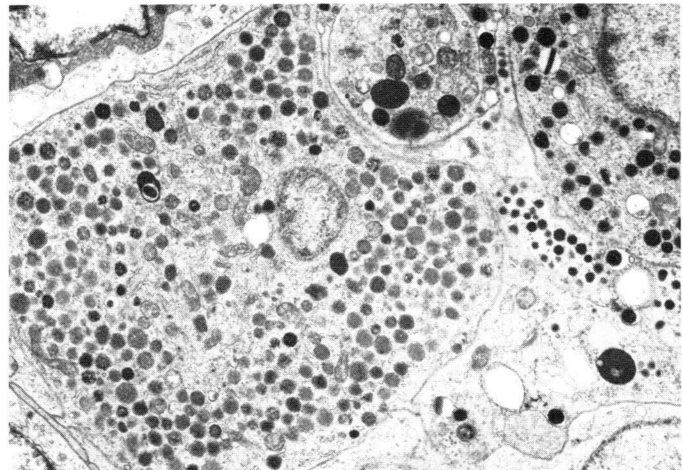

Fig. 11.3C. Electron micrograph showing a delta cell (somatostatin); note that there is a partial beta cell in the upper right corner (8,500x).

for transplantation, preparation of single cells suspensions, and assessment of BB function are described elsewhere and are not included in this chapter.[7]

FISH SUPPLIERS

Commercial suppliers for "research grade" tilapia or gourami are rare to nonexistent. We acquire our tilapia from Dr. Roger Doyle, the Director of the Dalhousie University Marine Gene Probe Laboratory. He breeds tilapia for DNA fingerprinting and other genetic studies but has also been able to supply our needs. On an individual basis, he is willing to supply and ship limited numbers of adult fish or larger numbers of fry. His address is: Dr. Roger W. Doyle, Professor of Biology, Director Marine Gene Probe Laboratory, Dalhousie University, Halifax, Nova Scotia, Canada B3H 4J1; (902) 494-6414, 494-3736 (fax).

Using aquaculture industry literature, I have compiled a list of commercial producers of tilapia nilotica (Table 11.1). However, this list is undoubtedly incomplete and is heavily biased toward North American sources; furthermore, some of these are probably rather large producers who may not be able to sell small numbers of fish for research. Additional information can be acquired by contacting the American Tilapia Association, c/o Curtis Stutzman, Secretary/Treasurer, 4943 Cosgrove Road SW, Kalona, Iowa 52247; (319) 683-2495, 683-2995 (fax).

Compiling a similar list for Osphronemus gourami was more difficult because this fish does not seem to be commercially produced in North America. However, I have identified two North American brokers that can obtain this species; I have also included both of Professor Schrezenmeir's sources (Table 11.2).

PISCINE HUSBANDRY

Our donor tilapia are maintained at 28°C in large fiberglass holding tanks in a fish housing facility located about a mile from our laboratory. They are fed a custom-made feed (Corey Mills, Fredrickton, New Brunswick, Canada) containing whey powder, soya bean meal, whole corn, whole wheat, her-

ring meal, corn oil, brewer's yeast, diocalcium phosphate, vitamin premix, mineral premix, binder, choline chloride, and DL-methionine (pellet size #3).

Several days prior to sacrifice, donor fish are moved to the laboratory. Methods for transporting live fish must be customized based on distances, climate, and the needs of the individual user. We transport five live tilapia (300 gm each) in about 4 gallons of fresh water by sealing then in 10 gallon plastic garbage bags placed inside of 6 gallon plastic buckets. If transporting multiple buckets of fish at one time, we do not seal the plastic bags until all the buckets are loaded with fish and ready for transport. Then we seal the bags by tying a knot in the middle-to-distal portion of the bag leaving a pocket of about one liter of air above the water. Once the bags are sealed, we quickly load them into the back of a truck or car and drive to the laboratory. Tilapia tolerate transportation in this manner for at least 15 minutes except on very hot days when the density of the fish per bucket should be decreased; this is necessary because, as the water temperature increases, its oxygen content decreases and because, at higher water temperatures, the oxygen becomes increasingly difficult for fish to extract.[16]

If longer periods of time are required for transportation, the size of the receptacles used to transport the fish should be increased and/or oxygen should be supplemented. A simple method to supplement oxygen is to flood the plastic bag with oxygen from a cylinder before sealing the bag; this oxygen will tend to diffuse into the water while driving. Another, slightly more complicated, method of oxygenating the water while driving is to bubble air into the buckets using a small portable compressor and a series of plastic hoses attached to a branched connector. On a relatively small scale, this can be accomplished using a compressor designed to inflate automobile tires powered by an automobile cigarette lighter.

Once in the laboratory, the fish are placed in 40 gallon aquariums containing distilled water. We use an AquaClear 300 filtration/aeration system (Rolf C. Hagen, Mansfield,

Table 11.1. Potential sources for *Tilapia niolotica**

North America

American Aquafarms, Inc.
3330 N. Causeway Blvd.
Suite 402
Metairie, LA 72002-3573
USA
800-448-5142/504-830-4848
FAX: 504-830-4704

Aquamar Ind. Inc.
1945 Pocomoke Beltway
Pocomoke City, MD 21851
USA
410-957-0206
FAX: 410-957-0206

ASI Consulting
RRI Box 23
Golden Valley, ND 58541
USA
701-983-4447

Caribbean Marine Research Ctr.
805 East 46th Place
Vero Beach, FL 32358
USA
407-234-9931
FAX: 407-234-9954

East Arkansas Fish Distributors
P.O. Box 361
Hasen, AR 72064
USA
501-255-3455
FAX: 501-673-7499

Gen-Al, Inc.
Box 97474
Raleigh, NC 27624
USA
919-846-8323

Hidrocultivos del Caribe
P.O. Box 1652
Juana Diaz, PR 00795
USA
809-837-5040
FAX: 809-837-5045

AquaFuture, Inc.
Industrial Road
P.O. Box 783
Turners Fall, MA 01376
USA
413-863-8905
FAX: 413-863-3575

Aquatech Int'l Fisheries, Inc.
P.O. Drawer 460
New Smyrna Beach, FL 32170
USA
904-423-1222
FAX: 904-423-1222

Awbrook Aqua Farms
33-08 Newton Sparta Road
Newton, NJ 07860
USA
201-383-5444
FAX: 201-383-8379

Cinvestau - IPN
Calle 21 - A #67
Frac. El Cedral
Merida Yucatan 97200
MEXICO
99-260835

The Fish Factory
312 W. Fresno
Ponca City, OK 74601
USA
405-762-2016

The Gila River Fishery
HCR 1, Box 47F
Dateland, AZ 85333
USA
602-454-2293

Hofstra University Marine Lab
Hofstra University
Hempstead, NY 11550
USA
516-463-5520

Hydrocynth
Route 1, Box 55
Halstad, MN 56548
USA
218-456-2583

Lake Geneva Fisheries
Rt. 1, Box 245
Geneva, AL 36340
USA
205-684-6473

Miami Aqua-culture, Inc.
4606 SW 74 Ave.
Miami, FL 33155
USA
305-262-4430
FAX: 305-262-6701

Oakview Fish Farms
5395 E. St. Rd. 119
Minster, OH 45865
USA
419-628-2474
FAX: 419-628-2472

Willow Branch Fish Farm
Rt. 61, Box 54
Tahlequah, OK 74464
USA
918-868-2802

South America
Acuagranja Ltd.
Avenida 13 No. 137-50
Santafe de Bogota, DC 90811
COLOMBIA, SA
(571) 6250665 - 2581513
FAX: (571) 6250996

Asia
P.T. Aquafarm Nusantara
P.O. Box 239
Solo 57101
INDONESIA
+62-271-48338
FAX: +62-271-42789

Inslee Fish Farm
P.O. Box 207
Connerville, OK 74836
USA
405-836-7150

Manatee Aquaculture, Inc.
P.O. Box 472
Myakka City, FL 34251
USA
813-322-2189
FAX: 813-531-7796

Mississippi Aquaculture
 Biotechnologies
613 Old Riffle Range Road
Petal, MS 39465
601-584-6044

Simaron Freshwater Fish
14019 SW Freeway #340
Sugarland, TX 77478
USA
713-242-3870
FAX: 713-242-3914

Sergio Zimmerman-Brazil
Lucas de Oliveira, 1061 #402
Porto Alegre, RS, 90440-011
BRAZIL
55-51-332-1222
FAX: 55-51-335-8121

San Miguel Foods, Inc.
2F PCPD Bldg.
Nichols Interchange, Makati
Metro Manila, Philippines 1385
PHILLIPPINES
819-4031
FAX: 810-4015

*Based on: Aquaculture Magazine Buyer's Guide '93 and Industry Directory, P.O. Box 2329, Ashville, NC 28802

Table 11.2. Potential sources for *Osphroneumus gourami*

North America		**Europe**	**Asia**
Capay Aquatics	World Wide Fish Farm, USA	Willy Gabert	Dr. Patanakamjorn
102 East Street	90 Lexington Ave.	Auf der Steig	Rajamanjala Institute
Woodland, CA 95695	Suite 7F	Hohenstein	of Techniques
USA	New York, NY 10016	GERMANY	Bangkok
916-662-2811	USA		THAILAND
FAX: 916-662-3762	212-686-6309		
	FAX: 212-685-5789		

MA) and a 300 watt Thermal Compact submersible aquarium heater (Rolf C. Hagen) set at 28°C in each aquarium. When the density of the fish in an aquarium is high, we will often bubble supplemental air into the water by placing a weighted hose connected to the laboratory air supply line. An aquarium set up in this manner will house up to 15-20 tilapia weighing 250-300 gm each for a few days.

Fish maintained in the laboratory are fasted for two reasons. First of all, we determine fasting plasma glucose levels on all donor fish. Secondly, fasted fish do not soil the water in the tanks nearly as quickly, thus saving the time required to clean the aquariums and change the water.

PISCINE ANESTHESIA

Several minutes prior to sacrifice, donor fish are placed in a bucket of water containing anesthesia. We use 2-phenoxyethanol (Sigma, St Louis, P1126) at a dose of roughly 1 ml/L; benzocaine (ethyl p-aminobenzoate, 4-aminobenzoic acid ethyl ester) (Sigma E1501) (200 mg/L) and tricaine (ethyl m-aminobenzoate, 3-aminobenzoic acid ethyl ester) methanesulfonate (Sigma A5040) (200 mg/L) are other popular piscine anesthetic agents. All three agents are quickly absorbed via the gills and the fish become deeply anesthetized in a matter of a few minutes. Fish are anesthetized when they turn "belly up." However, if the fish are returned to fresh water after a brief period of anesthesia, they will fully recover.

One of the benefits of working with tilapia pancreata is that the remainder of the fish is delicious. This creates a dilema because fish terminally anesthetized in this manner are not approved by the U.S. Food and Drug Administration for human consumption. If tilapia filets are desired as a byproduct of a particular donor, the unanesthetized fish can be immobilized by a hammer blow to the head.

HARVESTING BBs

The process of harvesting BBs is well-suited to an assembly line approach but will be described here as if one person is performing all of the steps.

Several donor fish are anesthetized at one time to increase the efficiency of the harvesting process; these are removed from the bucket one at a time for dissection. Immediately prior to dissection, each fish is weighed and given an identifying number. Next, the fish is placed on its left side in a dissecting tray and a blood sample is taken. The simplest method is to remove the tail, immediately proximal to the caudal fin, using a heavy pair of scissors; the blood sample can be collected from the dorsal vein, which runs along the ventral aspect of the vertebral column, using a heparinized capillary tube. The sample is labeled with the fish's identifying number and retained to determine donor plasma glucose levels at a later time.

The donor fish is then placed in a well-illuminated work space and killed by cutting the cervical spinal cord with a scalpel. The peritoneal cavity is widely exposed by cutting along the ventral surface from the anus to the pericardial cavity; this cut is extended dorsally caudal to the right operculum (gill flap) and then caudally along the dorsal aspect of the peritoneal cavity to the anus. Finally, the triangular flap of musculointegumentary tissue bounded by these three cuts is removed (Fig. 11.4A). Care should be exercised when removing this flap because the gallbladder, a useful anatomical landmark, is usually quite dilated and is easily punctured.

The "BB region" can be quickly located by reflecting the omentum, intestines, liver, and, in females, the right ovary away from the peritoneal cavity (Fig. 11.4B); this reveals a roughly triangular shaped region bounded anteriorly by the liver, superiorly by the stomach, and inferiorly by the spleen and gallbladder (Fig. 11.4C). The largest BB is usually embedded in mesentery adjacent to the bile duct near the head of the spleen and smaller BBs are usually scattered throughout the mesentery between the stomach and the spleen; however, BBs may be located anywhere in this triangular region. Identifying the BBs is greatly facilitated by

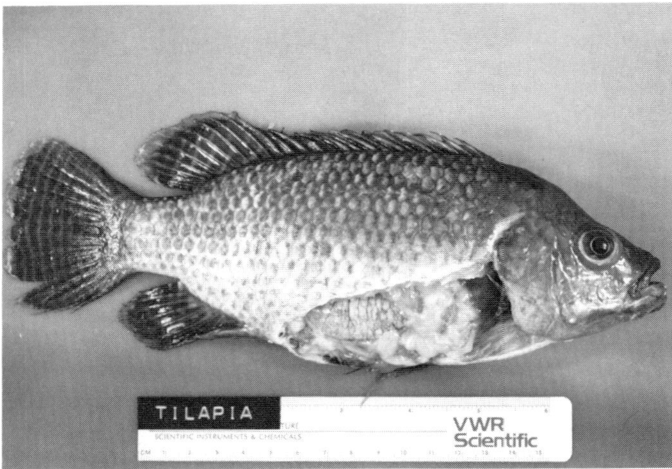

Fig. 11.4A. Tilapia with triangular musculointegumentary flap removed revealing viscera in situ.

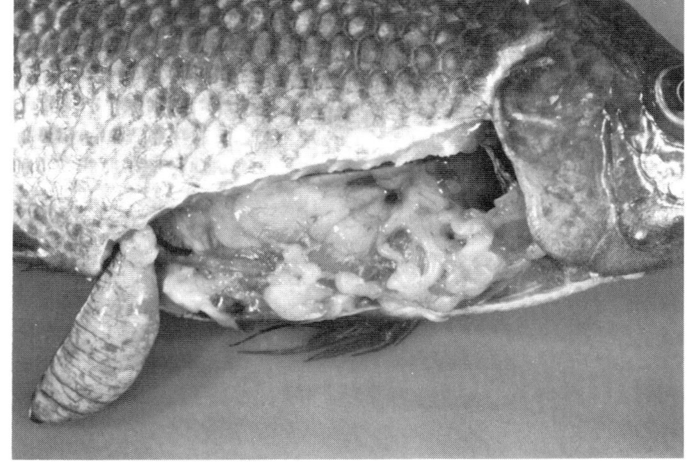

Fig. 11.4B. Layered dissection of a female tilapia with the right ovary reflected downward revealing a fatty omentum somewhat obscuring the remainder of the viscera.

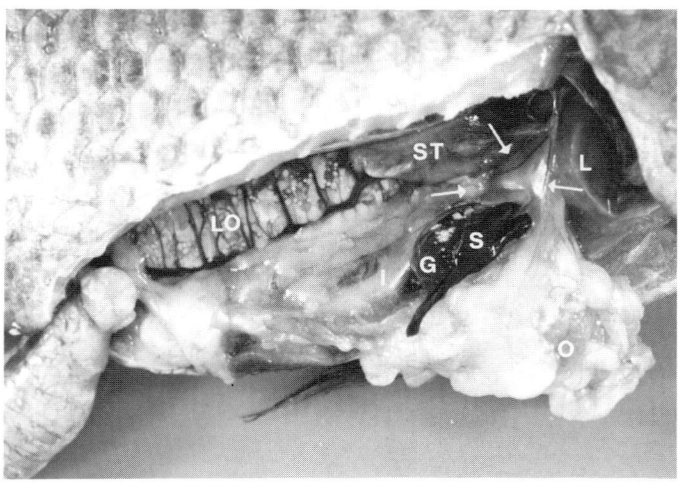

Fig. 11.4C. Layered dissection of female tilapia with the right ovary and the omentum (O) reflected downward. The roughly triangular BB region" is surrounded by the liver (L) anteriorly, stomach (ST) superiorly, and spleen (S) and gall bladder (G) inferiorly and is outlined with arrows. Also labeled is the left ovary (LO).

excellent illumination and, for the visually impaired, surgical loops may be helpful. Once the BBs are identified in situ, the mesentery containing them is excised and placed into a petri dish (Fig. 11.5A) containing Hanks balanced salt solution (HBSS) containing 27 mM HEPES, 200 U/mL penicillin, and 200 µg/mL streptomycin sulfate (Gibco, Grand Island, NY, USA). The dish is then labeled with the fish identifying number, placed in a laminar flow workstation used for micro-dissection (see below), and held at room temperature until any additional donor fish have been processed through these steps. An experienced technician, working alone, can harvest about 15 BB regions per hour.

PREPARATION OF BBs

Once the "BB regions" are harvested from the required number of donor fish (see below), the BBs are cleaned while visualized through a dissecting microscope equipped with both transmitted and incident light as well as a green filter.[17] The "BB regions" are composed of 2-6 BBs embedded in loose connective tissue, mostly adipose tissue. The BBs can be easily visualized within the connective tissue by transillumination. The "BB regions" are simply teased apart and then the BBs are micro-dissected. The only instruments required for this step are sterile microvascular scissors and jeweler's forceps.

Once cleaned (Fig. 11.5B), all BBs from a donor fish are transferred to a clean weighed dish of HEPES-HBSS and then the dish is reweighed; the total weight of the BBs is recorded by fish identifying number. Finally, the BBs are prepared for culture and transplantation by dividing the larger BBs with microvascular scissors to achieve a uniform size of <1mm. An experienced technician can clean and prepare 6-12 "BB regions" per hour.

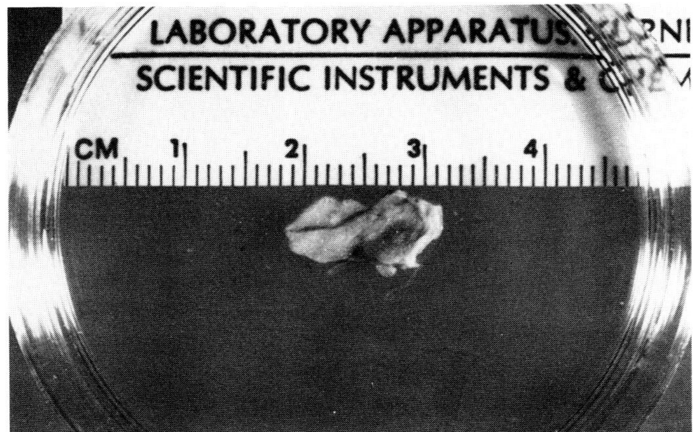

Fig. 11.5A. Excised "BB region" free-floating in petri dish containing HEPES-HBSS.

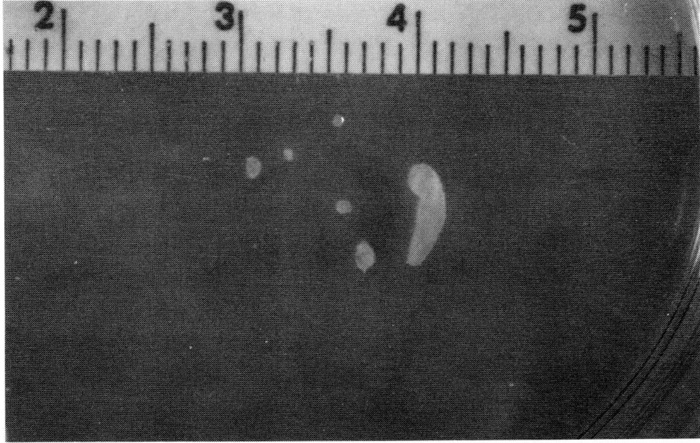

Fig. 11.5B. BBs after microdissection of "BB region" seen in Fig. 11.5A.

Both Fig. 11.5A and Fig. 11.5B are reproduced with permission from: Wright, JR., JR, Schrezenmeir J. Transplantation of fish islets. In C Ricordi, ed. Methods in Cell Transplantation. Austin: RG Landes, 1994 (in press).

DETERMINING NUMBER AND SIZE OF DONOR FISH

In most of our studies, we have transplanted tilapia BB fragments under the kidney capsules of diabetic mice.[3-5] In our hands, the optimal volume of tilapia BB fragments that will insure normoglycemia and minimize the chance of hypoglycemia immediately post transplantation is about 0.05 kg of donor fish body weight per gram of recipient mouse body weight, e.g., a 24 gm recipient mouse would require about 1.2 kg of donor tilapia. The total donor fish body weight can be supplied by one large fish or multiple small fish. For most of our murine transplants, we use 3-5 donor fish weighing 250-500 gm each.

Studies transplanting tilapia BBs into larger animals have not yet been performed. Therefore, no data is available on the numbers and size of donor fish required for these types of studies.

BB CULTURE

After the harvesting and preparing steps are completed, BB fragments from each donor are cultured free-floating in a 60 mm petri dish containing CMRL-1066 medium (Gibco, Grand Island, NY) with 10% fetal calf serum, 2.5 mg/mL D-glucose, 100 U/mL penicillin, and 100 μg/μL streptomycin sulfate. BB fragments are cultured overnight before transplantation at 37°C in a humidified incubator containing 5% CO_2. This allows insulin to leach out of any damaged cells and to permit any exocrine tissue attached to the BB fragments to degenerate prior to transplantation. Once all petri dishes are in the incubator, plasma glucose levels for each donor fish are determined and recorded by donor fish identifying number.

In most of our studies, BB fragments have been transplanted on the day after harvesting.[3-5] However, BB fragments, prepared as described above, will tolerate long-term culture as well as culture conditions commonly used for the purpose of immunomodulation. Specifically, we have cultured tilapia BBs for 1 week under the following conditions without loss of in vivo function after transplantation: (1) 37°C, 5% CO_2/95% air, 1 ATA (atmosphere absolute);

(2) 24°C, 5% CO_2/95% air, 1 ATA; and (3) 37°C, 5% CO_2/95% oxygen, 1 ATA.[18]

PREPARATION OF BBs FROM OSPHRONEMUS GOURAMI

The harvesting and culturing methods used by Schrezenmeir's laboratory in Mainz, Germany differ from our methods in several ways. First, they use a different donor species, Osphronemus gourami. Second, they use younger donor fish weighing 30-60 gm each and they harvest only the largest BB from each donor fish. The advantage of this method is that the BBs are of uniform size and, therefore, do not require subdivision. On the other hand, larger numbers of donor fish (70-100) are required per transplant. Finally, they culture BBs using HEPES rather than CO_2 to maintain an appropriate pH. Each BB is cultured in 2 mL of RPMI 1640 (Biochrom - Seromed, Berlin) containing 100 mg/dl glucose, 20 mM Hepes, 200 mg/L glutamine, 10% v/v fetal calf serum, 100 U/L penicillin, 10 mg/l streptomycin, and 10 mg/L ciprofloxacin (Bayer Leverkusen, Germany). They change the culture media every two days for long-term culture.[7]

SUMMARY

Brockmann bodies (BBs) offer an exciting new model for discordant islet xenotransplantation studies. Tilapia BBs are easily and inexpensively harvested and, when transplanted into diabetic nude mice, will uniformly reverse streptozotocin-induced diabetes, maintain normoglycemia, and produce a normal, mammalian-like glucose tolerance curve. When transplanted into immunocompetent diabetic mice, BBs reject in 7-8 days. Further charactrization of this model should provide many insights into the mechanism of discordant islet xenograft rejection.

ACKNOWLEDGMENTS

I would like to thank Prof. Roger Doyle of Dalhousie University and Mr. Jack Robinson of Mississippi Aquaculture Technologies for supplying tilapia for our studies and Profs. Michael Conlon, Sture Falkmer, Erika Plisetskaya, and Jürgen Schrezenmeir for help and/or advice.

REFERENCES

1. Hering BJ. Islet xenotransplantation. In: Ricordi C, ed. 1892-1992. One Century of Transplantation for Diabetes. Pancreatic Islet Cell Transplantation. Austin: RG Landes Co., 1992.

2. Wright JR Jr. Experimental transplantation using principal islets of teleost fish. In: C Ricordi, ed. 1892-1992. One Century of Transplantation for Diabetes. Pancreatic Islet Cell Transplantation, Austin: RG Landes Co., 1992, pp. 336-51.

3. Wright JR Jr, Polvi S, MacLean H. Experimental transplantation with principal islets of teleost fish (Brockmann bodies): Long-term function of tilapia islet tissue in diabetic nude mice. Diabetes 1992; 41: 1528-32.

4. Wright JR Jr, Kearns H, Polvi S, MacLean H, Yang H. Experimental xenotransplantation using principal islets of teleost fish (Brockmann bodies): Graft survival in selected strains of inbred mice. Transplant. Proc. 1994; 26:770.

5. Wright JR Jr, Kearns H, MacDonald AS. Leflunomide and cyclosporin-A prolong fish-to-mouse islet xenograft survival in balb/c mice. Transplant. Proc. - in press.

6. Falkmer S. Comparative morphology of pancreatic islets in animals. In: Volk BW, Arquilla ER, eds. The Diabetic Pancreas, 2nd ed., New York: Plenum Medical Book Co., 1985, pp. 17-52.

7. Wright JR Jr, Schrezenmeir J. Transplantation of fish islets. In C Ricordi, ed. Methods in Cell Transplantation. Austin: RG Landes, 1994 (in press).

8. Schrezenmeir J, Stürmer W, Gobel D, Krause U, Beyer J. Brockmann-bodies in hollow fibers may solve availability problems for islet transplantation. Life Support Syst. 1985; 3 (suppl. 1): 666-9.

9. Schrezenmeir J, Stürmer W, Gobel D, Boddin J, Laue Ch, Müntefering H, Dienes HP, Krause U, Beyer J. Brockmann bodies in hollow fibers: New way for islet transplantation. In: Brunetti P, Waldhausl WK, eds. Advanced Models for the Therapy of Insulin-Dependent Diabetes, New York: Raven Press, 1987, pp.331-340.

10. Schrezenmeir J, Laue Ch, Boddin J, Gobel D, Sturmer W, Stallmach T, Müntefering H, Beyer J. Brockmann bodies of tropical fishes: A model for islet transplantation. In: Shafrir E, Renold AE, eds. Frontiers in Diabetes Research: Lessons from Animal Diabetes II. London: John Libbey, 1988, pp. 229-232.

11. Schrezenmeir J, Lassak D, Laue Ch, Botens F, Bülow MV, Beyer J. Reversal of STZ-diabetes after transplantation of piscine principal islets to nude mice. Diabetes 1989; 38 (suppl. 1): 106A (abstract).

12. Laue Ch, Kaiser A, Wendl K, Beyer J, Schrezenmeir J. Piscine islet organs normalize fasting and postprandial blood-glucose levels of diabetic nude mice. Diabetes 40 (Suppl 1) 1991; 281A (abstract).

13. Nelson JS. Order Perciformes. Family Cichlidae - cichlids. In: Fishes of the World, 2nd ed., New York: John Wiley & Sons, 1984, pp. 315-317.

14. Jayaram KC. The Freshwater Fish of India, Pakistan, Bangladesh, Burma and Sri Lanka — A handbook. Calcutta, Zoological Survey of India, 1981, pp. 339-40.

15. Mohsin AKM, Ambak MA. Freshwater Fishes of Peninsular Malaysia. Malaysia: Penerbit Universiti Pertanian Malaysia, 1983, pp. 184-6.

16. Wetzl RG. Limnology. Philadelphia: WB Saunders, 1975, pp. 123-41.

17. Fink EH, Lacy PE, Ono J. Use of reflected green light for specific identification of islet in vitro after collagenase isolation. Diabetes 1979; 28: 612-3.

18. Wright JR Jr, Kearns H. Long-term culture, low temperature culture, and hyperoxic culture do not prolong fish-to-mouse islet xenograft survival. - submitted

CHAPTER 12

ISLET CRYOPRESERVATION

Ray V. Rajotte   Jonathan R.T. Lakey

Garth L. Warnock

The therapies presently being used for insulin-dependent diabetes mellitus (IDDM) patients are ineffective in preventing the late complications of the disease. In recent years, clinical islet transplantation has been realized with clear evidence of β-cell function following implantation.[1-5] The best success to date has been when a combination of fresh and cryopreserved islets were transplanted.[1] Cryopreservation of isolated islets is the only realistic way to store islets long-term. Low temperature banking allows for the collection of islets with a wide variety of HLA phenotypes, and also allows for transplantation of islets from multiple donors, which seems to be needed for patients with long-standing diabetes. In addition to storage, cryopreservation offers several other advantages: prolonged storage allows induction of relative allograft unresponsiveness by host manipulation;[6] reduces the requirement for immunosuppression by modulating donor tissue immunogenicity;[7,8] by selectively destroying the unwanted exocrine contaminants;[9] or by the down-regulation of class 1 expression.[10] In addition, low temperature banking allows for quality control testing to ensure the islets are sterile and viable before transplantation.[11]

SMALL AND LARGE ANIMALS

Since 1976 much work has been done on islet cryopreservation when we showed that frozen-thawed transplanted islets were able to normalize diabetic rats.[12] Using adult rat islets, a number of different freezing protocols have been proposed with viability demonstrated both in vivo and in vitro.[13,14]

In vivo success with rodent islets has been with both slow and fast cooling rates.[12,15,16-20] Culture after thawing was found to improve insulin release from the islets,[12,13,21] while Sandler[22] has shown similar effects of culture before freezing. We have found, however, this not to be the case for syngeneic islets transplanted into rats[23] and for human islets isolated from our local donors.[24] However, the use of a culture period before freezing was not found deleterious to in vivo function,[24] and it is reasonable to conclude that if the islets suffer some damage during the isolation procedure, then a prefreeze culture period may optimize survival, particularly with allografted islets.

Pancreatic Islet Transplantation Volume I: Procurement of Pancreatic Islets, edited by Robert P. Lanza, MD, William L. Chick, MD; ©1994 R.G. Landes Company.

We have found that slow cooling to -40°C with rapid thawing from -196°C gives a high percentage survival, with an identical clinical response regardless whether 3000 frozen-thawed or the same number of fresh islets were transplanted beneath the kidney capsule.[25] Using this freezing procedure, dog pancreatic microfragments can normalize carbohydrate metabolism when autografted into totally pancreatectomized dogs[19,26,27] and partially pancreatectomized pigs.[28,29] We found that the temperature of 25°C was important for equilibration of the 2M dimethylsulfoxide (DMSO).[27] Dogs autotransplanted with cryopreserved pancreatic microfragments have been rendered normoglycemic and have had nondiabetic glucose tolerance for up to 2.5 years after transplantation.[26] Using a similar freeze-thaw protocol for purified dog islets, the same number of fresh or cryopreserved syngeneic islets induced long-term normoglycemia.[30] However, an increased number of allogeneic frozen-thawed islets was needed to induce normoglycemia in combination with cyclosporine immunosuppression.[31] This effect could not be attributed to rejection, because insulin secretion persisted in the splenic vein during an intravenous glucose tolerance test 30 days post-transplant.[32] This problem was not observed in cryopreserved allografted mouse islets, which functioned as well as fresh islets when the same number were transplanted.[10] The cryopreserved allografts in this murine model did not appear to be less immunogenic, in contrast with cryopreserved xenografts,[7] although MHC class I expression was reduced.[10]

HUMAN

The methods used to isolate human islets have improved to the point where it is now possible to obtain in excess of 250,000 islets from a single cadaver pancreas.[33-38] When human islets were first frozen, then thawed, they responded to glucose in vitro[39-41] and survived when transplanted beneath the kidney capsule of nude athymic rats.[40] Using this freeze-thaw protocol it has been possible to produce insulin independence long-term when a combination of fresh and cryopreserv-

ed tissue was used as the donor tissue.[42]

Cryopreservation of islets has facilitated the clinical use of this technique. The freezing protocol outlined in this chapter has been used by the author for successful islet cryopreservation in mice[10] (Fig. 12.1), rats[25] (Fig. 12.2), dogs[30,31] (Fig. 12.3 and 12.4), humans[41,42] (Fig. 12.5 and 12.6), and for canine pancreatic microfragments[26] (Fig. 12.7). During freezing and thawing there are three distinct steps which are needed (Fig. 12.8): (1) a prefreeze phase during which the islets are equilibrated with the cryoprotectant; (2) freezing, storage, and thawing; and (3) return of the islets to a physiological medium.

CRYOPRESERVATION PROTOCOL

After isolation the islets are aliquoted into the freezing tube: mouse (300-500); rat (1000-3000); dog (5000-10,000); human (10,000-15,000); and pancreatic fragments (0.5 mL tissue). The final volume of media with cryoprotectant will vary from 0.8 mL to 4.0 mL depending on the number of islets being frozen.

Prefreezing Phase

Following islet isolation, mouse and rat islets are suspended at 22°C in 0.2 mL of Medium 199 (Gibco, Burlington, ON) which is supplemented with 25 mM HEPES, 10% fetal calf serum (v/v), penicillin (100 U/mL), and streptomycin (100 µg/mL). We have found that immediate cryopreservation is well tolerated without loss of islet viability in rats[23] and humans.[24] For dogs and humans, 10,000-15,000 islets are suspended in 1 mL of Medium 199. To these islets, DMSO is added stepwise as shown in Figure 12.9, with time allowed between the steps for equilibration with the cryoprotectant to occur.

For the mice and rats, groups of 500-3000 islets suspended in 0.2 mL Medium 199 with 25 mM HEPES, 10% fetal calf serum (v/v), penicillin (100 U/mL), and streptomycin (100 µg/mL) are aliquoted to each freezing tube. For dogs and humans, 10-15,000 islets suspended in 1.0 mL of the same medium are aliquoted to each tube. The 2M DMSO is then added in a volume of

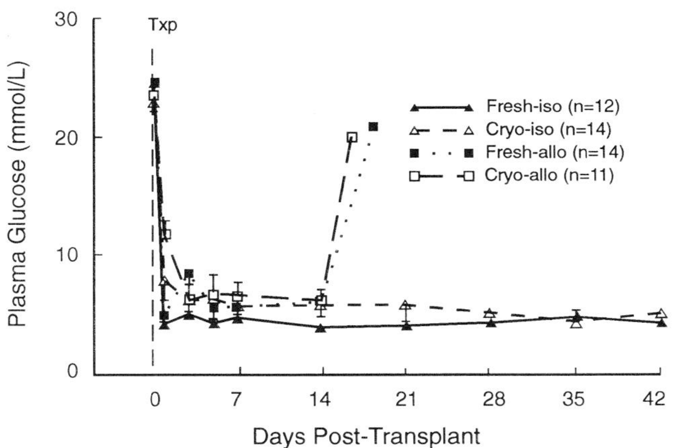

Fig. 12.1. Nonfasting blood glucose concentration (mean ± SEM) after transplantation of nonimmunosuppressed Balb/c mouse recipients of 400 fresh and frozen/thawed islet iso- and allografts. Txp, day of transplant.

Fig. 12.2. Plasma glucose (mg/dL) (mean ± SEM) of diabetic rats after syngeneic islet transplantation. Three thousand hand-picked islets were implanted beneath the kidney capsule immediately after isolation (n = 6) (O – O) or after cryopreservation (n = 7) (■ – ■). Txp = day of transplant. Sz, induction of diabetes.

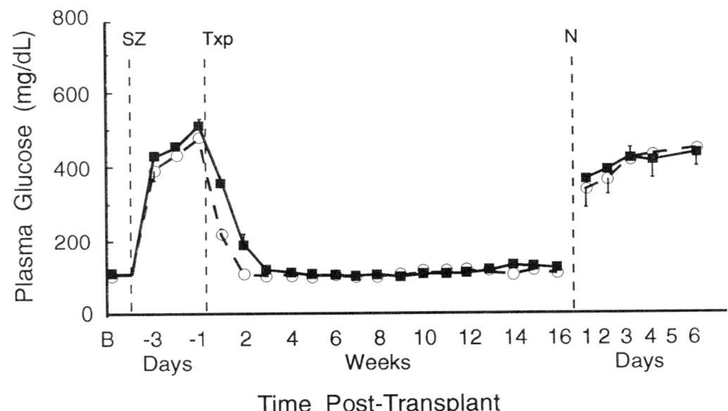

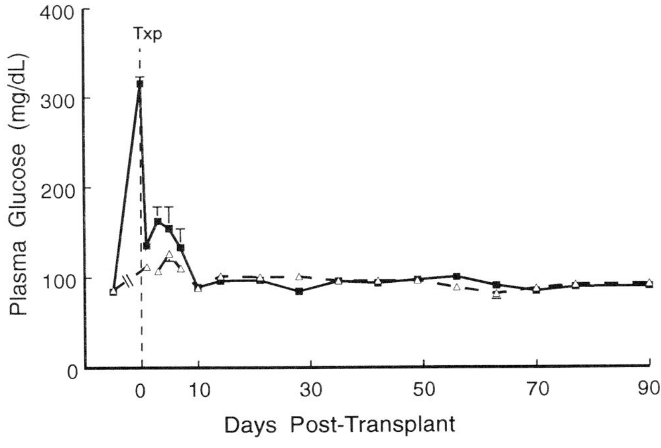

Fig. 12.3. Mean fasting plasma glucose (mg/dL) during the first 3 months after autoimplantation of cryopreserved pure islets into pancreatectomized dogs. The response in dogs that received cryopreserved islets (n = 7) (■ – ■) is similar to that observed in dogs that received a similar quantity of nonfrozen isolated islets (n = 7) (Δ – Δ). Txp, day of transplant.

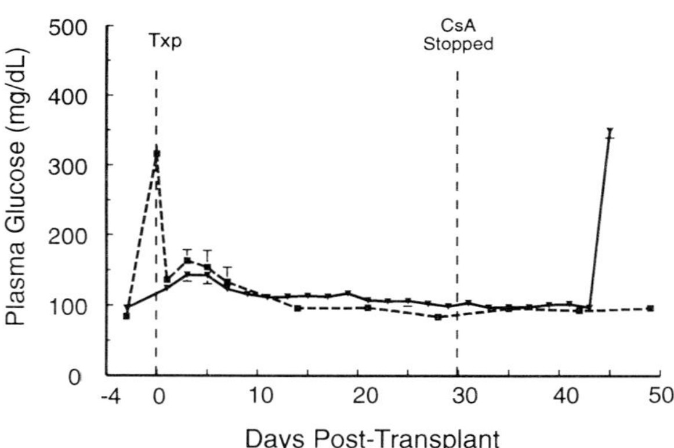

Fig. 12.4. Mean (± SEM) fasting plasma glucose concentration in five recipients of an autograft without cyclosporine A (■ − −■) and six immunosuppressed recipients of a multidonor allograft of augmented endocrine volume and cyclosporine A (▼ − ▼). Txp, day of transplant. CsA, cyclosporine A.

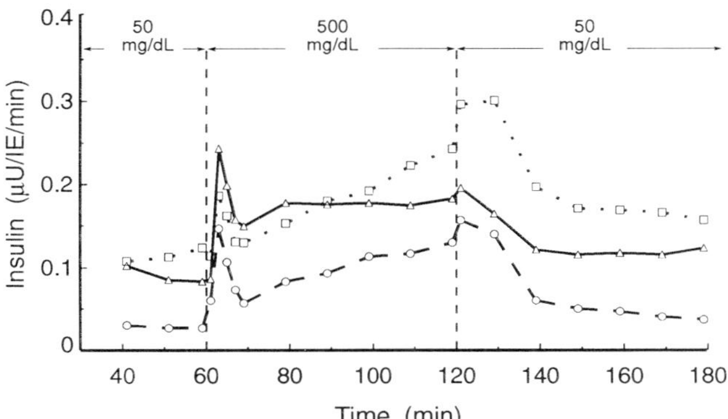

Fig. 12.5. Insulin release (µU/islet/ min, mean ± SEM) from frozen/ thawed islets of one human donor during periods of glucose stimulation (50 and 500 mg/dL). Islets immediately after thaw (❑− − −❑), and after 24 hours in tissue culture (Δ − Δ). For comparison, nonfrozen islets from same donor (O − O).

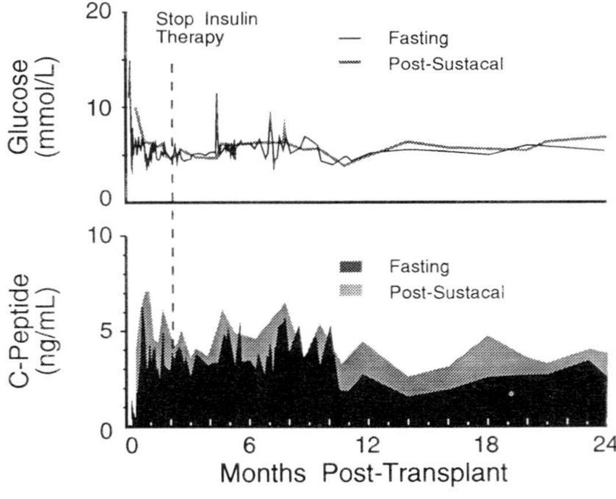

Fig. 12.6. Islet function (serum C-peptide levels) during 2 years of follow-up in a patient transplanted with approximately 600,000 islets (fresh plus cryopreserved). Insulin independence was achieved by 9 weeks, serum glucose remained in the normal range, except during therapy for renal rejection episodes at 18, 24, and 30 weeks.

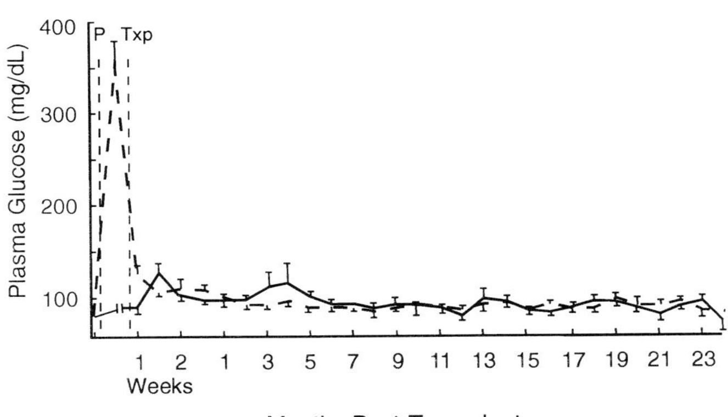

Fig. 12.7. Plasma glucose (mg/dL), mean ± SEM in pancreatectomized dogs who received intrasplenic autografts of pancreatic microfragments. Dogs transplanted with nonfrozen grafts (—) and cryopreserved tissue (----). P, Pancreatectomy; T, day of transplant.

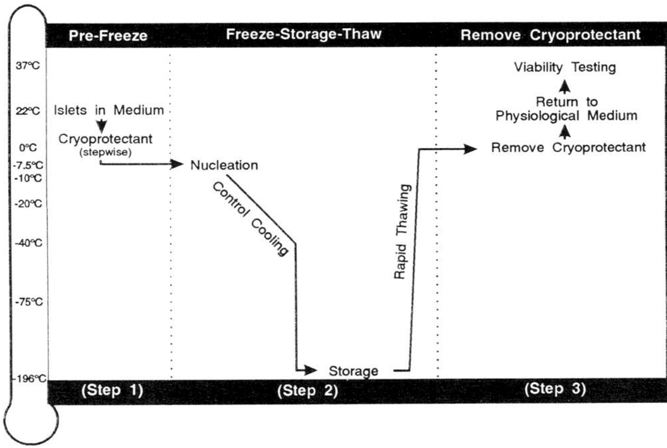

Fig. 12.8. Flow diagram indicating the three distinct steps that are needed for cryopreservation of islets.

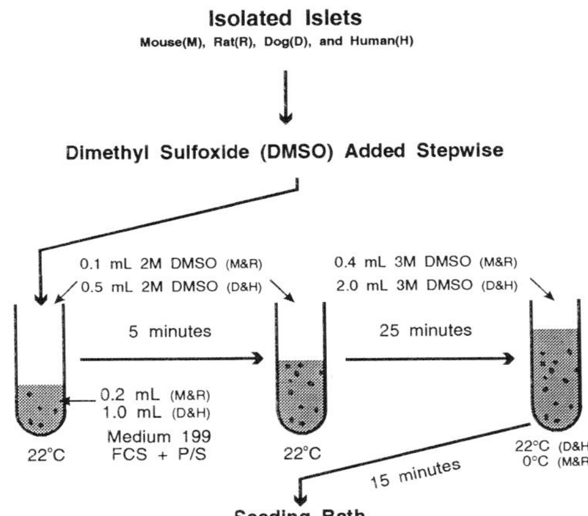

Fig. 12.9. Detailed protocol for addition of the cryoprotectant DMSO. M, mice; R, rats; D, dog; H, human.

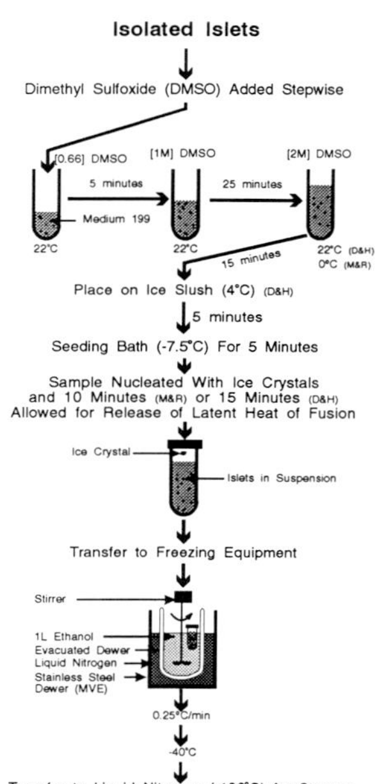

Fig. 12.10. Freezing protocol showing the addition of the cryoprotectant, nucleation and, after the release of the latent heat of fusion, transfer of the tubes to the freezing apparatus for control cooling of 0.25 °C/min.

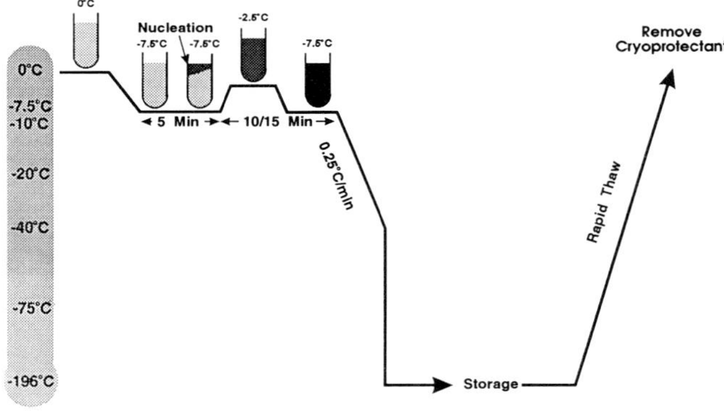

Fig. 12.11. Detailed protocol for nucleation step. After the final equilibration with the 2M DMSO, the samples are supercooled to -7.5 °C, held for 5 minutes at this temperature, and then nucleated with an ice crystal to ensure freezing of the samples. Following nucleation, the temperature of the samples rise back up to the freezing point of the 2M DMSO (≈ -2.5 °C) and remains there until all the latent heat of fusion is released. Only then will the temperature drop back down to -7.5 °C. After nucleation, mouse and rat islets are held at -7.5 °C for 10 minutes and the dog and human islets for 15 minutes. All the samples are then cooled slowly (0.25 °C/min) to -40 °C and then placed in liquid nitrogen for storage.

0.1 mL (mice and rats) and 0.5 mL (dogs and humans) (Fig. 12.9). The temperature is maintained at 22°C and 5 minutes is allowed for equilibration, then further aliquots of 0.1 mL (mice and rats) or 0.5 mL (dogs and humans) of 2M DMSO is added at 22°C and a further 25 minutes is allowed for equilibration. Finally, 0.4 mL for mice and rats or 2 mL for dogs and humans of 3M DMSO is added and 15 minutes allowed for final equilibration. During this step, the temperature is reduced to 0°C for mice and rats and is maintained at 22°C for dogs and humans; the latter are then transferred to 0°C for 5 minutes. All the tubes are then transferred to the seeding bath of 95% ethanol (-7.5° C).

Fig. 12.12. Detailed protocol for thawing and removal of cryoprotectant. When slow cooling of 0.25°C/min is used to −40°C, rapid thawing is needed from −196°C for maximal survival.

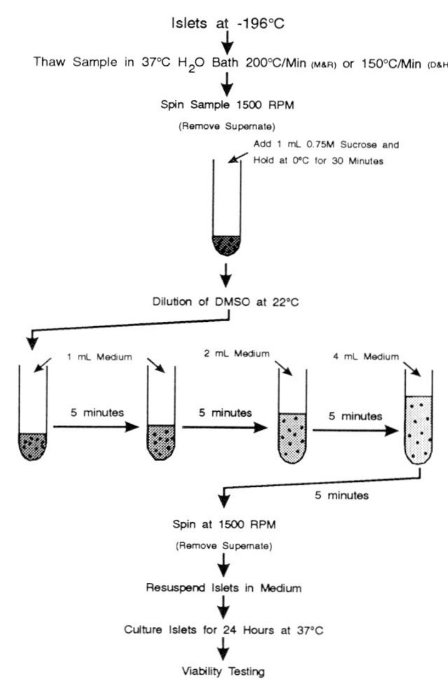

Fig. 12.13. Typical response when human islets are transplanted beneath the kidney capsule of diabetic streptozotocin-induced Balb/c nu/nu mice. When the human islets are transplanted, the plasma glucose returns to normal by 10–15 days post-transplant. When the kidney bearing the graft is removed (N) the animal becomes hyperglycemic proving conclusively that the transplanted islets had normalized the animal.

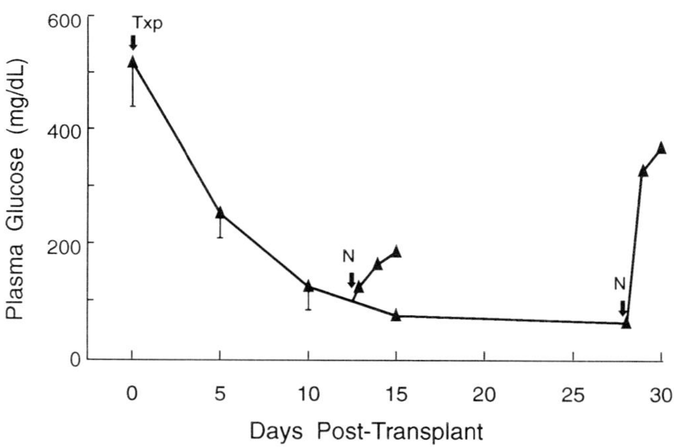

Freezing and Thawing

These steps are detailed in Figures 12.10-12.12. Once the tubes are transferred to the seeding bath, they are held at this temperature for 5 minutes. To ensure uniform cooling of all the freezing tubes, a nucleation step is used as outlined in Figure 12.11. Once the samples have supercooled to -7.5°C (approximately 5 minutes), the tube is gently agitated to suspend the islets in the freezing solution. Nucleation of mouse and rat islets is accomplished by touching the outside of the test tube at the meniscus of the solution with a metal rod which is taken from liquid nitrogen. For the dog and human islets (because of the larger number of tubes being frozen) nucleation is accomplished by touching the side of the freezing tube on a stainless steel coil that has liquid nitrogen circulating through it using an FTS pump (CP-10A-I; FTS System Inc., Stoneridge, NY, USA). After nucleation, the tubes are kept in the seeding bath (-7.5°C) for 10 minutes (0.8 mL tubes) and 15 minutes (4 mL tubes) for release of the latent heat of fusion.

When all the samples are frozen they are then transferred to an evacuated freezing dewar (manufactured at the University of Alberta, Edmonton), which gives a controlled cooling rate of 0.25°C/min from -7.5°C to -40°C (Fig. 12.10). The glass dewar is placed in an MVE (Model G-1, MVE; Cryogenics, New Prague, MN) stainless steel dewar which is filled with liquid nitrogen at roughly the 5 minute point during the step addition of the DMSO. Placing the dewar in the nitrogen at this point ensures that the temperature of the ethanol is at -7.5°C when the samples are transferred from the seeding bath to the freezing dewar. The tubes are placed in the freezing dewar and during controlled cooling the ethanol is mixed to ensure uniform cooling. Using this freezing device, a linear cooling rate of 0.25°C/min can be obtained from -7.5 to -40°C. Once -40°C is reached, the test tubes are removed from the freezing dewar and plunged into liquid nitrogen. For low temperature storage the test tubes are then placed on freezing canes, which identify the samples to facilitate retrieval from the storage vessels. The canes (with test tube) are then transferred to the liquid nitrogen storage vessel.

Figure 12.12 outlines the thawing procedure. When slow cooling of 0.25°C/min is used to -40°C, rapid thawing is needed from -196°C for maximal survival. The tubes are taken from storage and placed in a styrofoam container that is filled with liquid nitrogen. The level of the nitrogen is just below the cap to ensure the samples remain frozen and also prevent liquid nitrogen that may be trapped in the tube from boiling. When all the tubes are transferred to the styrofoam container, the caps are loosened and the liquid nitrogen is poured off. The tubes are recapped loosely and agitated quickly in a 37°C water bath just until the last piece of ice disappears (0°C), at which point they are transferred to an ice slush solution (0°C) until all the tubes are thawed. This procedure gives a thawing rate of 150-200°C/min (0.8 mL and 4 mL volume), which as mentioned is needed when a slow cooling rate of 0.25°C/min is used to -40°C.

REMOVAL OF THE CRYOPROTECTANT

Once all the tubes are thawed, they are centrifuged at 450*g* and the 2M DMSO removed as shown in Figure 12.12. One milliliter of 0.75M sucrose is added at 0°C and the tubes kept in an ice slush for 30 minutes. The sucrose is then serially diluted as shown in Figure 12.12 with 5 minutes allowed between steps. All the tubes are then centrifuged, the supernatant removed, and the islets transferred to an isotonic medium and readied for in vitro testing or transplantation.

VIABILITY TESTING AND QUALITY CONTROL

Viability testing is critical to ensure the islets have survived the freeze-thaw insult. There are several ways to assess islet function following cryopreservation. The two methods we use is to measure the dynamic response of the islets to glucose and the ability of the islets to normalize a diabetic recipient.

For in vitro measurement of insulin release, medium containing glucose is perifused around a known number of islets during three consecutive 60 minute periods as follows: initially 50 mg/dL glucose; then 500 mg/dL; and finally 50 mg/dL. Before in vitro viability testing we have found that a post-thaw culture period of 48 hours in RPMI (mice and rats) or CMRL 1066 (dogs and humans) supplemented with 10% fetal calf serum with penicillin and streptomycin at 37°C in a humidified atmosphere of 95% air plus 5% CO_2, optimizes the glucose mediated insulin response. In this culture system, the glucose concentration should be maintained at 8-10 mM/L .[43] This period of time at 37°C may allow for metabolic recovery of the islets. Using this approach a biphasic insulin response can be detected in response to high glucose levels (Fig. 12.5). Insulin secretion returns to basal levels when perifusate is returned to low glucose.

A second method of viability assessment is by transplantation. For mice (Fig. 12.1) and rats (Fig. 12.2), islets are transplanted as autografts or allografts into chemically-induced diabetic animals. After a period of hyperglycemia, a known number of islets are implanted into the liver via the portal vein or beneath the kidney capsule. The animals are examined daily (allograft) or weekly (autograft) for urine volume, urine glucose, plasma glucose, and body weight. For dogs (Fig. 12.3 and 12.4), a total pancreatectomy is performed before auto- or allotransplantation of the frozen-thawed islets which is carried out by reflux into the splenic vein.[44] For human islets, athymic nude mice are used to assess the in vivo function (Fig. 12.12). Quantitative studies of human islets that survived using this protocol show 80% of the original insulin content can be removed from the kidney of nude rats after implantation of cryopreserved islets.[45]

In carrying out our clinical trials of isolated human islets in which fresh and cryopreserved islets were used, pretransplant viability testing of the islets was by glucose perifusion and transplantation into diabetic nude mice. One tube which had 3000-5000 islets from each isolation was thawed and tested for viability and sterility before transplantation.[11]

CONCLUSION

Indefinite storage of islets is possible by cryopreservation. The methods outlined in this chapter have been used to successfully freeze islets from most species. When using a defined freeze-thaw protocol it is essential that all the steps be followed carefully as any change in one of the steps can and will affect the final outcome. It is also important that viability testing be carried out before clinical use to ensure the islets respond physiologically and have no microbiologic contamination. Cryopreservation of islets is the only reliable way for long-term storage, which will facilitate the clinical use of islet transplantation.

ACKNOWLEDGMENTS

The authors wish to thank Ms. C. Gardner for preparation of the manuscript. This work was supported by the Alberta Foundation for Diabetes Research, the Edmonton Civic Employees' Charitable Assistance Fund, the Muttart Diabetes Research and Training Center, and the Medical Research Council of Canada.

REFERENCES

1. Warnock GL, Kneteman NM, Ryan E, et al. Normoglycaemia after transplantation of freshly isolated and cryopreserved pancreatic islets in type 1 (insulin-dependent) diabetes mellitus. Diabetologia 1991; 34:55.
2. Scharp DW, Lacy PE, Santiago JV, et al. Results of our first nine intraportal islet allografts in type 1 insulin-dependent diabetic patients. Transplantation 1991; 51:76.
3. Socci C, Falqui L, Davalli AM, et al. Fresh human islet transplantation to replace pancreatic endocrine function in type 1 diabetic patient. Acta Diabetol. 1991; 28:151.
4. Gores PF, Najarian JS, Stephanian E, et al. Insulin independence in type I diabetes after transplantation of unpurified islets from single donor with 15-deoxyspergualin. Lancet 1993; 341:19.
5. Alejandro R, Burke G, Shapiro ET, et al. Long term survival of intraportal islet allografts in type I diabetes mellitus. In: Pancreatic Islet Cell Transplantation (Ricordi C, ed.). R.G. Landes, Austin, Texas, 1992; 410.
6. Gray DW, Reece-Smith H, Fairbrother B, et al. Isolated pancreatic islet allografts in rats rendered immunologically unresponsive to renal allografts: the effect of the site of transplantation. Transplantation 1984; 37:434.
7. Coulombe MG, Warnock GL, Rajotte RV. Prolongation of islet xenograft survival by cryopreservation. Diabetes 1987; 36:1086.

8. Bretzel RG, Blum BE, Holl E, Hering BJ, Federlin K. Rat islet allograft survival following different immunomodulative and immunosuppressive treatments. In: The Immunology of Diabetes Mellitus (Jaworski MA, Molnar GD, Rajotte RV, Singh B, eds.). Elsevier Science Publishers B.V., 1986; 181.

9. Evans MG, Rajotte RV, Warnock GL, et al. Cryopreservation purifies canine pancreatic microfragments. Transplant. Proc. 1987; 19:3471.

10. Cattral MS, Warnock GL, Kneteman NM, et al. The effect of cryopreservation on the survival and MHC antigen expression of murine islet allografts. Transplantation 1993; 55:159.

11. Lakey JRT, Warnock GL, Rajotte RV. Quality control issues for the maintenance of sterility in the human islet isolation laboratory. In: Methods in Cell Transplantation (Ricordi C, Warnock GL, eds.). R.G. Landes Company, Austin, Texas. IN PRESS.

12. Rajotte RV, Stewart HL, Voss WAG, et al. Viability studies in frozen-thawed rat islets of Langerhans. Cryobiology 1977; 14:116.

13. Schatz H (Chairman). In: Federlin K, Bretzel RG, eds. Islet isolation, culture and cryopreservation. Thieme-Stratton, Stuttgart, New York, 1981; 124.

14. Bank HL, ed. Cryobiology of isolated islets of Langerhans, Circa 1982. Cryobiology 1983; 20:119.

15. Rajotte RV, Scharp DW, Downing R, et al. Pancreatic islet banking: the transplantation of frozen-thawed rat islets transported between centers. Cryobiology 1981; 18:357.

16. Bank HL, Davis RF, Emerson D. Cryogenic presentations of isolated rat islets of Langerhans: effect of cooling and warming rates. Diabetologia 1979; 16:195.

17. Bretzel RG, Schneider J, Dobroschke J, et al. Islet transplantation in experimental diabetes of the rat: cryopreservation of rat and human islets. Horm. Metab. Res. 1980; 12:274.

18. Andersson A, Sandler S. Viability tests of cryopreserved endocrine pancreatic cells. Cryobiology 1983; 20:161.

19. Rajotte RV, Warnock GL, Kneteman NM. Cryopreservation of insulin-producing tissue in rats and dogs. World J. Surg. 1984; 8:179.

20. Rajotte RV, DeGroot TJ. Effects of warming rate on slowly cooled islets. Cryobiology 1986; 23:572.

21. Ferguson J, Allsopp RH, Taylor RMR, Johnston IDA. Isolation and presentation of islets from the mouse, guinea pig, and human pancreas. Br. J. Surg. 1976; 63:767.

22. Sandler S, Andersson A. The significance of culture for successful cryopreservation of isolated pancreatic islets of Langerhans. Cryobiology 1984; 21:503.

23. Warnock GL, Rajotte RV. Effects of precryopreservation culture on survival of rat islets transplanted after slow cooling and rapid thawing. Cryobiology 1989; 26:103.

24. Lakey JRT, Warnock GL, Kneteman NM, et al. Effects of pre-cryopreservation culture on human islet recovery and in vitro function. Transplant. Proc. (in press)

25. Coulombe MG, Warnock GL, Rajotte RV. Reversal of diabetes by transplantation of cryopreserved rat islets of langerhans to the renal subcapsular space. Diab. Res. 1988; 8:9.

26. Kneteman NM, Rajotte RV, Warnock GL. Long-term normoglycemia in pancreatectomized dogs transplanted with frozen/thawed pancreatic islets. Cryobiology 1986; 23:214.

27. Rajotte RV, Warnock GL, Bruch RC, Procyshyn AW. Transplantation of cryopreserved and fresh rat islets and canine pancreatic fragments: comparison of cryopreservation protocols. Cryobiology 1983; 20:169.

28. Wise MH, Gordon C, Johnson RWG. Intraportal autotransplantation of cryopreserved porcine islets of Langerhans. Cryobiology 1985; 22:359.

29. Wise MH, Yates A, Gordon C, Johnson RWG. Subzero preservation of mechanically prepared porcine islets of Langerhans: response to a glucose challenge in vitro. Cryobiology 1983; 20:211.

30. Evans MG, Warnock GL, Kneteman NM, Rajotte RV. Reversal of diabetes in dogs by transplantation of pure cryopreserved islets. Transplantation 1990; 50:202.

31. Cattral MS, Warnock GL, Evans MG, Rajotte RV. Transplantation of purified frozen/thawed canine pancreatic islet allografts with cyclosporine. Transplantation 1991; 52:457.

32. Daudi FA, Warnock GL, Cattral MS, et al. Islet banking: transplantation of cryopreserved canine islet auto- and allografts. 59th Annual Meeting of the Royal College of Physicians and Surgeons of Canada (Toronto, Ontario, September 14-17, 1990). Can. J. Surg. 33:322 (#262), 1990 (abstract).

33. Gray DWR, McShane P, Grant A, Morris PJ. A method for isolation of islets of Langerhans from the human pancreas. Diabetes 1984; 33:1055.

34. Scharp DW, Lacy PE. Human islet isolation and transplantation. Diabetes 1985; 34(Suppl.1):5A.

35. Rajotte RV, Warnock GL, Evans MG, et al. Isolation of viable islets of Langerhans from collagenase-perfused canine and human pancreata. Transplant. Proc. 1987; 19:918.

36. Warnock GL, Rajotte RV, Evans MG, et al. Isolation of islets of Langerhans following cold storage of human pancreas. Transplant. Proc. 1987; 19:3466.

37. Alejandro R, Mintz DH, Noel J, et al. Islet cell transplantation (TX) in type-I diabetes mellitus. Transplant. Proc. 1987; 19:2359.

38. Alderson D, Scharp DW, Kneteman NM. The isolation of purified human islets of Langerhans. Transplant. Proc. 1987; 19:196.

39. Kneteman NM, Rajotte RV. Isolation and cryopreservation of human pancreatic islets. Transplant. Proc. 1986; 18:182.

40. Warnock GL, Gray DWR, Morris PJ. Transplantation of cryopreserved isolated adult human islets of Langerhans into nude rats. Surg. Forum 1986; 37:334.

41. Warnock GL, Gray DWR, McShane P, et al. Survival of cryopreserved isolated adult human pancreatic islets of Langerhans. Transplantation 1987; 44:75.

42. Warnock GL, Kneteman NM, Ryan EA, et al. Long-term follow-up after transplantation of insulin-producing pancreatic islets into patients with type 1 (insulin-dependent) diabetes mellitus. Diabetologia 1992; 35:89.

43. Sandler S, Andersson A. The significance of culture for successful cryopreservation of isolated pancreatic islets of Langerhans. Cryobiology 1984; 21:503.

44. Warnock GL, Rajotte RV, Procyshyn AW. Normoglycemia after reflux of islet-containing pancreatic fragments into the splenic vascular bed in dogs. Diabetes 1983; 32:452.

45. Sutton R, Warnock GL, McWhinnie DL, et al. Expression of HLA in isolated human pancreatic islets and cryopreservation. Br. J. Surg. 1986; 73:1026.

CHAPTER 13

QUANTITATIVE AND QUALITATIVE ASSESSMENT OF ISLETS

Richard G. Bretzel   Bernhard J. Hering

Konrad F. Federlin

Replacement of the patient's islets of Langerhans either by pancreas transplantation or by isolated islet transplantation is the only treatment of Type 1 diabetes mellitus to achieve a constant normoglycemic state. The demonstration of insulin independence following intraportal adult islet allotransplantations into C-peptide negative diabetic patients has to be regarded as a major achievement in diabetes care, in transplantation and in human medicine in general.[1] Islet cell transplantation offers potential advantages over pancreas transplantation.[2,3] It is a minor rather than a major surgical procedure, and islet cells potentially can be altered in vitro or isolated in devices to obviate the need for post-transplant immunosuppression.[2,3] Furthermore, if animal islet cell transplantation proves successful, the supply of islet cells is potentially much greater than the supply of whole human glands. The outcome of either pancreas or islet transplantation has to be measured in several ways: patient life expectancy, graft functional survival, i.e., insulin independence, normalcy of the patient's metabolic state, impact on diabetic complications, and patient's quality of life.[3]

However, islet cell transplantation is still a clinical investigational procedure and several centers are currently at the early beginning of clinical islet isolation and transplantation programs. Therefore, guidelines were set for human islet quality control in order to facilitate clinical islet transplant programs, to make results from various centers more comparable and finally, and to facilitate future multicenter studies.[4]

Several quality control measures (Table 13.1) need to be evaluated to ascertain whether an islet preparation merits transplantation into a patient. Before organ donation, (pre-donation) factors such as pancreas procurement and distension have to be considered, and parameters such as islet yield in terms of islet number and islet volume, islet purity, islet viability, and islet sterility must be assessed. The most crucial point will be the transplantability, or what in vitro parameter best predicts the in vivo endocrine effect after islet transplantation?

Pancreatic Islet Transplantation Volume I: Procurement of Pancreatic Islets, edited by Robert P. Lanza, MD, William L. Chick, MD; ©1994 R.G. Landes Company.

Table 13.1. Islet quality control testing

- Islet Quantity
  - Counting by size
  - Islet equivalent count
  - Islet volume
- Islet Purity
  - Determined by dithizone stain
- Islet Viability and Function
  - Counting living and dead islets
  - In vitro
    - Perifusions
    - Insulin Stimulation Index
  - In vivo
    - Rodent Transplants
- Islet Sterility
  - Samples
    - Donor Pancreas
    - Reagents
    - Processing Steps
    - Preserved Islets
    - Culture Media
  - Testing
    - Filtration Culture
    - 24°C + 37°C
    - Bacteria + Fungus

PRE-ORGAN DONATION FACTORS, PANCREAS PROCUREMENT AND DISTENSION

The impact of pre-organ donation factors on the outcome of islet isolation has been addressed elsewhere and recently studied in a small number of organ donors.[5,6] It appeared that young (<21 yr) donor age, low body mass index (<21), blood glucose levels above 10 mM/L (it should be mentioned that hyperglycemia more often reflects insulin resistance and central dysregulation of the brain-death donor than does beta-cell failure), and prolonged intensive care management are associated with significantly reduced or lower islet yields, whereas increased serum amylase levels are not associated with low islet yields.[6-8]

Critical issues of human pancreas procurement are the warm ischemia time, which should be as short as possible; an in situ vascular perfusion with cold University of Wisconsin (UW) solution which appears superior to, e.g., Eurocollins; no overperfusion

and no intrapancreatic venous hypertension; cold ischemia time of no more than 12 hr and, interestingly, no less than 2 hr; and a well-preserved pancreatic capsule that allows subsequent intraductal collagenase distension.[5-12]

At present, most centers with experience in human adult islet isolations prefer to start the pancreas dispersion procedure with intraductal administration of collagenase followed by an automated digestion-filtration using recirculating collagenase solution.[13-16] A critical factor in the successful isolation of islets is the collagenase reagent but it will not be discussed in detail here. The persistent problems with and the lack of standardized formulations of collagenase preparations have been recently addressed.[17]

ISLET NUMBER AND VOLUME

Based on calculations from historical and more recent work the average human pancreas, weighing 70 g, contains between 305,000 and 1.5 million islets of 150 μm equivalent diameter (IEQ),[4] corresponding to between 0.5% and 4% of the total pancreatic volume.[18-21] In case of absence of any form of insulin resistance including diabetogenic immunosuppressive substances such as cortison and cyclosporine A, a minimum of 265,000 human adult islets (3500 kg body weight of the recipient) may be enough to produce insulin independence with perfect metabolic control (fasting blood glucose, glycated hemoglobin, oral glucose test) after intraportal islet autotransplantation as demonstrated in patients after undergoing total pancreatectomy.[22] However, islets to be transplanted into Type 1 diabetic patients more often will be confronted with an environment characterized by long-lasting glucose toxicity and microangiopathy (perhaps also in the portal system) insulin-resistance, and autoimmune disease recurrence. It is therefore not surprising that the minimal number of islets required to render an adult Type 1 diabetic patient insulin independent has been about 8000 IEQ/kg.[23]

The sampling technique represents a critical factor that could affect the results of an islet count as well as insulin content from any islet preparation. It is preferable to collect multiple samples, e.g., five aliquots of 100 μL after suspension of the islet preparation in a 200 mL flask. As a specific stain for islet tissue, dithizone (DTZ), which stains zinc in the insulin granules and results in a characteristic red stain, proved to be most appropriate. An easy and rapid way to stain islets is to add a few drops of freshly prepared and filtered (4 - 5 - 8 μ) solution. The solution is prepared as follows. Add 50 mg DTZ to 5 mL dimethylsulfoxide (DMSO) stock solution, and dilute 1 mL of this solution with 20 mL of Hanks with 2% fetal calf serum (FCS); add a few drops of the final solution to a sample contained in a petri dish. The addition of DMSO accelerates the staining process.

Stained islets are counted according to diameter classes using a calibrated grid in the eyepiece of the phase contrast microscope. Particles smaller than 50 μm are not considered and islets larger than 350 μm are no further subdivided. Table 13.2 gives the mean volume for each diameter class and the relevant conversion factor into islets of 150 μm diameter. The total islet volume of the final preparation also can be estimated and may be a further useful parameter to characterize an islet preparation. The potential use of automated methods using computerized imaging analyzers appears to be an attractive alternative to visual methods and may provide a more objective and standardized quantitative evaluation. Although this technology appears promising, it is expensive and too early in development to be proposed as a general standard.

ISLET PURITY

Transplanting highly purified islet preparations holds potential advantages of increased safety, reduced immunogenicity of the graft and probably improved islet implantation, although these issues recently have been questioned in light of new results obtained in a few diabetic patients using unpurified islet preparations.[24-27] However, reports of severe portal hypertension and in three deaths resulting from intraportal autotransplantation of unpurified islet tissue should be a warning to use only highly purified (i.e. >80%) islet preparations for transplantation purposes.[28-31]

Large-scale, continuous-gradient centrifugation established on a COBE 2991 cell processor using different or specifically designed gradient media is at present the preferred technique for rapid, effective, and reproducible human islet purification.[32,33] To run in parallel a test gradient for each individual pancreas may help to further increase islet recovery and islet viability.

Although many approaches for determination of islet purity have been proposed, including insulin/amylase ratio and algebraic equations, each approach has inherent problems that result in assessment variabilities that are not easily controlled. Again, it is possible that the

---

Table 13.2. Determination of islet volume for each 50 μm-diameter range and conversion into islet equivalents (IEQ) with a diameter of 150 μm

Islet Diameter Range (μm)	Mean Volume (μm³)	Conversion Factor (counted islet number x conversion factor)
50 - 100	294,525	x 0.16
100 - 150	1.145,373	x 0.66
150 - 200	2.977,968	x 1.7
200 - 250	6.185,010	x 3.5
250 - 300	11.159,198	x 6.3
300 - 350	18.293,231	x 10.4
> 350	27.979,808	x 15.8

automatic methods using either specific stains or highly specific monoclonal antibodies ultimately will be used. For now, however most investigators use the dithizone stain as an easy method to roughly estimate the approximate degree of purity of the islets in any preparation.

ISLET VIABILITY AND ENDOCRINE FUNCTION

Islet viability is a critical factor that determines the outcome of transplantation. However, there is currently no entirely reliable method for standardizing viability assessment. In vitro methods include light and electron microscopic morphology, fluorometric membrane integrity tests, colorimetric tests of mitochondrial function, and glucose-stimulated insulin release determined in static incubation or in continuous perifusion systems.[34-46] Moreover, in studies of basic islet physiology and responses to pharmacological agents insulin and protein synthesis and glucose utilizsation have also been used to assess vital islet functions.[44,46,47]

For rapid assessment of islet viability before islet transplantation, a fluorometric assay using inclusion and exclusion dyes that allow discrimination between intact and damaged cells is now widely used and recommended.[36,37] The combination of the inclusion and exclusion dyes acridin orange (AO) and propidium iodide (PI) have minimal background fluorescence, and when used in optimal concentrations (AO - 0.67 µmol/L; PI - 75 µmol/L), they stain living cells green and dead cells red. Using this fluorometric method, viable and non-viable whole islets may be differentiated, as may viable and non-viable components within an islet. The stability, cytotoxicity, and reproducibility of the assay has been demonstrated on animal and human islets.

It is crucial that the isolated islets be shown not only to be viable but also able to respond appropriately to a glucose challenge. The standard in assessing in vitro islet endocrine function is the perifusion of islets with glucose, which provides a dynamic profile of the characteristics of glucose-mediated insu-

lin release from pre-stored and newly synthesized insulin and of the ability of the islet endocrine cells to downregulate insulin secretion after the glycemic challenge is interrupted (return to baseline).[43,45] Technical details have been described previously.[4,48] In brief, duplicate groups of 200-300 islets of comparable size are perifused with Krebs-Ringer bicarbonate solution, which is maintained at 37°C and gassed with 95% O_2 and 5% CO_2. The perfusate is pumped through the chambers for three consecutive hours, during which time the glucose concentration is 50, 300 (500) and 50 mg/dL, respectively. The effluent from the chamber is sampled every 10 min after subjecting the islets to perifusion for 40 minutes to eliminate an artificial increase in insulin due to mechanical stimulation from the transfer procedure. During the second hour, samples are removed at 1, 2.5, 5, 7.5, 10, 20, 30, 40, 50, and 60 min, and during the final hour every 10 minutes. The samples are collected at 4°C and stored at -20°C until assay for insulin is initiated using a double-antibody radioimmunoassay technique.[49]

Standards for reporting results of perifusion studies are critical for the accurate comparison of data. The absolute levels of insulin secretion during the prechallenge baseline period, the high glucose challenge, and the last period of perifusion after return to low glucose concentration should be reported. The profile of insulin release is best reported as a plot that shows the release during the three consecutive periods.[50] Stimulation index estimated by determining the ratio between basal (last 15 minutes before high glucose and last 15 minutes after return to basal conditions) and stimulated insulin release (first 15 minutes and last 15 minutes of stimulation) identifies the secretory capacity but lacks details on basal insulin release, the quality of the biphasic response and return to basal secretion.[15] However, in-vitro insulin release does not necessarily predict in vivo transplant outcome, and the results of islet perifusion studies should therefore be interpreted with caution. Thus, cryopreserved rodent islets showed normal perifusion response but later failed to reverse diabetes, and vice versa, cryopreserved canine islets that failed to secrete insulin during perifusion induced normoglycemia after autotransplantation and it has been reported that a poor response from human islets during perifusion did not predict their in vivo function after transplantation.[51-53]

Therefore, the best index of viability is the ability of transplanted islets to withstand the rigors of engraftment in an ectopic site of a diabetic recipient until revascularisation is complete and to reverse diabetes in this recipient. In vivo endocrine function of human islets can be tested after transplantation (bioassay) of aliquots of the final islet preparation beneath the renal capsule of diabetic immunodeficient and athymic mouse or rat.[54-56]

ISLET STERILITY

Testing should start as usual with donor screening for viral antibodies (hepatitis A, B, and C; human immunodeficiency viruses 1 and 2; cytomegalo-virus). The demonstration that islets to be transplanted are free from bioburden risk is an important quality control test. This issue should be carefully considered because a period of tissue culture may amplify microbial contamination and the induction of an immunosuppressed state in islet transplant recipients may render them susceptible to infections. It has been demonstrated that 42% of human donor pancreas had low level contaminants, usually of gram positive bacteria, and 15% had fungal contaminants.[57] During islet isolation, 97% of these contaminants are eliminated and only some new environmental contaminants are added, mostly fungal. However, holding the islets for 7 days and culturing the samples both at 24°C and at 37°C has prevented contaminated islet preparations from being transplanted into immunosuppressed recipients.[58] By contrast, other centers transplanting freshly isolated islets have reported septicemia in two cases whereas another center observed no clinical apparent infection despite retrospectively demonstrable microbial contamination of the islet preparations.[59,60]

CONCLUSION

The various issues of the quality control program suggested should serve as guidelines for investigators going to initiate clinical islet transplantation programs. The main message should be that only an islet preparation with well-documented quantity, purity, viability, function, and sterility (Table 13.3) before transplantation fulfills the criteria of transplantability and merits transplantation into a patient.

Table 13.3. Minimal requirements to be met by islet preparations intended for clinical islet transplantations

• Islet Mass	> 6,000–8,000 IEQ/kg body wt in type 1 diabetic recipient > 3,500 IEQ/kg body wt in patients to be autotransplanted after pancreatectomy
• Islet Purity	> 80 % (percentage of the islet volume in the total cell volume)
• Islet Viability	> 80% (assessed by a microfluorometric membrane integrity test)
• Islet In Vitro Function	Documented biphasic response to a glucose challenge and return to baseline phenomenon
• Islet Sterility	Exclusion of microbial contamination

REFERENCES

1. Hering BJ, Browatzki CC, Schultz A, Bretzel RG, Federlin KF. Clinical islet transplantation - registry report, accomplishments in the past and future research needs. Cell Transplant 1993; 2:269

2. American Diabetes Association Pancreas transplantation for patients with diabetes mellitus. Diab Care 1993, 16 suppl 2:21

3. American Diabetes Association Technical review on pancreas transplantation for patients with diabetes mellitus. Diab Care 1992, 15:1668

4. Bretzel RG, Alejandro R, Hering BJ, van Suylichem PTR, Ricordi C Clinical islet transplantation:guidelines for islet quality control. Transplant Proc 1994, 26:388

5. Scharp DW The elusive human islet:variables involved in its effective recovery. In:van Schilfgaarde R, Hardy MA (eds), Transplantation of the Endocrine Pancreas in Diabetes Mellitus, Amsterdam, Elsevier, 1988, 97

6. Klitscher D, Brandhorst H, Hering B, Federlin K, Bretzel RG Can donor data predict human islet isolation outcome? Horm Metabol Res 1993, 25:60

7. Zeng Y, Torres MA, Thistlethwaite RJ Correlation between donor characteristics and human pancreatic islet yield and purity. Transplant Proc (in press)

8. Yao QX, Yao Z, Heintz R et al. Effect of donor age and cold ischemia time (CIT) on yield, purity and function of human islets isolated from fifty-four (54) consecutive pancreas donors. Transplant Proc (in press)

9. Brandhorst H, Klitscher D, Hering BJ, Federlin K, Bretzel RG Influence of organ procurement on human islet isolation. Horm Metabol Res 1993, 25:51

10. Kneteman NM, de Groot TJ, Warnock GL, Rajotte RV The evaluation of solutions for pancreas preservation prior to islet isolation. Horm Metabol Res 1990, Suppl Ser 25:4

11. Kneteman NM, Lakey JRT, Warnock GL, Rajotte RV Human islet isolation after prolonged cold storage. Diab Nutr Metab 1992, 5 suppl 1:33

12. Ricordi C, Mazzeferro V, Casavilla A, Scotti C, Pinna A, Tzakis A, Starzl TE Pancreas procurement from multiorgan donors for islet transplantation. Diab Nutr Metab 1992, 5 suppl 1:39

13. Gray DW, McShane P, Grant A, Morris PJ A method for isolation of islets of Langerhans from the human pancreas. Diabetes 1984, 33:1055

14. Horaguchi A, Merrell RC Preparation of viable islet cells from dogs by a new method. Diabetes 1981, 30:455

15. Ricordi C, Lacy PE, Finke EH, Olack BJ, Scharp DW Automated method for isolation of human pancreatic islets. Diabetes 1988, 37:413

16. Socci C, Davalli AM, Vignali A, Pontiroli AE, Maffi P, Magistretti P, Gavazzi F, de Nittis P, di Carlo V, Pozza G A significant increase of islet yield by early injection of collagenase into the pancreatic duct of young donors. Transplantation 1993, 55:661

17. Scharp DW Commentary. Cell Transplant 1993, 2:299

18. Ogilvie F A quantitative estimation of the pancreatic islet tissue. Quart J Med 1937, 6:287

19. Gepts W Method for the quantitative determination of islands of Langerhans. Can Roy Soc Biol 1958, 152:879

20. Hellman B The frequency distribution of the number and volume of the islets of Langerhans in man. 1. Studies on non-diabetic adults. Acta Soc Med Upsal 1959, 64:432

21. Saito K, Iwama N, Takahashi T Morphometrical analysis on topographical difference in size distribution, number and volume of islets in the human pancreas. Tohoku J Exp Med 1978, 124:177

22. Pyzdrowski KL, Kendall DM, Halter JB, Nakhleh RE, Sutherland DER, Robertson RP Preserved insulin secretion and insulin independence in recipients of islet autografts. N Engl J Med 1992, 327:220

23. Gores PF, Najarian JS, Stephanian E, Lloveras JJ, Kelley SL, Sutherland DER Insulin independence in type I diabetes after transplantation of unpurified cislets from single donor with 15-deoxyspergualin. Lancet 1993, 341:19

24. Gray DW The role of exocrine tissue in pancreatic islet transplantation. Transplant Int 1989, 2:41

25. Gores PF, Sutherland DER Commentary. Cell Transplant 1993, 2:291

26. Ulrichs K, Mueller-Ruchholtz W Mixed lymphocyte islet culture (MLIC) and its use in manipulation of human islet alloimmunogenicity. Horm Metabol Res 1990, Suppl Ser 25:123

27. Zeevi A, Rilo HLR, Fontes PA, Carroll PB, Behboo R, Ricordi C Effect of purity and culture on human islet immunogenicity in vitro. Transplant Proc (in press)

28. Memsic L, Busuttil RW, Traverso LW Bleeding esophageal varices and portal vein thrombosis after pancreatic mixed-cell autotransplantation. Surgery 1984, 95:238

29. Cameron JL, Mehigan DG, Broe PJ, Zuidema GD Distal pancreatectomy and islet autotransplantation for chronic pancreatitis. Ann Surg 1981, 193:312

30. Toledo-Pereyra LH, Rowlett AL, Cain W, Rosenberg JC, Gordon DA, MacKenzie GH Hepatic infarction following intraportal islet cell autotransplantation after near total pancreatectomy. Transplantation 1984, 38:88

31. Grodsinsky C, Malcolm S, Goldman J, Dienst S, Westrick P Islet cell autotransplantation after pancreatectomy for chronic pancreatitis. Arch Surg 1981, 116:511

32. Robertson GSM, Chadwick DR, Contractor H, James RFL, London NJM The optimization of large scale density gradient human islet isolation. Acta Diabetologica 1993, 30:93

33. London NJM, Robertson GSM, Chadwick DR et al. Purification of human pancreatic islets by large scale continuous density gradient centrifugation. Horm Metabol Res 1993, 25:61

34. Andersson A, Sandler S Viability tests of cryopreserved endocrine pancreatic islet cells. Cryobiology 1983, 20:161

35. Rajotte RV, Stewart HL, Voss WAC, Shnitka TK, Dossetor JB Viability studies on frozen-thawed rat islets of Langerhans. Cryobiology 1977, 14:116

36. Bank HL Assessment of islet cell viability using fluorescence dyes. Diabetologia 1987, 30:812

37. Bank HL Rapid assessment of islet cell viability using fluorescent dyes. In vitro 1988, 24:266

38. London NJM, Contractor H, Lake SP, Ancott GC, Bell RPF, James RFL A microfluorometric viability assay for isolated human and rat islets of Langerhans. Diab Res 1989, 12:141

39. Gray DW, Morris PJ The use of fluorescein diacetate and ethidium bromide as a viability stain for isolated islets of Langerhans. Stain Technol 1987, 62:373

40. Gutte N, Kuhn F, Matthes G, Georgi K, Gronau K, Braun K The MTT-dye test for the in vitro vitality control of fresh as opposed to cryopreserved rat pancreatic islets for syngeneic intraportal islet transplantation. Z Exp Chir Transplant Kuenstliche Organe 1989, 22:323

41. McKay DB, Karow AM Factors to consider in the assessment of viability of cryopreserved islets of Langerhans. Cryobiology 1983, 20:151

42. Kuhn F, Abri O, Lohde E, Gutte N, Schulz HJ, Jahr H In vitro rapid calorimetric assay for viability control of fresh isolated and deep-frozen huma pancreatic islets. Diabetes 1989, 38 suppl 1:278

43. Lacy PE, Walker BS, Fink CJ Perifusion of isolated rat islets in vitro:participation of the microtubular system in the biphasic release of insulin. Diabetes 1972, 21:987

44. Ashcroft SJH, Bassett JM, Randle PJ Isolation of human pancreatic islets capable of releasing insulin and metabolizing glucose in vitro. Lancet 1971, i:888

45. Lacy PE, Finke EH, Conant S, Naber S Long-term perifusion of isolated rat islets in vitro. Diabetes 1976, 25:484

46. Kneteman NM, Rajotte RV Isolation and cryopreservation of human pancreatic islets. Transplant Proc 1986, 18:182

47. Scharp DW, Lacy PE, Finke E, Olack B Low temperature culture of human islets isolated by the distension method and purified with Ficoll and Percoll gradients. Surgery 1987, 102:869

48. Ricordi C, Hering BJ, London NJM, Rajotte RV, Gray DWR, Socci C, Alejandro R, Carroll PB, Bretzel RG, Scharp DW Islet isolation assessment. In:Ricordi C (ed) Pancreatic Islet Cell Transplantation, Landes Company, Georgetown, 1992, 132

49. Morgan CR, Lazarow A Immunoassay of insulin:antibody system. Plasma insulin levels of normal, subdiabetic and diabetic rats. Diabetes 1963, 12:115

50. Warnock GL, Ellis D, Rajotte RV, Dawidson I, Baekkeskov S, Edebjerg J Studies of the isolation and viability of human islets of Langerhans. Transplantation 1988, 45:957

51. Rajotte RV, Evans MG, Warnock GL, Kneteman NM Islet cryopreservation. Horm Metabol Res 1989, Suppl Ser 25:72

52. Evans MG, Rajotte RV, Warnock GL, Kneteman NM Viability studies on cryopreserved isolated canine islets of Langerhans. Transplant Proc 1989, 21:3368

53. Socci C, Davalli AM, Vignali A et al. Evidence of in vivo human islet graft function despite a weak response to in vitro function. Transplant Proc 1992, 24:3056

54. Ricordi C, Scharp DW, Lacy P Reversal of diabetes in nude mice after transplantation of fresh and 7-day-cultured (24°C) human pancreatic islets. Transplantation 1988, 45:994

55. London NJ, Thirdborough SM, Swift SM, Bell PR, James RF The diabetic "human reconstituted" severe combined immunodeficient (SCID-hn) mouse:a model for isogeneic, allogeneic, and xenogeneic human islet transplantation. Transplant Proc 1991, 23:749

56. Lake SP, Chamberlain J, Bassett PD et al. Successful reversal of diabetes in nude rats by transplantation of isolated adult human islets of Langerhans. Diabetes 1989, 38:244

57. Scharp DW, Lacy PE, McLear M, Longwith J, Olack B The bioburden of 590 consecutive human pancreata for islet transplant research. Transplant Proc 24, 974, 1992

58. Scharp DW Islet quality control testing and the islet isolation laboratory. In:Ricordi C (ed), Pancreatic Islet Cell Transplantation, Landes Company, Georgetown, 1992, 82

59. Lakey JRT, Rajotte RV, Taylor GD, Kirkland T, Warnock GL,Microbial studies of a tissue bank of cryopreserved human islet cells. Transplant Proc 1994, 26:827

60. Lloveras J, Farney AC, Sutherland DER, Wahoff D, Field MJ, Gores PF Significance of contaminated islet preparations in clinical islet transplantation. Transplant Proc 1994, 26:579

CHAPTER 14

ISLET CELL PROLIFERATION

Jens Høiriis Nielsen

New pancreatic islet cells are formed either by differentiation of stem cells from the pancreatic duct epithelium, neogenesis, or by proliferation of already differentiated islet cells.[1] Both events seem to be rare in adult man and in human diabetics of either type.[2] In type 1 diabetes any attempt to regenerate β cells would lead to rapid destruction by the immune system although some long-term patients retain C-peptide production, which could be due to arrest of the autoimmune reaction leaving some β cells intact or regeneration of a limited number of β cells. It is not known whether the remission period often observed shortly after the onset and initial treatment with insulin is due to the recovery of the function of the remaining β cells or to actual formation of more β cells.

In type 2 diabetes associated with obesity the β-cell mass is lower when compared with obese non-diabetic individuals,[3] supporting the recent hypothesis, that low birth weight is a risk factor for the development of type 2 diabetes due to the lack of sufficient compensatory growth of the β-cell mass in response to the weight gain later in life.[4] In the young type 2 diabetics (MODY) mutations in the glucokinase gene have been discovered suggesting a functional defect in the β cells.[5] In gestational diabetes it is conceivable that the hyperplasia of β cells normally occurring during gestation is insufficient to compensate for the increased demand.[6]

Thus, the relative lack of normally functioning β cells in both types of diabetes warrants the search for means to increase their number either by induction of neogenesis and/or proliferation of endogeneous β cells or of exogenous β cells for transplantation.

After a discussion of the methodological aspect, the possibilities for induction of β cell proliferation will be reviewed on the basis of the numerous substances which have been studied both in vivo and in vitro. Focus will be on the more recent developments and references will be given to books and reviews where the original references may be found.[7-11]

METHOD TO STUDY ISLET CELL PROLIFERATION

Islet cell proliferation in experimental animals in vivo has been studied by classical techniques, i.e., injection of ^{3}H-thymidine (Tdr) and processing of the pancreas for autoradiography and identification of the cell type by

Pancreatic Islet Transplantation Volume I: Procurement of Pancreatic Islets, edited by Robert P. Lanza, MD, William L. Chick, MD; ©1994 R.G. Landes Company.

electron microscopy or immunochemical staining with dyes or specific antibodies to the hormones.[1] More recently injection or oral administration of the thymidine analogue 5-bromo-2'-deoxyuridine (BrdU) which is detectable with monoclonal antibodies is used.[12] The study of the embryonic or regenerating pancreas is hampered by the low expression of the hormones not allowing detection by conventional immunocytochemistry or in situ hybridization. In this case reverse transcription in situ followed by polymerase chain reaction (PCR) would be desirable.

Islet cell replication can readily be studied in isolated islets in culture. The choice of suitable culture media has been discussed elsewhere.[8,13-15] It can be mentioned that mouse islets have been cultured free floating in bacteriological plastic culture dishes with RPMI 1640 culture medium supplemented with 10% newborn calf serum for up to one year where they retained the ability to respond to glucose and theophyllin.[16] Human islets were kept for almost two years in culture in RPMI 1640 supplemented with either 10% newborn calf serum or 10% normal human serum and continued to release insulin to the medium.[17] The responsiveness to glucose was preserved for at least 9 months.[18] A marked species variation in the requirements for the maintenance of the insulin production should be noted. Thus rat and human islets can maintain a constant insulin production in a minimal serum or albumin supplement provided that the glucose concentration is high, i.e., 11 mM. Mouse islet however require at least 5% normal human serum in order to maintain constant insulin production. Attempts to identify the serum factor revealed that a protein with a molecular weight of 70-100 kD contained the activity, which was found to be higher in serum from type I diabetic patients.[8,19] The serum factor can be replaced with hormones like cortisol or human growth hormone (hGH) although their modes of action are different (see below). Thus stimulation by glucose, hormones and serum factors seems to be important for long-term maintenance of the β cell function of the islets.

If islets or dispersed islet cells are allowed to attach to uncoated plastic culture dishes or dishes coated with an extracellular matrix in the presence of high glucose, serum, IBMX or hGH they will spread out into a monolayer which allows the study of the morphology as well as replication directly or after labeling with ^{3}H-Tdr or BrdU and hormone staining.[20-23] As intact islets have to be processed for histology the uptake or incorporation of ^{3}H-Tdr into DNA has often been used as a measure of islet cell replication. There are however several pitfalls with this method.[24] The incorporation into DNA depends on a.o. transport, thymidine kinase activity, pool of cold Tdr, DNA damage and mycoplasma infection. As an example a very high uptake was seen in rat insulinoma (RIN) cells cultured in the presence of fresh human serum, but with no concomitant increase in cell number. The activity in serum was blocked by heat-inactivation or by heparin, but not further characterized.[25] In purified β cells from adult rat islets glucose was found to stimulate ^{3}H-Tdr incorporation, but no labeled nuclei were seen by autoradiography or by BrdU labeling.[26] However when grown on extracellular matrix a marked increase in BrdU labeling was reported in adult rat islet cells.[23] Thus cell replication should be assessed by cell counting or DNA measurement. However one should not rely on the latter alone as cells may have died during the culture period.[27] A higher cell number may thus be due to increased survival rather than cell proliferation as was pointed out in a recent study on β cell culture media.[28] The development of the confocal microscope allows the counting of BrdU labeled cells in the intact islet.[29]

Mitotic activity can also be assessed by the classical metaphase counting after colchicine treatment as has been described for islet cells.[24] Synchronization of islet cells by hydroxyurea of the S-phase has been used to determine the length of the cell cycle.[24] Hydroxyurea blockade can also be used to distinguish between ^{3}H-Tdr incorporation into DNA in the S-phase or by repair mechanisms.[24] Flow cytometry has been used to determine mitotic activity in islet cells.[30]

Quantitation of BrdU labeled islet cells can also be performed by flowcytometry.[31]

In conclusion the use of BrdU labeling and hormone staining is a reliable technique to assess islet cell replication both in vivo and in vitro. A 24-hours' chase period will furthermore allow the identification of doublets of BrdU-positive cells proving that they have undergone mitosis.[22] BrdU should however only be used for brief labeling experiments as it is known to affect the differentiation of cells in the pancreas.[32]

ISLET GROWTH BY NEOGENESIS

The organogenesis of the pancreas depends on the interaction between the primitive gut epithelium and the surrounding mesenchyme.[33] In the absence of mesenchymal cells differentiation to endocrine, mainly glucagon-producing cells, occurs, whereas addition of mesenchyme, or still unknown mesenchymal factor(s), results in proliferation and differentiation of the epithelium into the whole organ comprising both exocrine and endocrine cells suggesting the existence of a common stem cell.

Recent studies of the earliest detectable hormone gene expression has revealed insulin and glucagon mRNA already at 20 somites (8 days of gestation) in the mouse in the region of the foregut, from where the pancreas will be formed.[34] Thus, the initial differentiation takes place even before evagination of the dorsal foregut. Although the putative stem cells have not been identified it is believed that they are pluripotent cells which under the influence of common neuroendocrine transcription factors, express several neuroendocrine gene products[35] before they come under the influence of other combinations of transcription factors including IPF-1[36] and lmx-1.[37] During the differentiation, other genes may be turned off as shown in a cloned rat insulinoma cell line, serving as a model of a pluripotent stem cell of the neuroendocrine lineage, which mainly express the insulin genes when growing in vivo and partially loses this ability when grown in vitro.[38]

The exogenous factors which supposedly influence the expression of the transcription factors involved in the islet cell differentiation are not known. Several of the abundant growth factors like IGF-I, IGF-II, TGFα, TGFβ2, aFGF, and bFGF are expressed in the pancreas anlage in the mouse[39] but it is not clear to which extent these factors are involved in differentiation or in proliferation or both.

The regeneration of the pancreas after resection of 90% of the pancreas in the rat seems to have features in common with the embryonic development of the pancreas.[40] The sequential proliferation of ductular cells and the formation of acini and islets by neogenesis probably accounts for the major part of the regeneration whereas proliferation of already differentiated exocrine and endocrine cells plays a minor role.[40] A rise in the expression of IGF-1 was observed in the duct cells and endothelial cells, but not in the endocrine cells.[41]

Of potential interest is the recent finding that nicotinamide can induce differentiation or maturation of fetal human pancreatic cells by stimulating the out-growth of insulin-containing cells from apparently undifferentiated epithelial cell clusters. Also the content of glucagon and somatostatin in the clusters was increased.[42] Such an effect was reported for fetal porcine pancreas which after treatment with nicotinamide in vitro showed a marked acceleration of the islet development when transplanted into diabetic nude mice.[43] The mechanism of action may involve inhibition of poly ADP-ribosyl synthase and increase in the NAD(P)H level known to play an important role in normal β cell function. It is in accordance with the original observation that nicotinamide protects against the diabetogenic effect of streptozotocin in rats, but several months later develop insulin producing tumors, may be as a result of the inhibition of the repair of DNA damaged by alkylation and strand breaks by streptozotocin.[44] Even after partial pancreatectomy nicotinamide is able to enhance islet regeneration.[44] In the on-going and planned clinical trials treatment by individuals having islet cell antibodies not only a protective effect, but also the possible effect on β cell regeneration may be considered. The risk of development of insulinomas is probably only theoretical as it may depend on an extensive damage of the β cell genome. During the regenerative process a marked increase in the expression of the reg gene has been found.[44] However, the reg gene product is identical to the pancreatic stone protein, which is abundant in the exocrine pancreas, and as the molecule is homologous to mammalian lectins, it may be classified as a stress protein induced by any damage to the pancreas rather than playing a specific role in the islet cell regeneration.[45]

Based on the classical observation that ligation of the pancreatic duct causes fibrosis and atrophy of the exocrine pancreas without damage to the islets, it was found that simply wrapping the pancreas into cellophane resulted in marked islet neogenesis from the duct epithelium.[46] By extraction of the en-wrapped pancreas a protein "ilotropin" with a molecular weight of 29-44 kD was found to be able to stimulate islet cell differentiation in vivo.[46] The identity of this factor is not yet known.

In another model mice were made transgenic with the interferon-γ (IFN γ) gene under the insulin promoter. Besides a massive lymphocytic infiltration with profound β cell destruction, formation of new islets from the ductal epithelium was observed.[47] The islets budding into the lumen of the ducts were apparently protected against the immune destruction. These results suggest that even in autoimmune diabetes islet regeneration may occur at least in certain animal species.

Thus, neogenesis of islet cells by differentiation is certainly a potential source of β cells in both fetal and adult experimental animals in vivo and in vitro. In man it has only so far been reported in fetal issue, and it is not known whether the adult pancreatic duct cells retain the capacity to differentiate. However, induction of differentiation in fetal tissue either prior to or after transplantation is a potential method to obtain larger quantities of β cells for therapeutic use. Nicotinamide may prove to be useful in this respect, but the search for more potent physiological differentiation factors like "ilotropin" should be continued.

ISLET GROWTH BY REPLICATION

Numerous factors have been tested for their effect on proliferation of already differentiated islet cells. They include nutritional factors like glucose and amino acids, hormones like islet hormones, gastrointestinal hormones, pituitary hormones, steroid and thyroid hormones, secretagogues like methylxanthines and oral hypoglycemic drugs, growth factors like IGF-1, IGF-2, PDGF and NGF and cytokines like interleukin 1 (IL-1), TNFα, and IFNγ. Several of these factors may contribute to islet cell growth both by stimulating islet cell differentiation and islet cell replication. However, most of the studies discussed in this part are based on effects on isolated islets, where the islet cells have reached a high degree of differentiation although islets of fetal and newborn origin still may contain less differentiated cell types. It is therefore not always possible to draw firm conclusions from these studies, specially since the proliferating cells only in a few cases have been identified by specific staining. As the effects of several of the factors have been reviewed recently[7-11] only the factors which are considered of physiological importance for the β cell proliferation and function will be discussed here. Insulinoma cells and other transformed islet cells will therefore not be dealt with in this review.

NUTRIENTS

The β cell mass seems to be closely correlated with the insulin demand, which again is closely correlated with body mass, i.e., the number of insulin sensitive cells and the sensitivity of these cells to insulin. The main indicator for the β cell sufficiency is the blood glucose concentration. Glucose not only stimulated insulin release and synthesis, but also replication.[10] Thus in several animal models with hyperglycemia either genetically as in the ob/ob-mouse, the db/db mouse and the fa/fa-rat[7] or by partial pancreatectomy or by glucose infusion, insulin antibody injection, glucocorticoid treatment, alloxan and streptozotocin injection, a long-lasting or transitory increase in the mitotic activity in the β cells is observed.[1,7,9,48] Conversely reduction in the insulin demand by prolonged fasting or implantation of islets or insulin producing tumors results in suppression of the β cell activity and apparently also the number as indicated by a burst of mitotic activity after glucose infusion or removal of the tumor.[45,49,50] In the db/db mouse restriction of the food intake prevented the mitotic activity even before hypoglycemia was measured suggesting a fine tuning of the β cell replication by both glucose and amino acid supply as indicated by feeding experiments.[51] The latter is in accordance with the observation that protein malnutrition in pregnant rats results in marked reduction in β cell mass in relation to the body weight of the off-spring.[52]

These in vivo studies are confirmed in isolated islets in vitro, where both glucose and amino acids were found to stimulate islet cell replication not by changing the length of the cell cycle but by recruitment of more cells to enter the cell cycle.[10]

Several vitamins have been shown to influence the islet function, but only nicotinamide has been extensively studied with regard to islet cell differentiation and proliferation. As mentioned above it stimulates differentiation and replication of immature islet cells, but it does not affect adult human islet function.[53]

GASTROINTESTINAL HORMONES

Gastrointestinal hormones have long been known to stimulate the β-cell function.[54] In Zollinger-Ellison's syndrome islet cell hyperplasia has been described suggesting that gastrin may act as a growth factor.[55] In fact gastrin is detected in the developing pancreas.[56] CCK has been implicated in the islet hypertrophy in rats fed trypsin inhibitor or treated with CCK[57] and CCK is actually expressed in some rat insulinoma (RIN) cell lines.[58]

The truncated GLP-1 (7-36) amide (GLP-1) is now considered as the best candidate for "incretin" and specific GLP-1 receptors are abundant in the islets.[59] It has, however, not been reported to stimulate β cell replication, but as it stimulates adenylate cyclase it may do so. Although cAMP plays

an important role in the insulin formation and secretion its function in the mitotic activity is not clear.[10] Conflicting results have been obtained, e.g., the phosphodieterase inhibitor IBMX stimulates replication in low concentrations, but inhibits in higher concentration as does theophylline.[60] However these inhibitors may affect other pathways as well and cAMP may also affect the cell function through different pathways as has been described in the thyroid, where TSH stimulates both thyroid hormone production and proliferation,[61] and in the pituitary, where GRF stimulates both growth hormone production and proliferation.[62]

Oral hypoglycemic sulfonylurea drugs were earlier reported to induce β-cell hyperplasia in vivo. This has, however, not been confirmed in vitro, but the physiological ligand to the receptor which is identical or closely associated with the ATP-dependent channel, believed to play an essential role in the control of the insulin release, may affect β cell replication.[63]

PITUITARY HORMONES

The possible role of growth hormone and prolactin in the growth of the pancreatic islets has been discussed in recent reviews.[8,64,65] Growth hormone (GH) was originally recognized for its diabetogenic effect and both trophic and deleterious effects on the islets were considered as indirectly caused by the hyperglycemia following the insulin antagonistic effect on glucose metabolism. After it became possible to maintain isolated islets in culture for prolonged periods of time, both GH and prolactin (PRL) were found to stimulate both insulin synthesis and β cell replication. Specific receptors for both GH and PRL were demonstrated in the islets. Although the accumulation of insulin in the culture medium and the cells was increased, the acute insulin release in response to glucose was reduced. When either intact newborn rat islets or dispersed islet cells were cultured in the presence of hGH they continue to grow in monolayer culture for 2-3 months corresponding to a 10-20-fold increase in β cell number.[22] At this stage or after withdrawal of hGH the cells stopped growing and began to detach from the dish and rounded up into numerous islet-like clusters. The reason for this arrest is not known, but is in accordance with the decreased mitotic activity with age,[10] and with the hypothesis, that the number of mitotic events a β cell can undergo is limited and genetically determined.[1] Another possibility is the existence of a pool of less differentiated precursor cells which continue to replicate until their terminal differentiation. This is, however, less probable, as it has been reported that the consecutive mitotic events occur at different locations in cultured islet cells[66] which was confirmed by labeling the cells with BrdU where only one pair of labeled β cell nuclei was observed at each location after a prolonged chase period (Nielsen, unpublished observation). The chance for a cell to enter the S-phase seems thus to be stochastic although depending on trophic factors and receptors as well as the previous "history" of the cell. The effect of GH also depends on the species. It was already noted by Houssay and colleagues that GH was not diabetogenic in the intact rat, only when 90% of the pancreas was removed. Thus, the insulin antagonistic effect may be compensated by an increase in the β cell mass in the intact rat, but not when the initial number was diminished. In the adult dog GH was diabetogenic, but Young and colleagues noted that it was not the case in puppies and similarly in adult man GH causes hyperglycemia, whereas this is not the case in GH treated children suggesting that there is an age-dependent decrease in responsiveness of the islets to GH. In adult human islets GH has little, if any, effect on insulin production[8] and PRL has a limited effect on the replication.[67] Studies are in progress to determine whether the low responsiveness is due to changes in expression of GH and PRL receptors or the signaling pathways.

In conclusion GH and PRL may contribute to β cell proliferation in the growing individual, but may be of little use in vivo because of the insulin antagonistic effects. These hormones may, however, be useful in the expansion of the β cell number islets from certain animal species and human fetal islets for transplantation purposes.

PREGNANCY HORMONES

During pregnancy β cell hyperplasia has been described both in women and in rodents.[6,64,66] The increase in mitotic activity in the pregnant rat correlates with the rise in placental lactogens (PL)[29], and hPL as well as rPL-I and rPL-II have been shown to stimulate insulin production and β cell replication in cultured rat islets.[67] The increased mitotic activity is also correlated with an increase in the expression of PRL and GH receptors in the pancreas.[68] It is interesting to note that in male rats PRL receptors are expressed in the pancreas but not in the liver suggesting a different mode of regulation.

In isolated islets cultured in the presence of PRL, GH, progesterone, dexamethasone and testosterone, it was found that PRL and GH induced a marked increase in the expression of PRL but not GH receptor mRNA, whereas dexamethasone and progesterone induced a significant increase in the GH but not PRL receptor mRNA. Thus the two receptors are regulated differently. It is of particular interest that in pregnant women, the islets seem to become responsive to the mitogenic effect of PL, PRL, and GH which is in accordance with the early finding by Young and coworkers that GH did not cause diabetes in the pregnant dog. It is therefore of great interest to unravel the mechanisms whereby the islets become responsible to GH and PRL during pregnancy. It may then be feasible to render the human islets responsive in vitro, and thereby increase the number of β cells for transplantation.

STEROID AND THYROID HORMONES

Although treatment with glucocorticoid hormones in vitro results in β-cell hyperplasia and direct effects on glucose induced insulin release are demonstrated in vitro, only inhibition of the DNA synthesis has been reported.[69] Also sex steroid may influence islet function in vivo but progesterone inhibits the DNA synthesis in the islets whereas extradiol and testosterone had no effect.[6]

Thyroid hormones influence the β cell function both in vivo and in vitro,[14] but no effect on replication has been reported.

GROWTH FACTORS

A number of known growth factors has been tested for their effects on β cell replication and insulin production.[9-11] Several studies have dealt with the role of IGF-I, IGF-II and their binding proteins in islet cell replication in particular because many effects of GH are mediated via IGF-I. Although IGF-I may contribute to the growth of the fetal pancreas, it is not likely to be involved in the effect of GH on the already differentiated islet cells as IGF-I mRNA was not detected in GH stimulated newborn rat islets and neutralizing IGF-I antibodies did not block the effect of IGF-I.[70] Fetal islets prepared from rats just before birth were found to both produce and respond to IGF-I, IGF-II and four species of IGF binding proteins including IGFBP-2.[71] IGF-II and TGFα was found in the fetal human islets and suggested to be involved in the growth.[72] PDGF in particular in combination with IGF-1 was reported to stimulate DNA synthesis in fetal rat islets.[10] FGF and EGF were found to stimulate the DNA synthesis in newborn rat islets[25] but in several of these studies the proliferating cells were not identified. It may be that other cell types, i.e., endothelial cells, ductular cells or fibroblasts present in the islet preparations respond to the growth factors. Recently the NGF receptor trkA was identified in fetal rat islets suggesting a role of NGF in growth and/or differentiation of the islets cells.[73] It remains to be determined whether these factors influence or may act as maintenance factors of the differentiated function and thus preventing degeneration and programmed cell death.

CYTOKINES

Cytokines were originally considered as factors produced by cells of the hemapoietic lineage in particular cells in the immune system. They include the interleukines, tumor necrosis factors and lymphocyte stimulating factors. Today, however, it is known that several of these factors are produced in cells outside the immune system, and also act on many tissues as growth or differentiated factors or are cytotoxic to certain cells. With regard to the pancreatic β cells the effects of the cytokines IL-1α and β, TNFα and IFNγ have been studied extensively during the last few years. It was initially found that IL-1β was cytotoxic to rat β cells after prolonged exposure to picomolar concentrations. This finding formed the basis for the hypothesis that IL-1 is the effector molecule in the initial destruction the β-cell leading to the development of type 1 diabetes.[74] The effect of IL-1 is, however, bimodal, i.e., low concentration or short exposure time stimulate the insulin release and production whereas higher concentrations or long exposure result in inhibition and death of the β cells.[75] IL-1 also influences the β cell replication in a bimodal way, i.e,. short term inhibition followed by long-term stimulation.[76,77] This paradoxical effect may be due to preferential damage to the fully differentiated and/or most active β cells, and stimulation of the surviving less differentiated cells.

The insulin release from mouse and human islets is stimulated by IL-1 alone, but become inhibited by addition of TNFα and/or IFNγ.[78] This species difference may at least in part be due to a 10-20-fold higher expression of the type I IL-1 receptor in rat islets as compared with human islets.[79] Although the signaling pathways for the mitogenic effect of IL-1 is not known,[80] it may be that IL-1 and other cytokines could play a role as growth factors for the immature islet cells and thus used in recruitment of islet cells for transplantation.

CONCLUSIONS

In this chapter the effects of nutrients, hormones and growth factors on the differentiation and growth of the pancreatic islet cells have been reviewed. The method of choice to study islet cell replication both in vivo and in vitro is labeling with 5-bromo-2'-deoxyuridine. The growth of the islet cell mass is determined by the demand. The capacity to grow is dependant on of the existence and potential of islet stem cells in the duct epithelium as well as the capacity of the differentiated β cells to replicate. If the number of cell divisions is limited either genetically[11] or by fetal malnutrition[4] it may be important to reduce the demand for insulin by diet or prophylactic treatment with insulin or islet cell transplantation. If the growth is hampered by the lack of proper stimuli it may be possible to treat with growth or differentiation factors. Glucose is the most prominent regulator of the β cell function as it influences insulin secretion and biosynthesis as well as transcription of the insulin gene and cell replication. Some of these effects are potentiated by intestinal hormones of which GLP-1 and CCK seem to be the most important. The natural ligand for the sulphonyl urea receptor may also be found here. GH, PRL and PL are "islet trophic hormones" as they stimulate both proliferation and hormone gene transcription and biosynthesis. The cytokine IL-1 has both trophic and inhibitory effects on the beta-cells, which may be important in both normal and pathological condition. A model for

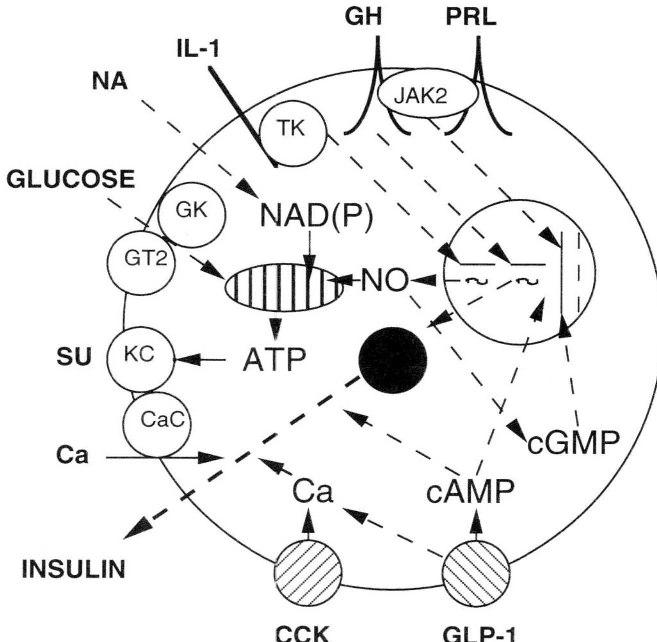

Fig. 14.1. β cell model with the site of action of factors involved in growth and function. GH (growth hormone) and PRL (prolactin) act via specific receptor dimers to activate a tyrosine kinase, JAK2, which initiates both the mitogenic pathway and a separate transcriptional pathway. IL-1 (interleukin-1) acts via the type I receptor by activating an unknown tyrosine kinase (TK) initiating transcription of the enzyme nitric oxide synthase which catalyzes the formation of NO radicals inhibiting the mitochondrial function but increasing the cGMP level, which may stimulate the cell proliferation. Nicotinamide (NA) contribute to NAD(P) formation both directly and by inhibition of poly ADP ribosesynthase. Glucose is transported by glucose transporter-2 (GT2) and via glucokinase (GK) metabolized to give a rise in the ATP formation. ATP will close the potassium channel (KC) as will sulfonylurea (SU) and depolarize the cell whereby a calcium channel (CaC) will open for extracellular calcium (Ca). CCK (cholecystokinin) acts via its receptor to mobilize intracellular calcium, which stimulates insulin release as does GLP-1 (7-36 glucagon-like peptide-1) which acts via its G-protein coupled receptor to increase the cAMP level resulting in increased insulin release and expression of the insulin gene and may be proliferation.

the site of action of these factors on the beta-cell is depicted in Fig. 14.1. The search for factors responsible for islet cell neogenises is still in its beginning, "ilotropin" may be one of them, nicotinamide another. For the procurement of insulin producing cells for transplantation further studies on the mechanism of action of these and other factors on fetal and adult islet cells are needed.

REFERENCES

1. Logothetopoulos J. Islet cell regeneration and neogenesis. In: Steiner DF, Freinkel N, eds. Handbook of Physiology, section 7: Endocrinology, vol. 1. Washington: American Physiological Society, 1972: 67-76.

2. Gepts W, LeCompte PM. The pathology of type 1 (juvenile) diabetes In: Volk BW, Arquilla ER, eds. The Diabetic Pancreas. 2nd ed. New York: Plenum, 1985: 337-65.

3. Rahier J. The diabetic pancreas: A pathologist's view. In: Lefebvre PJ, Pipeleers DG, eds. The Pathology of the endocrine Pancreas. Heidelberg: Springer-Verlag, 1988: 141-70.

4. Hales CN, Barker DJ. Type 2 (non-insulin-dependent) diabetes mellitus: the thrifty phenotype hypothesis. Diabetologia 1992; 35: 595-601.

5. Randle PJ. Glucokinase and candidate genes for type 2 (non-insulin-dependent) diabetes mellitus. Diabetologia 1993; 36: 269-75.

6. Nielsen JH, Nielsen V, Pedersen LM et al. Effects of pregnancy hormones on pancreatic islets in organ culture. Acta Endocr (Cph) 1986; 111: 336-41.

7. Hellerström C, Swenne I. Growth pattern of pancreatic islets in animals. In: Volk BW, Arquilla ER, eds. The Diabetic Pancreas. 2nd ed. New York: Plenum, 1985: 53-79.

8. Nielsen JH. Growth and function of the pancreatic beta-cell in vitro. Effects of glucose, hormones and serum factors on mouse, rat and human islets in organ culture. Acta Endocr (Cph) 1985; 108 (suppl 266): 1-39.

9. Hellerström C, Swenne I, Andersson A. Islet cell replication and diabetes. In: Lefebvre PJ, Pipeleers DG, eds. The Pathology of the endocrine Pancreas. Heidelberg: Springer-Verlag, 1988: 141-70.

10. Swenne I. Pancreatic beta-cell growth and diabetes mellitus. Diabetologia 1992; 35: 193-201.

11. Welsh M, Mares J, Öberg C et al. Genetic factors of importance for beta-cell replication. Diab Metab Rev 1993; 9: 25-36.

12. Parsons JA, Brelje TC, Sorenson RL. Adaptation of islets to pregnancy: increase in B-cell division and insulin secretion correlates with the onset of placental lactogen secretion. Endocrinology 1992; 130: 159-66.

13. Andersson A. Isolated mouse pancreatic islets in culture: effects of serum and different culture media on the insulin production of the islets. Diabetologia 1978; 14: 397-404.

14. Clark SA, Chick WL. Islet cell culture in defined serum-free medium. Endocrinology 1990; 126: 1895-1903.

15. King DL, Chick WL, Kitchen KC. Pancreatic beta cell replication. In: von Wasielewski E, Chick WL, eds. Pancreatic beta cell culture. Workshop Conferences Hoechst vol 5. Amsterdam: Excerpta Medica, 1977: 109-14.

16. Brunstedt J, Nielsen JH, Lernmark Å et al. Isolation of islets from mice and rats. In: Larner J, Pohl SL, eds. Methods in Diabetes Research, vol. 1: Laboratory Methods, part C. New York: John Wiley, 1985: 245-58.

17. Nielsen JH. Beta-cell function in isolated human pancreatic islets in long-term tissue culture. Acta Med Biol Germ 1981; 40: 55-60.

18. Nielsen JH, Brunstedt J, Andersson A et al. Preservation of beta-cell function in adult human pancreatic islets for several months in vitro. Diabetologia 1979; 16: 97-100.

19. Nielsen JH, Eff C, Deckert T et al. Stimulatory effect of serum from diabetic patients on beta-cell function of mouse pancreatic islets maintained in tissue culture. Diabetologia 1981; 20: 60-65.

20. Chick WL, King DL, Lauris V. Techniques for the preparation and maintenance of pancreatic beta cell monolayer culture. In: von Wasielewski E, Chick WL, eds. Pancreatic beta cell culture. Workshop Conferences Hoechst vol 5. Amsterdam: Excerpta Medica, 1977: 85-91.

21. Rabinovitch A. Pancreatic monolayer culture: Preparation of purified islet cell cultures and assessment of beta-cell replication. In: Larner J, Pohl SL, eds. Methods in Diabetes Research, vol. 1: Laboratory Methods, part C. New York: John Wiley, 1985: 309-16.

22. Nielsen JH, Linde S, Welinder BS et al. Growth hormone is a growth factor for the differentiated pancreatic beta-cell. Mol Endocrinol 1989; 3: 165-73.

23. Schuppin GT, Bonner-Weir S, Montana E et al. Replication of adult pancreatic beta-cells cultured on bovine endothelial cell extracellular matrix. In vitro 1993; 29A: 339-44.

24. Swenne I. The cell cycle and growth regulation of pancreatic beta-cells. In: Larner J, Pohl SL, eds. Methods in Diabetes Research, vol. 1: Laboratory Methods, part A. New York: John Wiley, 1985: 182-91.

25. Nielsen JH. Mechanisms of pancreatic beta-cell growth and regeneration: Studies on rat insulinoma cells. Exp Clin Endocrinol 1989; 93: 277-85.

26. De Vroede MA, In't Veld PA, Pipeleers DG. Deoxyribonucleic acid synthesis in cultured adult rat pancreatic B cells. Endocrinology 1990; 127: 1510-16.

27. McEvoy RC. Tissue culture of fetal rat pancreatic islets: Quantitation of changes in the number of islet cells during culture. In: Larner J, Pohl SL, eds. Methods in Diabetes Research, vol. 1: Laboratory Methods, part A. New York: John Wiley, 1985: 227-37.

28. Ling Z, Hannaert JC, Pipeleers D. Effects of nutrients, hormones and serum on survival of rat islet beta-cells in culture. Diabetologia 1994; 37: 15-21.

29. Brelje TC, Sorenson RL. Role of prolactin versus growth hormone on islet B-cell proliferation in vitro: implication for pregnancy. Endocrinology 1992; 128: 45-57

30. Larsen JK, Nielsen O. Flowcytometric evaluation of the DNA distribution in isolated pancreatic islets from normal and diabetic mice. Acta Histchem Cytochem 1979; 27: 410-12.

31. Stahl M, Nielsen JH. Effects of IL-1 and hGH on the DNA synthesis of rat pancreatic beta-cells in culture. Diabetologia 1991; 34(suppl 2): A95.

32. Githens S, Pictet R, Phelps P et al. 5-Bromodeoxyuridine may alter the differentiative program of the embryonic pancreas. J Cell Biol 1976; 71: 341-56.

33. Pictet R, Rutter WJ. Development of the embryonic endocrine pancreas. In: Steiner DF, Freinkel N, eds. Handbook of Physiology, section 7: Endocrinology, vol. 1. Washington: American Physiological Society, 1972: 25-66.

34. Gittes GK, Rutter WJ. Onset of cell-specific gene expression in the developing mose pancreas. Proc Natl Acad Sci USA 1992; 89: 1128-32.

35. Teitelman G, Alpert S, Polak JM, Martinez A et al. Precursor cells of mouse endocrine pancreas coexpress insulin, glucagon and the neuronal proteins tyrosine hydroxylase and neuropeptide Y, but not pancreatic polypeptide. Development 1993; 118: 1031-39.

36. Ohlsson H, Karlsson K, Edlund T. IPF-1, a homeodomain-containing transactivator of the insulin gene. EMBO J 1993; 12: 4251-59.

37. German MS, Wang J, Chadwick RB et al. Synergistic activation of the insulin gene by a LIM-homeo domain protein and a basic helix-loop-helix protein: building a functional insulin minienhancer complex. Genes & Dev 1992; 6: 2165-76.

38. Blume N, Pedersen JS, Andersen LC et al. Immature transformed rat islet beta-cells differentially express C-peptides from the genes coding for insulin I and II as well as a transfected human insulin gene. Mol Endocrinol 1992; 6: 299-307.

39. Nielsen JH, Gittes G. Expression of growth hormone and prolactin receptors in the developing mouse pancreas. J Cell Biochem 1992; Suppl 16F: 88.

40. Bonner-Weir S, Baxter LA, Schuppin GT et al. A second pathway for regeneration of adult exocrine and endocrine pancreas: a possible recapitulation of embryonic development. Diabetes 1993; 42: 1715-20.

41. Smith FE, Rosen KM, Villa-Komaroff L et al. Enhanced insulin-like growth factor-I gene expression in the regenerating rat pancreas. Proc Natl Acad Sci USA 1991; 88: 6152-56.

42. Otonkoski T, Beattie GM, Mally MI, Hayek A. Nicotinamide is a potent inducer of endocrine differentiation in cultured human fetal pancreatic cells. J Clin Invest 1993; 92: 1459-66.

43. Korsgren O, Andersson A, Sandler S. Pretreatment of fetal porcine pancreas in culture with nicotinamide accelerates reversal of diabetes after transplantation to nude mice. Surgery 1993; 113: 205-14.

44. Okamoto H. The molecular basis of experimental diabetes. In: Okamoto H, ed. Molecular Biology of the Islets of Langerhans. Cambridge: Cambridge University 1990: 209-31.

45. Chen L, Appel MC, Alam T et al. Factors regulating islet regeneration in the post-insulinoma NEDH rat.In: Vinik AI, ed. Pancreatic Islet Cell Regeneration and Growth. Adv. Exp. Med. Biol. vol 321. New York: Plenum, 1992: 71-80.

46. Rosenberg L, Vinick AI. Trophic stimulation of the ductular-islet cell axis: A new approach to the treatment of diabetes. In: Vinik AI, ed. Pancreatic Islet Cell Regeneration and Growth. Adv. Exp. Med. Biol. vol 321. New York: Plenum, 1992: 95-104.

47. Sarvetnick NE, Gu D. Regeneration of pancreatic endocrine cells in interferon gamma transgenic mice.In: Vinik AI, ed. Pancreatic Islet Cell Regeneration and Growth. Adv. Exp. Med. Biol. vol 321. New York: Plenum, 1992: 85-89.

48. Weir GC, Leahy JL, Bonner-Weir S. Experimental reduction of the B-cell mass: Implications for the pathogenesis of diabetes. Diab Metab Rev 1986; 2: 125-61.

49. Bonner-Weir S, Deery D, Leahy JL et al. Compensatory growth of pancreatic beta-cells in adult rats after short-term glucose infusion. Diabetes 1989; 38: 49-53.

50. Montana E, Bonner-Weir S, Weir G. Beta cell mass and growth after syngeneic islet transplantation in normal and streptozotocin diabetic C57BL/6 mice. J Clin Invest 1993; 91: 780-87.

51. Chick WL, Like AA. Studies in the diabetic mutant mouse: III. Physiological factors associated with alterations in beta-cell replication. Diabetologia 1970; 6: 243-51.

52. Pakri S, Snoeck A, Reusen-Billen B et al. Islet function in offsprings of mothers on low-protein diet during gestation. Diabetes 1991; 40(suppl 2): 115-20.

53. Sandler S, Hellerström C, Eizirik DL. Effects of nicotinamide supplementation on human pancreatic islet function in tissue culture. J Clin Endocr Metab 1993; 77: 1574-76.

54. Kofod H. Secretin and the endocrine pancreas. Acta Endocr (Cph) 1992: 126 (suppl 1): 1-41

55. Larsson L-I, Nielsen JH, Rehfeld JF. Presence and physiological significance of pancreatic gastrin. Diabetologia 1976; 12: A404.

56. Gittes GK, Rutter WJ, Debas HT. Initiation of gastrin expression during the development of the mouse pancreas. Am J Surg 1993; 165: 23-25.

57. Bonnevie-Nielsen V. The endocrine pancreas: Aspects of beta-cell function in relation to morphology, insulin secretion and insulin content. Scand J Clin Lab Invest 1986; 46 (suppl 183): 1-46.

58. Madsen OD, Larsson L-I, Rehfeld JF et al. Cloned cell lines from a transplantable insulinoma are heterogeneous and express cholecystokinin in addition to islet hormones. J Cell Biol 1986; 103: 2025-34.

59. Thorens B, Waeber G. Glucagon-like paptide-I and the control of insulin secretion in the normal state and in NIDDM. Diabetes 1993; 42: 1219-25.

60. Nielsen JH. Dissociation between insulin secretion and DNA synthesis in cultured pancreatic islets. Biomed Biochim Acta 1985; 44: 161-66.

61. Dumont JE, Lamy F, Roger P et al. Physiological and pathological regulation of thyroid cell proliferation and differentiation by thyrotropin and other factors. Physiol Rev 1992; 72: 667-96.

62. Billestrup N, Swanson LW, Vale W. Growth hormone releasing factor stimulates proliferation of somatotrophs in vitro. Proc Natl Acad Sci USA 1986; 83: 6854-57.

63. Henquin JC. The fiftieth anniversary of hypoglycaemic sulphonamides. How did the mother compound work? Diabetologia 1992; 35: 907-12.

64. Nielsen JH, Møldrup A, Billestrup N et al. The role of growth hormone and prolactin in beta-cell growth and regeneration. In: Vinik AI, ed. Pancreatic Islet Cell Regeneration and Growth. Adv. Exp. Med. Biol. vol 321. New York: Plenum, 1992: 9-17.

65. Nielsen JH, Billestrup N, Møldrup A et al. Growth of the endocrine pancreas: the role of somatolactogenic hormones and receptors. Biochem Soc Transact 1993; 21: 146-49.

66. Fischer EJ, Meisinger M. Time lapse cinematography of endocrine pancreatic cells in monolayer culture. In: von Wasielewski E, Chick WL, eds. Pancreatic beta cell culture. Workshop Conferences Hoechst vol 5. Amsterdam: Excerpta Medica, 1977: 115-18.

67. Brelje TC, Scharp DW, Lacy PE et al. Effect of homologous placental lactogens, prolactins and growth hormones on islet B-cell division and insulin secretion in rat, mouse, and human islets: Implication for placental lactogen regulation of islet function during pregnancy. Endocrinology 1993; 132: 879-87.

68. Møldrup A, Pedersen ED, Nielsen JH. Effects of sex and pregnancy hormones on growth hormone and prolactin receptor gene expression in insulin-producing cells. Endocrinology 1993; 133: 1165-72.

69. Nielsen JH. Hormonal regulation of growth and function of insulin-producing cells in culture. In: Fischer G, Wieser RJ, eds. Hormonally defined Media. A Tool in Cell Biology. Berlin: Springer-Verlag, 1983: 264-73.

70. Billestrup N, Nielsen JH. The stimulatory effect of growth hormone, prolactin, and placental lactogen on beta-cell proliferation is not mediated by insulin-like growth factor-I. Endocrinology 1991; 129: 883-88.

71. Hogg J, Han VKM, Clemmons DR et al. Interactions of nutrients, insulin-like growth factors (IGFs) and IGF-binding proteins in the regulation of DNA synthesis by isolated fetal rat islets of Langerhans. J Endocr 1993; 138: 401-12.

72. Miettinen PJ, Otonkoski T, Voutilainen R. Insulin-like growth factor-II and transforming growth factor-alpha in developing human fetal pancreatic islets. J Endocrinol 1993; 138: 127-36.

73. Scharfmann R, Tazi A, Polak M et al. Expression of functional nerve growth factor receptors in pancreatic beta-cell lines and fetal rat islets in primary culture. Diabetes 1993; 42: 1829-36.

74. Mandrup-Poulsen T, Helqvist S, Wogensen LD et al. Cytokines as effector molecules in the destruction of pancreatic beta cells. In: Bækkeskov S, Hansen BA, eds. Human Diabetes: Genetic, environmental and autoimmune etiology. Current Topics in Microbiology 164. Berlin: Springer-Verlag, 1990: 169-93.

75. Spinas GA, Hansen BS, Linde S et al. Interleukin-1 dose-dependently affects the biosynthesis of (pro)insulin in isolated rat islets of Langerhans, Diabetologia 1987; 30: 474-80.

76. Sjöholm Å. Differential effects of cytokines on long-term mitogenic and secretory responses of fetal rat pancreatic beta-cells. Am J Physiol 1992; 263: C114-20.

77. Stahl M, Petersen RO, Nielsen JH. Effect of interleukin-1 on 5-bromodeoxyuridine incorporation into rat pancreatic beta cells in culture. Diabetes 1991; 40 (suppl 1) A151.

78. Corbett JA, McDaniel ML. Does nitric oxide mediate autoimmune destruction of beta-cells? Diabetes 1992; 41: 897-903.

79. Nielsen JH, Jensen D, Pedersen JA et al. Regulation of type 1 interleukin-1 receptor expression in pancreatic islets in culture. Diabetologia 1993; 36 (suppl. 1): A96.

80. Sjöholm Å. Intracellular signal transduction pathways that control pancreatic beta-cell proliferation. FEBS Lett 1992; 311: 85-90.

GENETIC ENGINEERING OF INSULIN SECRETING CELL LINES

Hector BeltrandelRio   Wolfgang J. Schnedl

Sarah Ferber   Christopher B. Newgard

Diabetes mellitus has a prevalence of 1% in the United States, with approximately 20% of that classified as insulin dependent diabetes mellitus or IDDM.[1] The traditional treatment of choice for IDDM has been insulin injection. Although sophisticated treatment programs have been developed using a combination of regular, intermediate (lente) and long-acting (ultralente) insulins, these approaches do not allow for the precise moment-to-moment changes in insulin secretion that are provided by the islets and that guarantee glucose homeostasis. A second approach to the treatment of IDDM is islet transplantation. While the foregoing chapters provide evidence for the considerable promise of this approach, the high cost and complexity of islet isolation, as well as the inability of these cells to grow in vitro, make the broad applicability of this therapy uncertain.

Considering these problems, an alternative solution is to identify and develop cells that secrete insulin in response to glucose and other secretagogues in a manner similar to islets and that can be propagated in a laboratory or industrial setting in unlimited supply. Recently, we and other investigators have been working towards this goal with cells of islet origin, (mostly β-cell tumor lines), as well as cells of neuroendocrine non-islet origin.[2] Important advances have been made in the last few years in understanding the regulation of insulin secretion, and in the application of molecular approaches for the development of cells that could potentially be used for the treatment of IDDM. In the present chapter we will review these advances and the problems that are yet to be solved.

MECHANISM OF INSULIN SECRETION FROM ISLET β-CELLS

Blood glucose levels are controlled within a narrow range in normal humans despite constant variations in the rate of glucose intake and disposal. During postprandial states, islet β-cells are able to sense increases in blood glucose and to respond rapidly by secreting the precise amount of insulin required to prevent hyperglycemia. The mechanism(s) by which β-cells are

Pancreatic Islet Transplantation Volume I: Procurement of Pancreatic Islets, edited by Robert P. Lanza, MD, William L. Chick, MD; ©1994 R.G. Landes Company.

able to sense changes in glucose concentration over the physiological range (4-9 mM), and how this translates into stimulation of insulin secretion are not fully understood. Glucose metabolism appears to be required, since insulin secretion is not elicited by nonmetabolizable glucose analogs, or by glucose in the presence of inhibitors of glycolysis.[3,4]

Glucose Metabolism and Insulin Secretion

Glucose is transported into β-cells mainly by GLUT-2,[5] a glucose transporter with V_{max} and K_m values well above those of the other members of the family of facilitated glucose transporters.[6,7] Glucose transport does not appear to be rate limiting for β-cell glucose metabolism, since it has been demonstrated that the rate of glucose transport can be reduced significantly with the use of inhibitors without affecting glucose utilization or glucose-stimulated insulin secretion.[8] Furthermore, rapid equilibration of glucose occurs in β-cells (but not in α-cells) with nearly identical concentrations of intra- and extracellular glucose found over a wide range of glucose concentrations.[9,10]

Upon entry into the cell, glucose is rapidly phosphorylated by hexokinases. Two isozymes of hexokinase are expressed in β-cells at similar levels, hexokinase I and hexokinase IV (also known as glucokinase[3]). Hexokinase I has a low K_m for glucose (50 μM), while glucokinase has a high K_m (8 mM).[3,11] Since the glucose concentration dependence of islet glucose utilization and insulin secretion is almost identical to that of glucokinase from islet extracts, glucokinase-catalyzed glucose phosphorylation is considered the rate limiting step in β-cell glycolysis.[3] Furthermore, the use of inhibitors of glucokinase like alloxan[12] and mannoheptulose[13] block both glycolysis and insulin secretion. Taken together, these data have led to the suggestion that glucokinase represents the "glucose sensor" of the pancreatic β-cell, regulating changes in the rate of glucose metabolism in response to changes in external glucose.[3] To prevent insulin secretion at low glucose concentrations, most of the low K_m hexokinase I activity appears

to be inhibited in the intact cell, resulting in a very low rate of glucose utilization at submillimolar concentrations.[14,15]

How glucose metabolism translates into insulin secretion is not clear at the present time. β-cells have ATP-sensitive K^+ channels that appear to control the membrane potential and that are closed upon glucose administration.[16,17] The membrane potential in the absence of glucose is about -70 to -80 mV, and about -55 mV in the presence of non-stimulatory glucose concentrations.[18] A commonly quoted hypothesis is that ATP produced by the metabolism of glucose changes the ATP:ADP ratio, thus closing these channels and causing depolarization. However, this model has not been fully reconciled with recent studies in which changes in glucose concentration were found to have little effect on this ratio in whole islets.[19] The depolarization of the membrane activates voltage-gated channels to promote the entry of Ca^{++} into β-cells.[20,21] Insulin exocytosis in response to increases in intracellular Ca^{++} is thought to be mediated by activation of protein kinase C[20,21] or possibly by members of the Ca^{++}/calmodulin class of protein kinases.[22] Consistent with an important role for calcium is the finding that calcium-channel blockers like nitrendipine markedly reduce or eliminate insulin secretion in response to glucose.[20,21]

TYPES OF INSULIN SECRETING CELLS

Cells Derived from β-Cells

There are a number of insulin-secreting cell lines derived from β-cell tumors of rodents and small animals that have been produced by viral transformation of isolated islets (HIT cells),[23] by X-irradiation of whole animals and propagation of cell lines from resultant insulinoma tumors (RIN cells),[24] or by expression of oncogenes in β-cells of transgenic mice (β-TC or MIN cells).[25,26] These cell lines have widely variant phenotypes, particularly with regard to their capacity for glucose-induced insulin release. A short summary of the properties of the growing number of lines is in order to provide context for discussion of molecular approaches for modifying their function.

The SV40-transformed hamster insulinoma cell line (HIT) exhibits glucose-stimulated insulin secretion, but this response is to subphysiologic glucose concentrations.[26] Furthermore, the magnitude of the response is dependent on the expression of GLUT-2, which seems to be regulated by the amount of glucose in the media.[26] Unlike islet β-cells, glucose transport appears to be the rate-limiting step for glycolysis in HIT cells.

RIN cells are insulin secreting cells that were produced from a serially transplantable radiation-induced rat islet cell tumor.[24] The glucose-stimulated insulin secretion response in currently available RIN cell lines varies widely. RINm5F cells do not respond to glucose[27,28] even though their maximal rate of glucose metabolism is equivalent to that of islets. The difference between islets and RINm5F cells is that glucose metabolism is increased in proportion to the media glucose concentration over the range of 5-50 mM in islets, but is already maximal at submillimolar concentrations of glucose in RINm5F cells. RINm5F cells express GLUT-1 rather than GLUT-2[5] and hexokinase rather than glucokinase[28] as their primary glucose transporter and glucose phosphorylating isoforms, respectively. This may contribute to the failure of glucose to stimulate insulin secretion.

Other lines derived from radiation-induced insulinomas such as RIN1046-38 cells exhibit glucose-stimulated insulin secretion, albeit with maximal response at subphysiological glucose concentrations.[29] This glucose responsiveness is lost with time in culture[29] in parallel with the loss of expression of GLUT-2 and glucokinase.[30] Thus, RIN1046-38 cells that have been carried though 35 passages or more in culture are generally completely unresponsive and exhibit absent or sharply diminished expression of GLUT-2 and glucokinase.[29,30]

Insulin-secreting cell lines have also been created with the use of transgenic technology. This has been achieved by injection of fertilized mouse eggs with a vector containing the insulin promoter driving T-antigen expression to produce β-cell tumors.[25,26] Some of the cell lines created using this method, such as the βTC-1, βTC-3, or MIN-7 cell lines either lack glucose-stimulated insulin release or respond to subphysiological concentrations of the sugar.[25,26,31] Glucose metabolism appears to regulate the secretory response in these cell lines, since the glucose utilization curve is shifted to the left.[31,32] Other transgenic lines such as MIN-6 or βTC-7 exhibit a glucose-stimulated insulin secretion similar to that of normal mouse islet cells.[26,33] Interestingly, the glucose responsive MIN-6 line and the glucose unresponsive MIN-7 line differ in that MIN-6 cells express GLUT-2 predominantly, while MIN-7 cells express mostly GLUT-1.[26] βTC-7 cells express GLUT-2 at high levels and contain a glucokinase:hexokinase ratio similar to that of normal islets.[33] With time in culture, the glucose concentration dependence of insulin release shifts such that the cells become maximally responsive to subphysiological levels of glucose. This change is accompanied by a sharp increase in hexokinase activity, with little change in GLUT-2 or glucokinase expression.[33]

INSULIN-SECRETING CELL LINES OF NON-β-CELL ORIGIN

Cell lines of neuroendocrine origin derived from ACTH-secreting corticotrophs of the anterior pituitary gland have been stably transfected with the human proinsulin cDNA and designated AtT-20ins cells.[34] Since these cells express the peptidases PC2 and PC3[35,36] that are thought to process proinsulin to insulin, mature insulin is their primary secreted product.[34,37] While insulin release from AtT-20ins cells is stimulated by agents that increase cAMP such as forskolin,[34,38] glucose-stimulated insulin release is completely lacking.[38] AtT-20ins cells express the islet isoform of glucokinase,[39] but at low levels compared to their expression of hexokinase I. They also lack expression of GLUT-2,[38-40] instead expressing low levels of GLUT-1.[38]

MOLECULAR ENGINEERING OF INSULIN SECRETING CELLS

In recent years our laboratory has focused on applying molecular approaches for the engineering of glucose-stimulated insulin secretion in insulin secreting cell lines. The ultimate goals of this work are to achieve a better understanding of the role of glucose transport and phosphorylation in the regulation of insulin release and to investigate whether engineered cells might represent a new mode of cell-based insulin delivery in IDDM. Progress in these areas is summarized below.

STABLE TRANSFECTION OF AtT20 AND RIN CELLS

We have prepared AtT20ins cell lines that have been stably transfected with GLUT-1 or GLUT-2.[39,40] Using immunofluorescence and glucose transport assays, it has been confirmed that the cell localization and the function of these introduced glucose transporters are normal. As shown in Figure 15.1A, expression of GLUT-2, but not GLUT-1, confers glucose-stimulated insulin secretion to AtT20ins cells.[40] Secretion was studied by perifusion of the various cell lines, showing that the insulin secretory response to glucose in GLUT-2 expressing lines occurred within minutes, and just as importantly, that removal of glucose from the media resulted in rapid cessation of insulin release, indicating that the dynamics of the secretory response are similar to that of normal islets. Surprisingly, overexpression of either GLUT-2 or GLUT-1 did not affect total glucose utilization relative to un-transfected cells as measured by [5-^{3}H] glucose metabolism (Fig. 15.1B). These data suggest that GLUT-2 plays a role in glucose sensing that goes beyond the increase in glucose transport, possibly involving physical coupling of this transporter with other components of the signaling apparatus.[40] As is the case for many rodent insulinoma cell lines, maximal insulin release from GLUT-2 expressing AtT-20ins cells was achieved at subphysiologic concentrations of glucose, consistent with the fact that these cells have

higher hexokinase activity and lower glucokinase activity than islet cells.[39]

As mentioned above, RIN 1046-38 cells show glucose-stimulated insulin secretion at subphysiologic concentrations of glucose, and lose this responsiveness with time in culture.[29,30] Stable transfection of glucose unresponsive intermediate passage, but not high passage RIN 1046-38 cells with GLUT-2 results in restoration of the glucose response.[30] Interestingly, transfected intermediate passage, but not high passage cells, also exhibited a 4-fold increase in total glucokinase activity compared to untransfected cells of the same passage number.[30] Despite the increase in glucokinase activity in the intermediate passage number cells, glucose-stimulated insulin release is still maximal at submillimolar glucose concentrations. These cells have high levels of hexokinase expression, and their subphysiologic glucose dose response may be explained by a dominant effect of the low Km enzyme on regulation of glucose metabolism. The shift in dose-response occurring in parallel with the sharp increase in hexokinase activity as a function of passage number in βTC-7 cells described by Efrat and colleagues is also consistent with this model.[33]

We have used a chemical approach to test whether the lower threshold of glucose responsiveness in engineered RIN cells is explained by their high levels of hexokinase I. Inhibition of hexokinase activity was achieved by preincubation of cells with 50 mM 2 deoxyglucose (2-DOG), which accumulates in cells as 2 deoxyglucose-6-phosphate, resulting in inhibition of hexokinase but not glucokinase. Incubation of RIN cells with 2-DOG for 30 minutes prior to measuring glucose-stimulated insulin secretion caused a shift in the maximal response from 50 μM glucose in untreated cells to 5 mM glucose in pretreated cells.[30] These data suggest that stable inhibition of hexokinase activity by molecular means could provide cell lines with a glucose-stimulated insulin secretion response that resembles that of the normal islet.

Panel A

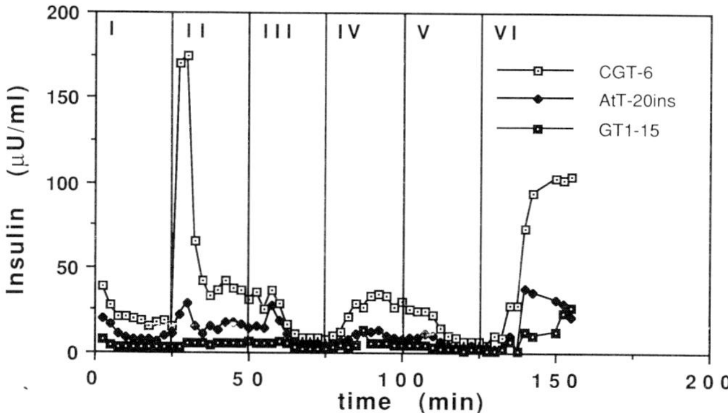

Panel B

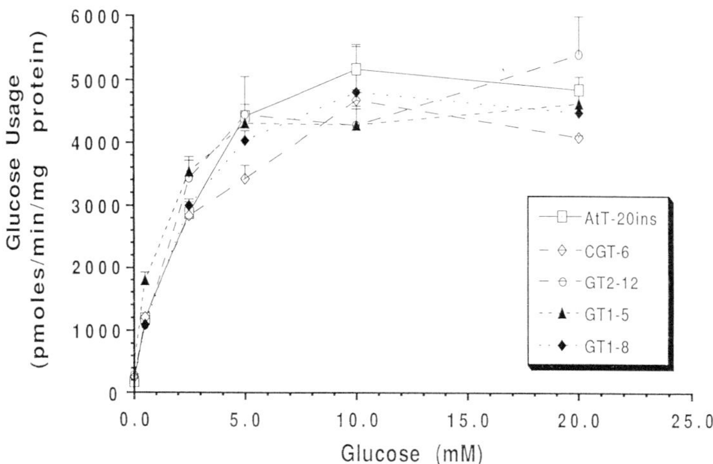

Fig. 15.1. Glucose-stimulated insulin secretion and glucose usage in AtT-20ins cell lines. Panel A: Glucose-stimulated insulin release from perifused AtT-20ins cell lines. The cells were exposed to the following: Phase I, Hanks Balanced Salt Solution (HBSS) without glucose; Phase II, HBSS with 5 mM glucose; Phase III, HBSS without glucose; Phase IV, HBSS with 5 mM glucose; Phase V, HBSS without glucose; Phase VI, HBSS with 5 mM glucose + 0.5 µM forskolin. Panel B: Glucose usage in AtT-20ins cell lines as a function of glucose concentration. Glucose usage was measured by administration of 5-^{3}H glucose to intact cells as described.[40] Symbol legends to the right of each panel refer to the following cell lines: CGT-6 and GT2-12 are GLUT-2 transfected lines; GT1-5, GT1-8, and GT1-15 are GLUT-1 transfected lines; AtT-20ins are untransfected control cells. Data adapted from Hughes, et al.,[40] with permission.

UTILITY OF ADENOVIRUS-MEDIATED GENE TRANSFER FOR STUDIES IN INSULIN SECRETING CELL LINES

Introduction of genes via stable transfection has provided insight into the relative contributions of glucose transport and phosphorylation in regulation of the glucose response in insulin secreting cell lines. There is, nevertheless, much more to be learned, and the pace of progress could be enhanced by application of gene transfer techniques that circumvent the time consuming process of selection and propagation of stable cell lines. To this end, we have recently investigated the utility of recombinant adenovirus for rapid evaluation of the effects of introduced genes.[30,41] Our previous studies have indicated that this system is highly effective for studies on metabolic regulation in hepatocytes[42] and primary islet cells.[43] Recombinant virions are prepared by cloning the gene of interest into a plasmid containing a promoter and a portion of the adenovirus genome. This plasmid is then contransfected into the permissive kidney cell line 293 with a second plasmid containing the remainder of the adenovirus genome. Recombination within the 293 cells results in virions that are infectious but replication-defective, meaning that they can be used to transfer genes with high efficiency without harming the target cells. We have tested the efficiency of this method with a virus containing the gene for β-galactosidase (AdCMV-βGAL[44]). As shown in Figure 15.2, the β-galactosidase gene is expressed in nearly 100% of RIN cells in culture 48 hours after a 1 hour exposure to the virus. These results are similar to our experiences with isolated islets (>70% efficiency[43]) and hepatocytes (86% efficiency[42]). In light of these promising results we have constructed a variety of recombinant viruses containing GLUT-2 (AdCMV-GLUT2), the islet and liver isoforms of glucokinase (AdCMV-GKI and AdCMV-GKL, respectively) and hexokinase I in both sense and antisense orientation (AdCMV-HKI and AdCMV-HKIrev, respectively).

The utility of these recombinant adenoviruses for rapid testing of concepts can be illustrated by two examples. The increase in glucokinase activity achieved by stable transfection of RIN cells with GLUT-2[30] was suprising in comparison to AtT-20ins cells, where no effects of GLUT-2 on glucokinase activity were observed.[39] We have used the AdCMV-GLUT2 virus to achieve independent confirmation of GLUT-2 dependent increases in glucokinase activity in RIN cells. Infection of intermediate, but not high passage insulinoma cells with the virus resulted in a time-dependent increase in glucokinase activity that became evident at 24 hours and that reached statistical significance 72 hours after viral treatment.[30] This experiment establishes that the increased glucokinase activity is a direct consequence of the expression of GLUT-2 and not due to clonal selection or variability. A second example of the application of recombinant adenovirus serves as a complement to the 2-deoxyglucose experiments for inhibition of hexokinase mentioned above. While the chemical studies suggest that inhibition of hexokinase activity may be an important step in achieving physiologically relevant glucose sensing, conformation of this principal by a rapid molecular approach would provide the motivation to investigate more permanent solutions such as hexokinase gene knock-out. To this end, molecular reduction of hexokinase activity was achieved with the recombinant adenovirus containing the rat hexokinase I cDNA in antisense orientation (AdCMV-HKIrev). Incubation of GLUT-2 expressing intermediate passage RIN cells with AdCMV-HKIrev resulted in a reduction of immunodetectable hexokinase I to 25% of that in uninfected cells, and 15% of that in cells infected with AdCMV-βGAL. In preliminary studies, we have detected a shift in glucose dose-response similar to that observed in the 2–deoxyglucose experiments in cells treated with AdCMV-HKI. (BeltrandelRio, H. and Newgard, C.B., unpublished observations). These data provide support for the concept of a dominant role for hexokinase in dictating the glucose dose response in cell lines. It should be pointed out that adenovirus does not allow permanent modulation of function, since the virus does not integrate effectively into host cell

A

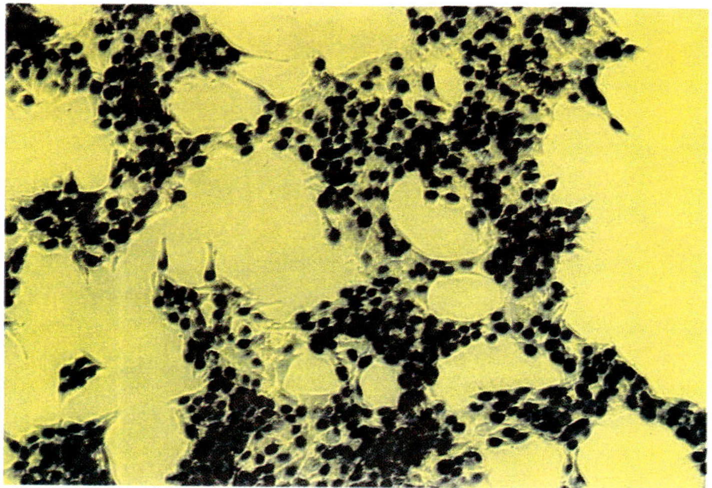

B

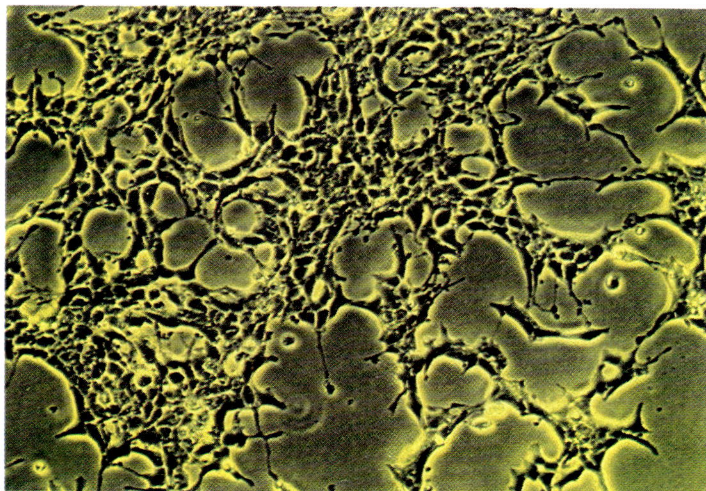

Fig. 15.2. Adenovirus-mediated gene transfer into insulinoma cells. Panel A: Intermediate passage RIN cells 48 hours after 1 hour of exposure to the AdCMV-bGal recombinant adenovirus. Panel B: Untreateded control cells. Both groups of cells were exposed to a chromogenic solution designed for visualization of b-galactosidase activity. The authors thank Richard Noel for providing these photographs.

DNA. Nevertheless, these early observations provide encouragement for future studies in which permanent expression of antisense hexokinase or hexokinase gene knockout by homologous recombination will be attempted.

EARLY TRANSPLANT STUDIES

We have recently initiated studies in which various RIN and AtT-20ins cell lines are transplanted into rodents. These early studies have been performed in athymic nude rats to avoid complications associated with rejection of xenografts. Even though currently available cell lines secrete insulin in response to subphysiological glucose concentrations (see above), the implantation studies have provided important information regarding the performance of insulin secreting cell lines in vivo.

Athymic Fisher nude rats (strain F344/NCr-rnu) received cell implants at 8-12 weeks of age, at which time they weighed between 130-210 grams. Various cell lines were injected subcutaneously (50-100 x 10^6 cells per injection) between the shoulder blades of recipient animals under sodium pentobarbital anesthesia. Both RIN and AtT-20ins cells grew as solid tumors in nude rats and produced insulin in increasing amounts proportional to the increase in tumor mass. Figures 15.3A-B provide information about the blood insulin and C-peptide levels between 14-20 days after cell implantation. Implantation of line CGT-6, a GLUT-2 expressing, glucose sensitive AtT-20ins cell line[39,40] actually caused a significant decrease in the circulating insulin level relative to unimplanted control animals, but did cause an approximate 3-fold increase in insulin levels relative to animals implanted with line D16-1, an AtT-20 cell line that lacks the transfected insulin gene. The CGT-6 cell line[39,40] is derived by GLUT-2 transfection of the AtT-20ins cell line, which was in turn produced by stable transfection of D16-1 cells with a DNA fragment consisting of a viral LTR sequence driving expression of the human proinsulin cDNA.[34] The same DNA fragment was independently introduced into D16-1 cells to produce line H23p, which

secretes approximately 15 times more insulin than either the AtT-20ins or CGT-6 cell lines.[45] Implantation of H23p cells (a gift from Drs. J-C. Irminger and P. A. Halban, Geneva) into nude rats resulted in a 1.8-fold increase in the circulating insulin levels relative to unimplanted controls, and a 4.2-fold and 12.1-fold increase relative to animals implanted with CGT-6 or D16-1 cells, respectively. Animals implanted with the GLUT-2 transfected rat insulinoma cell line RIN 36-7 or the untransfected line RIN 39 exhibited increases in circulating insulin levels that were similar to those caused by implantation of H23p cells.

To prove that the changes in insulin levels in implanted animals were due to enhanced rates of insulin production, we also measured C-peptide levels. Human C-peptide was measured only in unimplanted control rats and in animals receiving AtT-20ins cells producing human insulin. As shown in Figure 15.3B, CGT-6 cells caused a 2-fold increase in human C-peptide levels relative to unimplanted controls, while the increase caused by implantation of the H23p cell line was nearly 8-fold. These data are consistent with long-term proinsulin processing and insulin secretion from the implanted AtT-20-derived cell lines

As seen in Figure 15.4A, nude rats that did not receive cell implants maintained their blood glucose levels at approximately 100 mg/dL and insulin at near 25 µU/mL with no significant deviations throughout a 5-week observation period. Implantation of RIN 36-7 cells caused a decline in blood glucose such that the animals began to become frankly hypoglycemic (blood glucose of near 50 mg/dL) approximately 10 days after cell implantation (Fig. 15.4B). Experiments were terminated at day 12, a point at which the animals were becoming severely hypoglycemic (blood glucose of less than 25 mg/dL). The decrease in glucose correlated with an approximate 3-fold increase in insulin levels over the course of the experiment. In marked contrast, implantation of H23p cells did not cause a significant decrease in circulating glucose levels, even when experiments were carried out to 5 weeks, despite

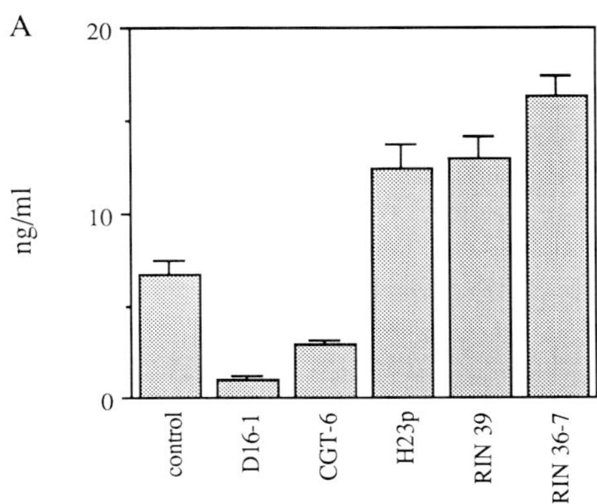

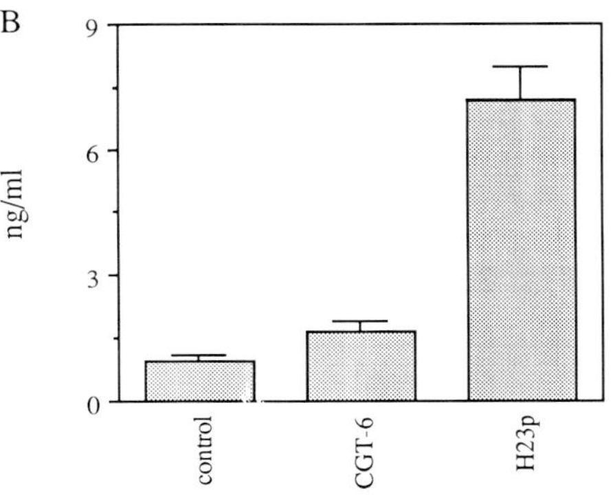

Fig. 15.3. Plasma insulin and C-peptide levels in nude rats implanted with insulin secreting cell lines. Panel A: Plasma insulin levels measured 2-3 weeks after implantation of cell lines. Panel B: Human C-peptide levels in plasma of nude rats containing AtT-20ins cell implants. The following cell lines were included: D16-1, AtT-20 cells lacking insulin expression; CGT-6, AtT-20ins cells engineered for GLUT-2 expression;[38] H23p, AtT-20ins cells with high insulin content;[44] RIN 39, RIN 1046-38 cells, passage 39; RIN 36-7, RIN 1046-38 cells, passage 36, engineered for GLUT-2 expression.[30] Data represent the mean ±S. E. M. for 2-3 animals per cell line.

the fact that these cells caused an increase in insulin levels that was indistinguishable from that achieved with the insulinoma line. Furthermore, while animals implanted with RIN cells gained weight throughout the study (from 188 grams at day 1 to 208 grams at day 12), animals that received the AtT-20ins line lost weight (from 168 grams at day 1 to 145 grams at 5 weeks) and appeared cachexic. This phenomenon was also noted during the experiments of Figure 15.1 in which other AtT-20 lines such as CGT-6 and D16-1 were implanted.

Implantation of insulinoma tissue is known to cause a sharp reduction in β-cell mass and insulin expression,[46,47] while injection of steroids such as dexamethasone causes insulin resistance, compensatory β-cell hyperplasia, and a sharp increase in pancreatic insulin release.[48] Consistent with the fact that AtT-20ins cell lines produce ACTH as

a major endocrine product, implantation of these cells caused more than a 10-fold increase in adrenal mass and dissipation of the normally well-defined boundary between the adrenal cortex and medulla (data not shown). The suggestion that the implanted AtT-20ins cells produced a steroid-induced insulin resistance is supported by the data of Figure 15.4C, in which high insulin levels are shown to have no effect on glucose concentrations. Further support is provided by the finding that AtT-20 cells causes a 3.5-fold increase in β-cell mass relative to animals that did not receive a cell implant. Implantation of RIN cells, in contrast caused a 2-fold decrease in β-cell mass and a clear diminution in insulin content within the islets (data not shown).

In summary, our early studies indicate that insulinoma or AtT-20ins cells are capable of producing insulin for prolonged periods of time in the in vivo environment. These studies have also been useful in that they have steered us toward insulinoma cells as the model system of choice for continuing studies on modulation of the glucose dose response by molecular manipulations. This conclusion is based on the metabolic side-effects induced by implantation of AtT-20ins cells that may be due to their expression of ACTH, but that could also be related in part to cytokines or other factors that may be produced by these cells. Work from other laboratories with insulinoma cell lines also provide encouragement. In one such study, transgenically derived βTC-1 cells attached to collagen coated microcarriers were transplanted into nude rats two weeks after induction of streptozotocin diabetes.[49] The βTC-1 cells caused a rapid decrease in blood glucose levels from 400 mg/dL to approximately 200 mg/dL and then a further gradual decrease to levels of approximately 100 mg/dL over the ensuing 40 days. Over this time period, severe hypoglycemia was not observed, despite the fact that insulin release from βTC-1 cells in response to glucose is maximal at subphysiological levels of the sugar,[49] as is also the case with the our GLUT-2 expressing RIN or AtT-20ins cell lines. The explanation for the lack of severe hypoglycemia in the foregoing study may instead be that the βTC-1 cells did not form tumors and were therefore restrained in their rate of growth.[49] Future work will focus on transplantation of insulinoma cell lines in the context of immunoprotective, permselective devices that will control the cell mass, and thereby the insulin production capacity.

PROBLEMS AND PROSPECTS FOR THE FUTURE

In this chapter, we have attempted to summarize progress in the area of development of insulin secreting cell lines with a glucose-stimulated insulin secretion response that resembles that of the normal islets. It appears that expression of GLUT-2 in cell lines, coupled with modulation of the glucokinase:hexokinase ratio may lead to cells that respond to glucose concentrations that are within or nearly within the physiological range. Once available such engineered cells may have several advantages relative to isolated islets as a vehicle for insulin delivery in IDDM. These advantages include, (1) cell lines can be grown at relatively low cost and in essentially unlimited numbers under pathogen-free conditions, (2) engineering of a clonal population of cells with genes that are expressed at a fixed level over time in culture should ensure that such lines have highly reproducible functional characteristics, as opposed to islets, which can be quite variable on a batch-to-batch basis, (3) new features can be introduced or eliminated more readily in a rapidLy growing population of cells than in primary islets.

These positive features must of course be balanced against the sizeable obstacles that remain before stable cell lines with fuel-mediated insulin secretion responses similar to those of the normal islet are available. Titration of the glucose dose response in engineered cells has been addressed above. Overexpression of GLUT-2 and glucokinase in cell lines has been achieved and appears to be quite stable, since expression of these genes is maintained in cell lines in continuous culture for many months. There is evidence to suggest, however, that viral promoters may not be suitable for maintenance of high levels of expression in cell lines implanted in vivo.[50] We are currently investigating this point, but are confident that other promoters can be used for long-term expression in the event that viral promoters are suppressed. Long-term down-regulation of hexokinase will be more difficult than overexpression of GLUT-2 and glucokinase. Approaches to this problem will include stable expression of hexokinase in antisense orientation, especially since the 2-deoxyglucose and adenovirus experiments have provided encouragement that such a manuever can lead to a desired change in glucose dose response (see above), or alternatively, knock-out of hexokinase by homologous recombination. It must also be recognized that engineered cells that ultimately embody a "physiological" glucose reponse may not respond to other positive and negative modulators of insulin secretion such as glucagon-like peptide-1 or catechola-

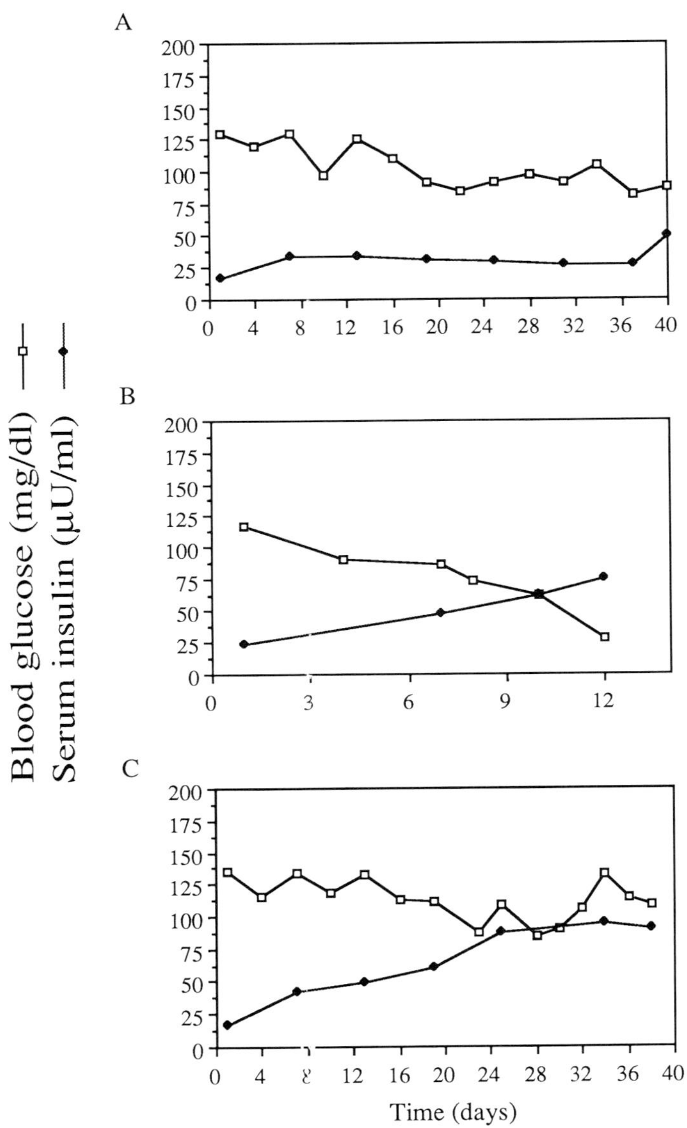

Fig. 15.4. Plasma insulin and glucose levels in nude rats implanted with AtT-20ins or RIN cell lines.
Panel A: Nude rats without a cell implant (control group).
Panel B: Nude rats implanted with RIN cell line 36-7 (passage 36, engineered for GLUT-2 expression).
Panel C: Nude rats implanted with AtT-20ins cell line H23p.[45]
Data represent the mean of two experiments per panel.

mines in a manner analagous to the islets. If so, careful monitoring of cell performance under a variety of experimental conditions will be required to ensure adequate control of glucose homeostasis. Another problem is that the AtT-20ins and insulinoma cell lines reported on in this chapter secrete only a fraction of the insulin that is produced by β-cells. The solution to this problem is to overexpress human insulin, and we have in

fact recently prepared new insulinoma lines derived from RIN 1046-38 cells that secrete approximately 20 times more insulin than the parental cells (Ferber, S., Clark, S., Constandy, H., and Newgard, C. B., unpublished observations). It remains to be determined whether this marked enhancement in human insulin expression will impact the expression of the rat insulin gene. If not, use of such cells for human therapy may require elimination of rat insulin expression by methods similar to those proposed for down-regulation of hexokinase activity. Furthermore, while it is known that insulinoma cell lines can thrive and produce insulin in syngeneic hosts[51] or in immunocompromised animals such as the nude rat,[49,52] it remains to be determined whether these cells can be grown and protected in permselective devices in the context of autoimmune diabetes. Finally, it is as yet unclear whether cellular proteins other than insulin will escape from encapsulation devices in sufficient quantity to cause adverse immunological or biological responses. This issue pertains not only to transplantation of rodent cell lines but also to transplantation of isolated islets from non-human sources such as dogs or pigs.

In summary, early studies on molecular engineering of insulin secreting cell lines provide hope for eventual sucess in conferring a physiologically relevant glucose response into such lines. We are rapidly approaching a phase in which the long term stability, in vivo function and viability of cell lines in the context of full-blown autoimmune diabetes must be evaluated. Only by these approaches can it be determined whether cell engineering technology will ultimately be applicable for therapy in human IDDM.

Acknowledgments

Studies from our laboratory relevant to this article were supported by National Institutes of Health Grants PO1-DK-42582 and RO1-DK-46492 and a sponsored research agreement with BetaGene Inc., Dallas, TX. W.J.S. is supported by a grant from the Austrian Science Foundation-Schrödinger, # J0730-MED.

References

1. Foster D W: Diabetes mellitus. In: Wilson J D, Braunwald E, Isselbacher K J, Petersdorf RG, Martin J B, Fauci A S, Root R K, eds. Principles of Internal Medicine. 12th ed. New York: Mc Graw Hill, 1991: 1739-59.

2 . Newgard C B: Cellular engineering for the treatment of metabolic disorders: prospects for therapy in diabetes. Bio/Technology 1992; 10: 1112-20.

3. Meglasson, M D, Matschinsky, F M: Pancreatic islet glucose metabolism and regulation of insulin secretion. Diabetes/Metabolism Rev 1986; 2: 163-214

4. Ashcroft, S J H: Metabolic controls of insulin secretion. In: Cooperstein, S J, Watkins, D, eds. The Islets of Langerhans. London, Academic Press, 1981: 117-48.

5. Thorens, B, Sarkar, H K, Kaback, H R, Lodish, H F: Cloning and functional expression in bacteria of a novel glucose transporter present in liver, intestine, kidney, and beta-pancreatic islet cells. Cell 1988; 55: 281-90.

6. Johnson, J H, Newgard, C B, Milburn, J L, Lodish, H F, Thorens, B: The high Km glucose transporter of islets of Langerhans is functionally similar to the low affinity transporter of liver and has an identical primary sequence. J Biol Chem 1990; 265: 6548-51.

7. Gould, G W, Thomas, H M, Jess, T J, Bell, G I: Expression of human glucose transporters in Xenopus ooctyes: kinetic characterization and substrate specificities of the erythrocyte, liver and brain isoforms. Biochemistry 1991; 30: 5139-45.

8. Hellman, B, Lernmark, A, Sehlin, J, and Taljedal, I-B: Effects of phlorizin on metabolism and function of pancreatic β-cells. Metabolism 1972; 21: 60-6.

9. Matschinsky, F M and Ellerman, J E: Metabolism of glucose in the islets of Langerhans. J Biol Chem 1968; 243: 2730-36.

10. Gorus, F K, Malaisse, W J, Pipeleers, D G: Differences in glucose handling by pancreatic A- and B-cells J Biol Chem 1984; 259: 1196-1200.

11. Wilson, JE: Regulation of mammalian hexokinase activity. In: Beitner R ed. Regulation of Carbohydrate Metabolism. Boca Raton: CRC Press, 1984: 45-85.

12. Meglasson, M D, Burch, P T, Berner, D K, Najafi, H, Matschinsky, F M: Identification of glucokinase as an alloxan-sensitive glucose sensor of the pancreatic β-cell. Diabetes 1986; 35: 1163-1173.

13. Coore, H G, Randle, P J: Inhibition of glucose phosphorylation by mannoheptulose. Biochem.J 1964; 91: 56-59.

14. Trus, M D, Zawalich, W S, Burch, P T, Berner, D K, Weill, V A, Matschinsky, F M: Regulation of glucose metabolism in pancreatic islets. Diabetes 1981;30: 911-22.

15. Giroix, M-H, Sener, A, Pipeleers, D G, Malaisse, W J: Hexose metabolism in pancreatic islets. Biochem J 1984; 223: 447-53.

16. Cook, D L, Hales, C N: Intracellular ATP directly blocks K$^+$ channels in pancreatic B-cells. Nature 1984; 311: 271-73.

17. Ashcroft, F M, Harrison, DE, Ashcroft, S J H: Glucose induces closure of single potassium channels in isolated rat pancreatic islets. Nature 1984; 312: 446-48.

18. Carroll PB. Anatomy and Physiology of Islets of Langerhans. In: Ricordi C. ed. Pancreatic Islet Cell Transplantation. Austin: RG Landes, 1992: 7-18.

19. Ghosh, A, Ronner, P, Cheong, E, Khalid, P, Matschinsky, F M: The role of ATP and free ADP in metabolic coupling during fuel-stimulated insulin release from islet β-cells in the isolated perfused pancreas. J Biol Chem 1991; 266: 22887-92.

20. Prentki, M, Matschinsky, F M: Ca^{2+}, cAMP, and phospholipid-derived messengers in coupling mechanisms of insulin secretion. Physiol Rev 1987; 67: 1185-1248.

21. Turk, J, Wolf, B A, McDaniel, M L: The role of phospholipid-derived mediators including arachidonic acid, its metabolites, and inositoltrisphosphate and of intracellular Ca^{2+} in glucose-induced insulin secretion by pancreatic islets. Prog Lipid Res 1987; 26: 125-81.

22. Ashcroft, S J H, Hughes, S J: Protein phosphorylation in the regulation of insulin secretion and biosynthesis. Biochem Soc Trans 1990; 18: 116-18.

23. Santerre, R F, Cook, R A, Crisel, R M D, Sharp, J D, Schmidt, R J, Williams, D C, Wilson, C P: Insulin synthesis in a clonal cell line of simian virus 40-transformed hamster pancreatic beta-cells. Proc Natl Acad Sci U S A 1981; 78: 4339-43,

24. Gazdar, A F, Chick, W L, Oie, H K, Sims, H L, King, D L, Weir, G C, Lauris, V: Continuous, clonal, insulin- and somatostatin-secreting cell lines established from a transplantable rat islet cell tumor. Proc Natl Acad Sci U S A 1980; 77: 3519-23.

25. Efrat, S, Linde, S, Kofod, H, Spector, D, Delannoy, M, Grant, S, Hanahan, D and Baekkeskov, S Beta-cell lines derived from transgenic mice expressing a hybrid insulin gene-oncogene. Proc Natl Acad Sci U S A 1988; 85: 9037-41.

26. Miyazaki, J-I, Araki, K, Yamato, E, Ikegami, H, Asano, T, Shibasaki, Y, Oka, Y, and Yamamura, K-I Establishment of a pancreatic β-cell line that retains glucose-inducible insulin secretion: Special reference to expression of glucose transporter isoforms. Endocrinology 1990; 127: 126-32.

27. Halban, P A, Praz, G A, Wollheim, C B: Abnormal glucose metabolism accompanies failure of glucose to stimulate insulin release from a pancreatic cell line (RINm5F). Biochem J 1983; 212: 439-443.

28. Shimizu, T, Knowles, B B, Matschinsky, F M: Control of glucose phosphorylation and glucose usage in clonal insulinoma cells Diabetes 1988; 37: 563-68.

29. Clark, S A, Burnham, B L, and Chick, W L: Modulation of glucose-induced insulin secretion from a rat clonal β-cell line. Endocrinology 1990; 127: 2779-88.

30. Ferber, S, BeltrandelRio, H, Johnson, J H, Noel, R, Becker, T, Cassidy, L E, Clark, S, Hughes, S D, Newgard, C B: Transfection of rat insulinoma cells with GLUT-2 confers both low and high affinity glucose-stimulated insulin release: relationship to glucokinase activity. J Biol Chem 1994; 268:11523-11529.

31. Whitesell, R R, Powers, A C, Regen, D M, and Abumrad, N A: Transport and metabolism of glucose in an insulin-secreting cell line, βTC-1. Biochemistry 1991; 30: 11560-11566,

32. D'ambra, R, Surana, M, Efrat, S, Starr, R G, Fleischer, N: Regulation of insulin secretion from β-cell lines derived from transgenic mice insulinomas resembles that of normal β-cells. Endocrinology 1990; 126: 2815-22.

33. Efrat, S, Leiser, M, Surana, M, Tal, M, Fusco-Demane, D, and Fleischer, N: Murine insulinoma cell line with normal glucose-regulated insulin secretion. Diabetes 1993; 42: 901-907.

34. Moore, H-P, Walker, M D, Lee, F, Kelly, R B: Expressing a human proinsulin cDNA in a mouse ACTH-secreting cell. Intracellular storage, proteolytic processing, and secretion on stimulation. Cell 1983; 35: 531-38.

35. Smeekens, S P, Steiner, D F: Identification of a human insulinoma cDNA encoding a novel mammalian protein structurally related to the yeast dibasic processing protease Kex2. J Biol Chem 1990; 265: 2997-3000.

36. Hakes, D J, Birch, N P, Mezey, A, Dixon, J E: Isolation of two complementary deoxyribonucleic acid clones from a rat insulinoma cell line based on similarities to Kex2 and furin sequences and the specific localization of each transcript to endocrine and neuroendocrine tissues in rat. Endocrinology 1991; 129: 3053-63.

37. Gross, D J, Halban, P A, Kahn, R C, Weir, G C, Villa-Komaroff, L: Partial diversion of a mutant proinsulin (B10 aspartic acid) from the regulated to the constitutive secretory pathway in transfected AtT-20 cells. Proc. Natl. Acad. Sci. U. S. A. 1989; 86: 4107-11.

38. Hughes, S D, Quaade, C, Milburn, J L, Cassidy, L C, Newgard, C B: Expression of normal and novel glucokinase mRNAs in anterior pituitary and islet cells. J Biol Chem 1991; 266: 4521-30.

39. Hughes, S D, Johnson, J H, Quaade, C, Newgard, C B: Engineering of glucose-stimulated insulin secretion and biosynthesis in non-islet cells. Proc Natl Acad Sci USA 1992; 89: 688-692.

40. Hughes, SD, Quaade, C, Johnson, J H, Ferber, S, Newgard, C B: Transfection of AtT-20ins cells with GLUT-2 but not GLUT-1 confers glucose-stimulated insulin secretion: relationship to glucose metabolism. J Biol Chem 1993; 268: 15205-12.

41. Becker, T C, Noel, R J, Coats, W S, Gomez-Foix, A M, Alam, T, Gerard, R D, Newgard, C B: Use of recombinant adenovirus for metabolic engineering of mammalian cells. Methods in Cell Biology 1994; 43:161-189.

42. Gomez-Foix, A M, Coats, W S, Baque, S, Alam, T, Gerard, R D, Newgard, C B: Adenovirus-mediated transfer of the muscle glycogen phosphorylase gene into hepatocytes confers altered regulation of glycogen metabolism. J Biol Chem 1992; 267: 25129-34.

43. Becker, T, Noel, R, Johnson, J H, and Newgard, C B: Divergent effects of glucokinase hexokinase and glucokinase mutants associated with MODY on glucose-induced insulin release. J Cell Biochem 1994; Suppl. 18A: 133

44. Herz, J and Gerard, R D: Adenovirus-mediated transfer of low density lipoprotein receptor gene acutely accelerates cholesterol clearance in normal mice. Proc Natl Acad Sci U S A 1993; 90: 2812-2816.

45. Irminger, J-C, Vollenweider, F, Halban, P A: Characterization of human proinsulin conversion in the regulated and the constitutive pathway of transfected AtT20 cells. J. Biol. Chem. 1994; in press.

46. Bedoya, F J, Matschinsky, F M, Shimizu, T, O'Neil, J J, Appel, M C: Differential regulation of glucokinase activity in pancreatic islets and liver of the rat. J. Biol. Chem. 1990; 261: 10760-10764.

47. Miyaura, C, Chen, L, Appel, M, Alam, T, Inman, L, Hughes, S D, Milburn, J L, Unger, R H, Newgard, C B: Expression of reg/PSP, a pancreatic exocrine gene: relationship to changes in islet β-cell mass. Mol. Endocrinol. 1991; 5: 226-234.

48. Ogawa, A, Johnson, J H, Ohneda, M, McAllister, C T, Inman, L, Alam, T, Unger, R H: Roles of insulin resistance and β-cell dysfunction in dexamethasone-induced diabetes. J. Clin. Invest. 1992; 90: 497-504.

49. Hicks, B A, Stein, R, Efrat, S, Grant, S, Hanahan, D, Demetriou, A A: Transplantation of β- cells from transgenic mice into nude athymic diabetic rats restores glucose regulation. Diabetes Res Clin Practice 1991; 14: 157-64.

50. Scharfmann, R, Axelrod, J H, Verma, I M: Long term in vivo expression of retrovirus-mediated gene transfer in mouse fibroblast implants. Proc. Natl. Acad. Sci. U. S. A. 1991; 88: 4626-4630.

51. Madsen, O D, Andersen, L C, Michelsen, B, Owerbach, D, Larsson, L-I, Lernmark, A, and Steiner, D F: Tissue-specific expression of transfected human insulin genes in pluripotent clonal rat insulinoma lines induced during passage in vivo. Proc Natl Acad Sci U S A 1988; 85: 6652-6656.

52. Ferber, S, Schnedl, W, BeltrandelRio, H, Irminger, J-C, Halban, P, Newgard, C B: Molecular strategies for the treatment of diabetes. Transplantation Proc, 1994; 26: 363-365.